Dreeben-Irimia's

# INTRODUCTION TO
# Physical Therapy
# Practice

## Mark Dutton, PT
**OrthoRecovery Specialists**
**Pittsburgh, Pennsylvania**

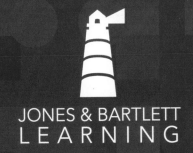

JONES & BARTLETT
LEARNING

*World Headquarters*
Jones & Bartlett Learning
25 Mall Road
Burlington, MA 01803
978-443-5000
info@jblearning.com
www.jblearning.com

Jones & Bartlett Learning books and products are available through most bookstores and online booksellers. To contact Jones & Bartlett Learning directly, call 800-832-0034, fax 978-443-8000, or visit our website, www.jblearning.com.

Substantial discounts on bulk quantities of Jones & Bartlett Learning publications are available to corporations, professional associations, and other qualified organizations. For details and specific discount information, contact the special sales department at Jones & Bartlett Learning via the above contact information or send an email to specialsales@jblearning.com.

30018-5

**Production Credits**

Vice President, Product Management: Marisa R. Urbano
Vice President, Content Strategy and Implementation: Christine Emerton
Director, Product Management: Matthew Kane
Product Manager: Whitney Fekete
Director, Content Management: Donna Gridley
Manager, Content Strategy: Orsolya Gall
Content Strategist: Colleen Joyce
Content Coordinator: Samantha Gillespie
Director, Project Management and Content Services: Karen Scott
Manager, Intellectual Properties: Kristen Rogers
Project Manager: Belinda Thresher
Senior Digital Project Specialist: Carolyn Downer
Marketing Manager: Mark Adamiak
Content Services Manager: Colleen Lamy
Product Fulfillment Manager: Wendy Kilborn
Composition: S4Carlisle Publishing Services
Project Management: S4Carlisle Publishing Services
Media Development Editor: Faith Brosnan
Rights & Permissions Manager: John Rusk
Rights Specialist: Robin Silverman
Cover Image (Title Page and Chapter Opener): © filo/Getty Images
Printing and Binding: Sheridan Kentucky

**Library of Congress Cataloging-in-Publication Data**

Names: Dutton, Mark, author. | Barrett, Christina M., 1967- Dreeben-Irimia's introduction to physical therapist practice for physical therapist assistants.
Title: Dreeben-Irimia's introduction to physical therapy practice / Mark Dutton.
Other titles: Introduction to physical therapy practice
Description: Fifth edition. | Burlington, MA : Jones & Bartlett Learning, [2026] | Preceded by Dreeben-Irimia's introduction to physical therapist practice for physical therapist assistants / Christina M. Barrett. Fourth edition. [2021] | Includes bibliographical references and index.
Identifiers: LCCN 2024010355 | ISBN 9781284289725 (paperback)
Subjects: MESH: Physical Therapy Specialty--methods | Physical Therapy Modalities | Physical Therapist Assistants
Classification: LCC RM725 | NLM WB 460 | DDC 615.8/2--dc23/eng/20240528
LC record available at https://lccn.loc.gov/2024010355

6048

To Julie and my daughters—Leah and Lauren—for their encouragement, understanding, and love.

# Brief Contents

# Contents

## CHAPTER 4 **The Physical Therapist Assistant as a Member of the Healthcare Team**. . . . . . . . . . . . . . . . **57**

## CHAPTER 5 **Examination, Evaluation, Plan of Care, and Intervention**. . . . . . . . . . . . . . . . **79**

## CHAPTER 6 **Ethics and Professionalism**. . . . . . . . . . . . . . . . . **113**

# Preface

I was 16 when I first learned about the physical therapy profession following a sports injury. I was impressed by the physical therapist's (PT's) knowledge, their attention to detail, and how they involved me in goal-setting. It was some years before I could enroll in a physical therapy program. Over the years, I have learned that the privilege of helping another person is just as life-changing for the PT as it is for the patient and, as an educator and consultant, I have enjoyed discussing and promoting physical therapy.

The fifth edition of *Dreeben-Irimia's Introduction to Physical Therapy Practice* is a culmination of my physical therapy experiences, and I hope it guides others. This introductory text provides a detailed overview of the entire profession, including the many practice areas, job duties, roles, and relationships of the PT/physical therapist assistant (PTA) team, and the professional attributes necessary to work as a team.

## Structure of the Text

This textbook is organized into 13 chapters:

- Chapter 1, "Student Learning Success," encourages students to understand the dedication necessary to complete a PT/PTA program and provides practical suggestions to create skills for success in school and beyond.
- Chapter 2, "The Physical Therapy Profession," is a historical overview and describes the progression of the profession in the skills it demands and in creating its unique identity, two aspects that separate it from other professions.
- Chapter 3, "Physical Therapist Clinical Practice," examines practice issues to assist students in understanding patient-related components of physical therapy practice and management. Employment settings and areas of practice are explained to foster in students an appreciation of the many opportunities available.
- Chapter 4, "The Physical Therapist Assistant as a Member of the Healthcare Team," introduces students to each of the healthcare team members and describes what role each has in the team. A detailed discussion of the relationship between the PT and PTA describes the supervisory and collaborative role the two have in patient care.
- Chapter 5, "Examination, Evaluation, Plan of Care, and Intervention," explains the components of the physical therapy experience. An understanding of the process and terminology of physical therapy will assist students in being more effective in treating patients.
- Chapters 6, "Ethics and Professionalism," and 7, "Laws and Regulations," address healthcare services' ethical, legal, and professional components. Understanding confidentiality, cultural competence, laws, and expectations of conduct for a PT/PTA provides the basis for patient interaction.
- Chapter 8, "Communication," lays the groundwork for learning the skills of successful verbal and nonverbal communication with patients and with colleagues.
- Chapter 9, "Teaching and Learning," discusses teaching techniques for patient instruction that will benefit students in several settings and their interactions with various patients, including patients with learning challenges.
- Chapter 10, "Introduction to Documentation and the Medical Record," introduces the basics of effective documentation and appropriate written communication for various audiences.
- Chapter 11, "Reimbursement and Research," helps students understand reimbursement by various payer sources and examines restrictions that may be in place. A discussion of research basics, levels of evidence, and the importance of evidence-based practices complete this chapter.
- Chapter 12, "Examination and Intervention of the Body Systems," provides an in-depth look at the specialized examinations for musculoskeletal, neurologic, cardiopulmonary, and integumentary systems.
- Chapter 13, "Lifelong Success," discusses successful people's attributes and tips for creating a résumé, preparing for a job interview, and creating lifelong success.

# New to the *Fifth Edition*

Key changes for the *Fifth Edition* include the following:

- Chapter 5 has been expanded to include details about the pediatric and geriatric populations and issues concerning Women's Health.
- Chapter 8, "Communication," now includes situational communication basics to help manage difficult people and those with dementia and cultural differences. A discussion of emotional intelligence also improves students' ability to understand their emotions and behaviors.
- Chapter 11, "Reimbursement and Research," features a rewritten research section that explains levels of evidence, reliability and validity, and the importance of evidence-based practice.
- Chapter 12 has been added to provide the reader with a detailed look at the examination and intervention processes for various body systems, including the musculoskeletal, neurologic, cardiopulmonary, and integumentary.

- Revised Table of Contents. The chapters of this text were reordered to improve the flow of information. Students begin by understanding what they are undertaking in studying the profession and its practice. The text concludes with information to help the student understand what it will take to be successful in the profession.
- Addition of Knowledge Checks. Within the reading, the text is interrupted by Knowledge Check questions that encourage students to pause and reflect on what has been read.
- Case studies have been added to provide examples of clinical practice.
- Data updates and visual enhancements. The data throughout the text have been updated since the previous edition. Further, current practice strategies and references to online resources have been included to reflect the ever-changing challenges relevant to health care today. Students will also appreciate the addition of graphics and charts to improve learning outcomes.

# Features of This Text

In each chapter of the text, students will find learning tools developed specifically to aid their understanding of the concepts presented. Each chapter includes the following:

- **Learning Objectives** focus student learning on the core concepts of the chapter.

- **Key Terms** are listed at the beginning of each chapter and defined in the **end-of-text Glossary** to provide students with a quick guide to important terminology.

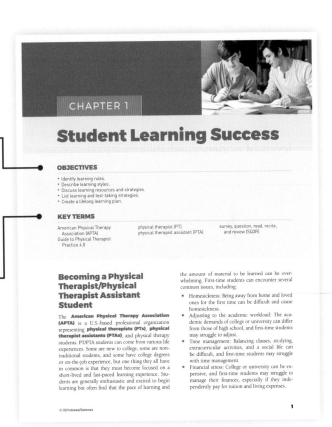

measurements should be taken before and after treatment to assess the patient's response to physical therapy interventions on the symptoms. These treatments may include physical modalities and agents, relaxation training, and patient education for behavioral modification (such as reinforcing proper body mechanics during ADLs). Pain is the most common symptom for which patients seek help. Two major pain measurements are used in physical therapy:

- The **Visual Analog Scale (VAS)** consists of a 10-cm unmarked line, either vertical or horizontal, with verbal or pictorial anchors indicating a continuum from no pain at one end to severe pain at the other. The patient is asked to mark on the line the pain they are experiencing (e.g., How bad is your pain?). This mark is then measured with a ruler and expressed in centimeters, with 10 cm representing severe pain.
- The Numerical Rating System (NRS) is easier to use than the VAS. The NRS uses a range of numbers (e.g., 0–5, 0–10) to reflect increasing degrees of pain. The patient is asked, "If zero is no pain and 10 is the worst pain imaginable, how would you rate your pain?"

Several social, biological, and psychological factors can influence how pain is experienced, interpreted, and expressed. Thus, it is common to find emotional overtones in the presence of pain, which likely result from an inhibition of the pain-control mechanisms of the central nervous system (CNS) from such causes as the side effects of medications, grief, or fear of re-injury. Nociplastic pain (called central sensitization) is the semantic term used to describe augmented CNS pain, maladaptive sensory processing, and altered pain modulation. In patients with nociplastic pain, increased activity is present in the brain areas involved in acute pain sensations and emotional representations, which can result in heightened pain levels in chronic conditions [2–5]. With these patients, it becomes more important to draw their attention away from a structural bias and help them become more aware of the biopsychosocial components involved in the pain experience [6]. A patient-reported questionnaire, the OSPRO-YF 10-Item Assessment Tool (Optimal Screening for Prediction of Referral and Outcome), is designed to estimate the multiple dimensions of psychological distress that adversely influence how people respond to musculoskeletal pain [7, 8]. OSPRO efficiently identifies yellow flags (e.g., negative mood, negative pain-coping).

## Systems Review

The systems review is a limited examination that provides additional information about the patient's general health and the continuum of patient/client care throughout their life span. The purpose of the systems review is to:

- Help determine the anatomic and physiologic status of all systems (musculoskeletal, neurologic, cardiovascular, pulmonary, integumentary, gastrointestinal, genitourinary, and genitoreproductive)
- Provide information about communication skills, affect, cognition, language abilities, education needs, and learning style of the patient
- Narrow the focus of subsequent tests and measures
- Define areas that may cause complications or indicate a need for precautions during the examination and intervention processes
- Screen for physical, sexual, and psychological abuse
- Determine the need for further physical therapy services based on an evaluation of the information obtained
- Identify problems that require consultation with, or referral to, another healthcare provider

## Tests and Measures

The tests and measures portion of the examination involves a physical examination of the patient and provides the PT with objective data to accurately determine the accuracy of the hypothesis and the degree of specific function and dysfunction [9]. Objective data collection is an important examination function to create a clear picture of the patient's problems. The type and number of the tests and measures used are modified based on the history and the systems review (see Chapter 12).

**KNOWLEDGE CHECK**

Where does the physical therapist obtain information for the examination?
What is the difference between an examination and an evaluation?

### Environmental Examination

The environmental examination is done at the patient's home or the institution where the patient lives. For example, the institutional environmental examination checks the patient's room for clutter or unsafe furniture, whether the lighting is bright enough

- **Knowledge Checks** encourage students to stop and reflect on what they have read, improving learning outcomes. An **answer key** is included at the end of the text.

- **Discussion Questions** push student learning further with questions that assess and expand upon the knowledge gained throughout the chapter.

- **Learning Opportunities** present additional activities for students to deepen their understanding.

**Discussion Questions**

1. List the values and culture of the physical therapy profession.
2. A second-year student member of the APTA is developing a presentation for incoming students. What should the student highlight as the purpose and value of becoming a member of the APTA?
3. List contributions that PTAs can make to the profession.
4. Identify the role and benefits of being a PTA.

**Learning Opportunities**

1. Go online at www.apta.org and research information about becoming a PTA.
2. Create a brochure identifying the vision, mission, and function of the APTA and the benefits of belonging to the APTA.
3. Participate in a district or chapter/subchapter meeting of the APTA.

**References**

1. American Physical Therapy Association: Guide to Physical Therapist Practice 3.0. Alexandria, VA, American Physical Therapy Association, 2014
2. Neumann DA: Polio: its impact on the people of the United States and the emerging profession of physical therapy. J Orthop Sports Phys Ther 34(8):479–492, 2004
3. DeLorme T, Watkins A: Techniques of Progressive Resistance Exercise. New York, Appleton-Century, 1951
4. Moffat M: The history of physical therapy practice in the United States. J Phys Ther Educ 17(3):15–25, 2003
5. Moffat M: Three quarters of a century of healing the generations. Phys Ther 76(11):1242–1252, 1996
6. Vogel EE: The beginning of "modern physiotherapy." Phys Ther 56(1):15–21, 1976
7. Murphy W: Healing the Generations: A History of Physical Therapy and the American Physical Therapy Association. Alexandria, VA, American Physical Therapy Association, 1995
8. Wright J: Physical and occupational therapy in poliomyelitis. Pediatr Clin North Am 1(1A):26–34, 1953
9. Woods EN: PTAs their history and development. PT Mag Phys Ther 4(1):34–39, 1993
10. American Physical Therapy Association: RC 11-14 Membership Value for the Physical Therapist Assistant, in House of Delegates Minutes. Alexandria, VA, American Physical Therapy Association, 2014
11. Goldstein M: Positive employment trends in physical therapy. PT Mag Phys Ther 9, 2001
12. American Physical Therapy Association House of Delegates: Vision 2020, in HOD P06-13-18-22. Alexandria, VA, American Physical Therapy Association, 2014
13. American Physical Therapy Association: APTA Strategic Plan 2022–2025 [Internet]. [cited 2023 Jan 31]. Available from: https://www.apta.org/apta-and-you/leadership-and-governance/vision-mission-and-strategic-plan/strategic-plan

# Instructor's Resources

Instructors also have access to a robust set of ancillaries, including the following:

- **Clinical Scenarios** present real-world examples of the concepts introduced in the text and include questions that instructors can utilize to assess students' application of those concepts.

- **Slides in PowerPoint format** provide a starting point for teaching the content in their course.
- **Test Banks** are available for each chapter and include new and revised test questions.
- **Practice Activities** provide additional questions that can be used for in-class activities to improve student understanding.

# About the Author

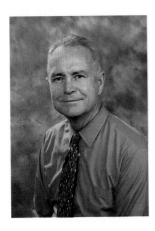

**Mark Dutton** is the author of many physical therapist and physical therapist assistant texts. He received his bachelor's degree in physical therapy from the University of Pittsburgh, and in 25 years in physical therapy practice and academia, he has taught hundreds of students while working in clinical practice, spending time in various practice settings.

# Reviewers

**Jeffrey Coon, PT, MPT**
PTA Program Director
Morgan Community College

**Julie Feeny, PT, MS**
Program Director PTA Program
Illinois Central College

**Tamey Howard-Feltner, PT, DPT**
PTA Program Director
Atlanta Technical College

**Amanda Wismer, PT, DPT, MSA**
Director of PTA Program
Mid Michigan College

**Sayda Ruelas, MPT**
South Texas College

**Renee Pruitt PT DPT, MHA**
Lone Star College

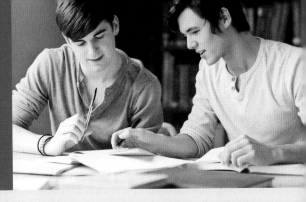

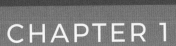

# CHAPTER 1

# Student Learning Success

## OBJECTIVES

- Identify learning rules.
- Describe learning styles.
- Discuss learning resources and strategies.
- List learning and test-taking strategies.
- Create a lifelong learning plan.

## KEY TERMS

American Physical Therapy
  Association (APTA)
Guide to Physical Therapist
  Practice 4.0

physical therapist (PT)
physical therapist assistant (PTA)

survey, question, read, recite,
  and review (SQ3R)

## Becoming a Physical Therapist/Physical Therapist Assistant Student

The **American Physical Therapy Association (APTA)** is a U.S.-based professional organization representing **physical therapists (PTs)**, **physical therapist assistants (PTAs)**, and physical therapy students. PT/PTA students can come from various life experiences. Some are new to college, some are non-traditional students, and some have college degrees or on-the-job experience, but one thing they all have in common is that they must become focused on a short-lived and fast-paced learning experience. Students are generally enthusiastic and excited to begin learning but often find that the pace of learning and the amount of material to be learned can be overwhelming. First-time students can encounter several common issues, including:

- Homesickness: Being away from home and loved ones for the first time can be difficult and cause homesickness.
- Adjusting to the academic workload: The academic demands of college or university can differ from those of high school, and first-time students may struggle to adjust.
- Time management: Balancing classes, studying, extracurricular activities, and a social life can be difficult, and first-time students may struggle with time management.
- Financial stress: College or university can be expensive, and first-time students may struggle to manage their finances, especially if they independently pay for tuition and living expenses.

- Making new friends: Starting college or university can be a great opportunity to make new friends, but it can also be challenging, especially if you are shy or introverted.
- Balancing independence and dependence: First-time students may struggle with finding the right balance between independence and dependence as they navigate their new environment.
- Finding your place: Finding a sense of belonging and community can be challenging for first-time students, especially if they are in a new city or away from home for the first time.
- Mental health: Students can face various mental health challenges during their academic journey, including stress, anxiety, depression, substance abuse, eating disorders, and sleep disturbances. Students need to seek help if they are struggling with their mental health, and many colleges and universities offer counseling services, mental health resources, and support groups. Students can also contact family, friends, or local mental

health providers for help and support. Seeking help is a sign of strength; taking care of your mental health is essential for overall well-being and success.

This chapter will explain some strategies for learning and exam taking that will assist the PT/PTA student during school and eventually to prepare for the National Physical Therapy Examination (NPTE)/ National Physical Therapist Assistant Examination (NPTAE).

# Learning

There are basic understandings of learning, and researchers constantly study how we learn to assist students. Several principles help us understand learning (see **Figure 1-1**).

1. The brain can adapt. The brain constantly processes incoming information to make sense of it. The processing of a person's thoughts, sensory

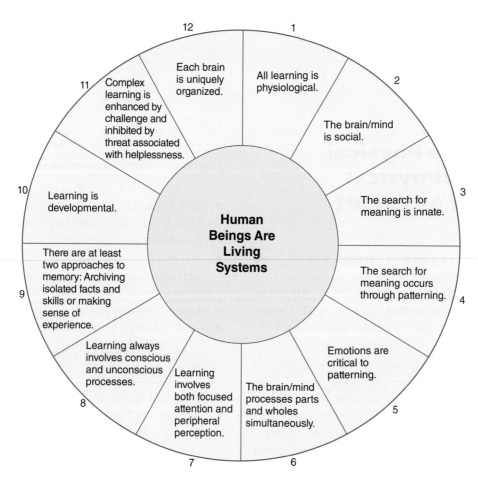

**Figure 1-1** Learning Principles
Copyright © Caine and Caine, 2000

information, and emotions influences how someone perceives what is occurring. Students should know that their perception differs from the person presenting the information and the others in the room.

2. The brain is social. The need to interact with others is innately within each of us, so students need to connect with others as they learn.

3. The brain looks for patterns. As the brain searches for ways to make sense of information, using similarities allows learners to connect the information to the pattern they already comprehend.

---

### KNOWLEDGE CHECK

Which positive learning traits do you employ?
Which negative learning traits do you have?

---

## Learning Styles

Learning styles are methods to gain, process, and store information. Research on personality and brain function (especially related to the differences in left and right hemispheric functions) indicates that each person gains, stores, and communicates information in a preferred way. Each person has a predominant learning style. Some people use a combination of learning styles, but most have at least one preferred one.

There is no best learning style, but some exchange information more effectively than others. Teachers always strive to identify and adapt their teaching styles to their students' preferred learning styles, especially in the sciences. As students and clinicians, PTs and PTAs are also trying to identify their and their patients' learning styles and adapt these to the learning and teaching processes. However, although the effectiveness of learning styles as a concept has been debated in academic circles, some research suggests that tailoring instruction to a student's learning style may not significantly improve their learning outcomes. Thus, it is generally recommended that students use a variety of approaches to learning to reinforce their understanding and improve their retention of information.

Because learning occurs in various ways—visual, auditory, via movement, and so on—students should not limit their learning to their preferred style.

### Visual Learning Style

The visual learner prefers seeing the information. The learner prefers symbols, charts, diagrams, pictures (including motion, such as in videos), and colors. Sometimes the learner may be easily distracted by images and not concentrate on the lecture. Highlighting the information; organizing the material as acronyms or mnemonics; and using CD-ROMs, videotapes, or photographs may be helpful [1].

The visual learner should utilize mind mapping to study, use graphic organizers by replacing words with symbols, turn phrases into images, and reconstruct images differently. For the visual learner, the written words will have less significance without visual aids. As study aids, the visual learner can utilize visual aids by:

- Drawing diagrams/pictures, graphs, and symbols
- Creating flashcards to identify concepts
- Practicing imaging techniques (by turning visual images into words or concepts)
- Recollecting mental pictures of their notes
- Utilizing the learning objectives to identify the learning task

### Auditory Learning Style

The auditory learner prefers to hear lectures and is eager (if not shy) to discuss any topic. The learner prefers to use a tape recorder instead of taking notes because they are too involved in the auditory part of the lectures. The learner works well in groups. For better learning, the information must be stated out loud, all important facts must be verbally reviewed, and sequences must be written out [1].

As study aids, the auditory learner may read text aloud to themselves to enhance understanding or may listen to lecture tapes. The auditory learner should study where auditory distractions are minimal. Working with a partner can assist the auditory learner because the student can explain concepts and problem-solve out loud, which helps to improve understanding and retention of information.

The auditory learner should:

- Explain concepts out loud
- Record lectures to listen to again
- Utilize repetition to help with retention
- Utilize study groups rather than solitary study

### Kinesthetic Learning Style

The kinesthetic learner prefers to learn by doing, often using trial and error. The learner prefers laboratory work, field/clinical activities, and manipulating objects or things. The learner prefers to read the instructions as a last resort. They prefer not to listen to lectures, take notes, or read the material. The learner prefers "hands-on" experience. Also, the learning process can be reinforced by using gestures or certain movements [1]. The learner should be cautious when learning procedures, as it is difficult to "unlearn" an incorrect technique.

The kinesthetic learner should:

- Use illustrations and note-taking during lectures to stay focused
- Talk or study with another kinesthetic learner
- Role-play the case studies (or scenarios)
- Write practice answers
- Utilize a motion when learning, such as counting on fingers to learn a list of symptoms
- Study in shorter blocks of time rather than marathon study sessions

The kinesthetic learner should read all the material (including the introduction and the summary). The kinesthetic learner should not make hasty decisions when choosing the right answers during tests. For example, answer A may be correct, but "all of the above" might be better.

### Analytic (Linear) Learning Style

The left-hemisphere-dominant analytic (linear) learner prefers to read, think about it, reread, organize, think about it again, rewrite, and reorganize. The learner prefers details and has difficulty seeing the "big picture." The learner uses many reference materials. They prefer clearly stated goals, lists, patterns, practice sets, and homework [1]. These students will have more difficulty in clinical situations where they must be aware of factual information and the social aspects of patient care.

The analytic learner should:

- Study by writing words and lists over and over
- Rewrite ideas in different ways
- Use organization charts

The analytic (left-hemisphere-dominant) learner should not spend too much time studying unnecessary concepts or details. When taking tests, the analytic learner should not get stuck on one question but continue to answer all questions.

### Spatial Learning Style

The right-hemisphere-dominant spatial learner prefers to learn by recognizing the sequencing of symbols, objects, and events. The learner sees the "big picture" first before the details. Learning is typically informal, spontaneous, and creative [1].

The spatial (right-hemisphere-dominant) learner should:

- Study by processing the information from whole to parts
- Use additional study time
- Work with others
- Learn to apply the new material

The spatial (right-hemisphere-dominant) learner should first look at the similarities of the information and form a total picture of the material before evaluating the details. Also, allowing more time to assimilate the new ideas and writing them down can be very helpful for this learner.

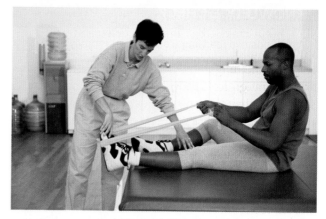

© Keith Brofsky/Photodisc/Getty Images

### KNOWLEDGE CHECK

What are the five learning styles?
Which learning style is most comfortable for you?

# Learning Resources
## Guide to Physical Therapist Practice 4.0

The **Guide to Physical Therapist Practice 4.0** ("the Guide") [2] was written to provide a comprehensive description of accepted PT practice, to reduce unwarranted variation in physical therapy treatments, improve the quality of physical therapy practice, enhance consumer satisfaction by maintaining and improving function and movement, promote appropriate utilization of healthcare services, and reduce the cost of treatment. The Guide introduces the patient and client management model, which comprises the elements involved in patient/client management: examination, evaluation, diagnosis, prognosis, intervention, and outcomes.

## Textbooks

Textbooks are intended to be a primary resource for student learning. The advent of electronic versions can make finding information very easy, and the organization of notes can be done with the click of a button. Learning how to use a textbook is important and can make learning easier.

One technique used for years is the SQ3R, which stands for **Survey, Question, Read, Recite, and Review**. Students should begin by surveying the chapter to be read. Looking at how the author has outlined the chapter and the objectives intended to be met helps the reader be prepared for the reading process. Second, the student should think about questions the reading can answer, an important step many skip, but it makes the difference between reading and understanding. Students must connect the information to something they know to understand and learn. In preparation for this process, students should consider what they already know and what questions they might have about the subject. Finally, the student is ready to read the chapter. Students should consider if their questions are being answered as they read. Looking at the pictures and figures can help bring clarity to the reading. At the end of each passage, the student should recite what they have learned from the reading to help organize the information in the student's mind and lead to memory retention.

Additionally, if the student does not understand a passage, they should reread the section, discuss it with classmates, and ask questions to the instructor. Taking notes during this activity can assist the student in reviewing the material later. Students should plan to review their notes daily to make sure that they remember the material. Students can quiz themselves by covering up the material and using keywords to recite the important concepts in their notes.

## The Internet

The internet has changed the way we live our lives and how we learn. It has been said that you can find anything on the web; however, just because you find anything does not mean it is true. Students must learn how to identify credible websites that can be trusted to give accurate information. The first thing to do is to identify the source of the information on the website. Credible sources can include universities and colleges (.edu), government webpages (.gov), medical organizations (.org), or hospital-related sites (.org). The website should have identified authors with expertise or provided a bibliography for the information

presented. Students should be cautious of commercial websites that endorse or sell products from the website. Students should also look for current information by identifying when the webpage was last updated.

## The Library

Libraries exist in every university and college and many cities. Librarians are excellent resources to help students find relevant and useful materials and answer questions. They can assist with selecting the correct database to perform research in and suggest relevant words and terminology when performing research queries. This assistance can save valuable time by helping to limit the available data to those most relevant to the project the student is working on. Librarians can also assist the student in ordering materials that may not be located in that library or on the internet.

## Student Services

Every university or college has a student service center to assist students in being successful. One common offering is tutoring. Tutoring is sometimes group tutoring or consists of review sessions with a graduate student or individual tutoring. The center usually offers study skill instruction and can assist students with test-taking skills. Students should not overlook those offerings. Students should not wait until they struggle in a class to seek assistance, either. Learning these skills early in a student's academic career can save the student anxiety and money.

## Instructor Assistance

Go early, go often. Instructors have office hours for students to come and get further assistance in the learning process. Students should ask the instructor specific questions rather than vague statements that no one understands. When students explain what they understand and what does not make sense to the instructor, the instructor can better focus the answers on the specific topic. Students who read the assigned material and attend class will be more successful with this learning strategy than those who expect the instructor to explain all the material again.

## Schedules and Calendars

Generally, students underestimate the time instructors expect them to spend studying outside class. Students may be used to instructors handing them the material to learn and memorize for the exam. Application and problem-solving require more than memorization. Manipulating the information in your mind, using it to solve problems, and formulating a rationale for choices are much better strategies. They prepare the student for comprehensive exams, clinical work, and the NPTE/NPTAE.

Students often juggle school, jobs, and families, requiring them to be very organized and to develop efficient use of their time. By utilizing a calendar, students can identify upcoming examinations and assignments so that they have adequate time to prepare. Additionally, students may need to utilize a calendar that helps them plan out each day more specifically to schedule study time; time for relaxation; time for exercise; and time for work, school, or chores. Busy schedules can be overwhelming when they are not planned out. Decreasing anxiety by being aware and prepared makes students feel calmer and in control of their daily lives.

Students should plan to study in blocks of time. A 50-minute study session should be followed by 10 minutes of another activity as a break. Students should set a timer to ensure adequate breaks for movement, food, and drink and that the 10-minute break does not become longer.

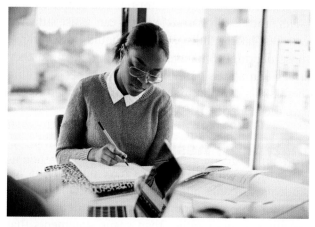

© Maskot/Getty Images

**KNOWLEDGE CHECK**

What does SQ3R stand for?
What college resources should a student look for when studying?

# Strategies for Success in PT/PTA School

Students will find that they are most successful when they do not just consider their learning styles but reflect on their learning as a whole. How successful have their strategies been? How organized is their studying? How committed have they been to learning the information, applying the information, and problem-solving? When students identify their motivation, effort, and strategies, they are better able to choose new strategies that will help them improve their learning skills.

## Learning Strategies

Several learning strategies exist (**Box 1-1**). It is important to note that different learning strategies may work better for different people and different types of information. Experimenting with different strategies can help determine which ones work best. Additionally, combining different strategies can be an effective way to reinforce learning and improve retention.

Important learning strategies include the ability to:

- Create a preferred learning environment. Students should consider the time of day, the type of lighting, surrounding sounds, temperature, type of seating, and snacks/drinks needed. Students who pay attention to these preferences will create a setting that improves their learning abilities by removing distractions and creating comfort.
- Read with a purpose and recognize the value of note-taking. Taking notes from reading or lectures helps to organize the information from the student's perspective and will help the student to

---

**Box 1-1 Learning Strategies**

- Active learning: This involves actively engaging with the material, such as through taking notes, summarizing information, and asking questions.
- Practice and repetition: Practicing and repeating information helps to reinforce learning and improve retention.
- Elaboration: This involves connecting new information to what you already know, making connections, and creating mental associations.
- Self-explanation: Explaining material to yourself, either out loud or in your mind, helps you better understand and remember the information.
- Chunking: Breaking information into smaller, manageable chunks can make it easier to learn and remember.
- Spaced repetition: Spacing out study sessions over time, rather than cramming all of the information into a short period, can help to improve long-term retention.
- Mental imagery: Creating mental images to help associate new information with a visual representation can improve recall.

understand the information better. Students who do not have good note-taking skills should devise a shorthand to help them become faster at note-taking. Utilize the lecture's organization to create an outline for the notes.

- Create mnemonics to help remember lists of information. Creating rhymes or incorporating information into music can also assist the mind in long-term recall.
- Develop supportive relationships; this is the easiest way to improve learning skills.
- Recognize the strengths of one's personal learning style and build on them; at the same time, value other learning styles.
- Create a study habit. Students should consider reading through their classroom notes every day. For example, a student takes notes on Monday and that same evening reads through their notes. On Tuesday evening, they read both Monday's and Tuesday's notes. On Wednesday, they read the notes from Monday, Tuesday, and Wednesday. This pattern continues for the rest of the week. This continuous review will make exam preparation much easier and decrease the tendency to "cram" at the last minute.
- Do not solve problems alone; learning power can be increased when working with others. In addition, working with people with opposite learning styles can add more to the learning process.
- Relate classwork to clearly defined long-range goals. Motivated students with clear goals will see their learning as a stepping stone to becoming a PT/PTA.
- PT/PTA school and clinical practice require a strategy and thought process different from what those students may have encountered. Because every patient is different, students must appreciate that not every answer is black and white. In reality, students will be expected to show competency in skills and the ability to rationalize when it is appropriate to deviate from the norm. In addition, students should learn to use research evidence to justify their reasoning. Recognize the need for active learning strategies. Memorization of information typically does not lead to a long-term recall of the data unless the student creates some personal meaning to the information. Students should practice skills and review material repeatedly to learn and know the necessary information. Secondly, students should understand the information well enough to explain it to others. Students should be able to provide examples to relate the information to the "bigger picture."

And finally, students should use the information to solve a problem, make a recommendation, or explain the rationale for a selected choice. Advanced thinking requires anticipating problems and considering possible solutions.

- Utilize review questions from the textbook to deepen learning and test understanding. The questions can be reviewed in a group setting to allow discussion of the answers or individually to test the student's preparedness for an exam. Such a review can be a valuable way to identify errors or omissions in understanding and generate questions that the student can discuss with the instructor.
- When studying for an exam, consider predicting questions. Review the concepts the instructor emphasized in the classroom and the learning resources. Consider what questions will be asked— definitions, application, and problem-solving. This activity may work best in a group to allow various ideas to be considered.
- Reflect on learning errors and successes. Students who actively seek to understand their mistakes will be more likely to feel in control, avoid negative feelings, and have better resilience. Students who actively engage in self-assessment, have control of their emotions, are resourceful, and set realistic goals will be more successful. Students should practice mindfulness. Mindfulness is an awareness technique for any given moment. Mindful meditation can include awareness of breathing, movements, and surroundings.
- Students should practice self-discipline in their studies. The instructor will offer information, resources, and guidance in learning, but the students should recognize that they must actively seek the answers instead of waiting for the information. Adequately preparing for class, fully participating in classroom activities, and asking questions/looking for answers are all critical components for long-term learning and understanding. Students can employ the following strategies to learn more effectively and deeply. Students should test themselves by putting away their books and notes and practice recalling and applying the information.
- Utilize online resources for learning.
  - Quizlet.com is an online learning platform that allows students or instructors to create study guides or quizzes for learning. Students can format their quizzes to match the material that they are learning. A search feature may reveal that other students or instructors have already created a quiz on the

material to be studied. This resource may work best for memorization work rather than problem-solving.

- Studyblue.com is similar to Quizlet in that you can create flashcards, study guides, and quizzes. It is touted as the largest crowd-sourced study library on the internet. One unique feature allows students to search for content already created by students from any specific school or university. This is one way to jump directly into the study mode and not have to spend time entering the information into the website. Another feature of this website allows students to ask specific questions and get multiple answers from different sources to aid in understanding the concepts.
- Brainscape.com allows users to access flashcards that have already been created in their subject area or to create their own. Repetition of terminology seems to be the best use of flashcards in this online tool.
- Simplemind.eu is an online mind-mapping tool allowing students to visualize overlapping concepts. The use of mind maps can be a valuable tool for considering the relationships between the materials the student is learning. The website has a free version and a paid subscription, offering more versatility.
- Dragon Anywhere is a mobile note-creating app that allows students to dictate their notes rather than type them. It can be used anywhere and is good for students who do not type quickly.

## KNOWLEDGE CHECK

Why should a student review and organize their classroom notes?

What is the value of reviewing the mistakes made on an exam?

What strategies help students learn deeply?

## Test-Taking Skills

Students who do not learn good test-taking skills work with an unseen disadvantage. In almost every objective test (such as in physical therapy), these students give up points needlessly because of undisciplined testing behaviors, irrational responses to test items, or a variety of other bad habits. As in other sciences, successful test-taking in physical therapy involves applying critical reading and thinking skills to the test to avoid making careless mistakes. These careless mistakes can be any of the following:

- Not reading the directions carefully: Students should not be in a hurry to start the test but should read the instructions first.
- Not monitoring the test time: Students should monitor their progress periodically to avoid getting caught in a time crunch.
- Changing the original answers due to second-guessing: Students should keep their original answers—research shows that the first intuition is more likely to be correct. Students should change their answers only when they strongly feel the original answer was incorrect or the question was read incorrectly.
- Not allowing enough time to go through the test: Students should leave time to check that no items are left blank or could be misread by a computerized grading program.
- Not identifying what the question is asking: Students should underline or highlight important words that help to answer the question or help to provide context to the question.

The three phases of test-taking strategies for students are as follows:

- In the first phase, the student should go through the test and answer only those items they are confident about; the other questions can be skipped momentarily. This strategy builds up confidence and ensures the student will get credit for what they know if they run low on time.
- In the second phase, the student should go through the test and focus on items they skipped in the first phase. The student should identify incorrect answers and eliminate choices that are definitely wrong or unlikely.
- In the third phase, the student should think critically by doing the following:
  - Being cautious of items that contain absolute terms, such as always, never, invariably, none, all, every, and must
  - Substituting a qualified term, such as frequently or typically, for an absolute term, such as always or most, to see if the statement is more or less valid than the original one
  - Looking for grammatical cues. If two answers are similar, they are usually not the correct answers. It is likely incorrect if the grammar in the stem does not match the grammar in the answer.

- When taking multiple-choice tests, a good strategy is to read only the "stem" of the question and not the multiple choices to see if the correct answer can be determined without being prompted by the choices. If no answer can be found, the student can read each multiple-choice answer separately and consider whether it is a "true" or "false" choice. The answer that seems most valid should be the final choice. Sometimes, teachers are limited in their supply of decoy answers and, as a result, will make up terms to use for that purpose. For a student who missed classes or has not studied, the decoy is hard to detect; however, if the student has been attending classes regularly and has done a good job of preparing for the test, the student will not choose an answer that sounds new.

- When taking a test with true–false items, students generally have difficulty reading and considering the choices carefully. A slight alteration in the phrasing of the item can make a big difference. The basic ground rule for answering true–false items is that the student should select false as the answer if any part of the statement is false. At the same time, true–false items can be overanalyzed to the point that the student goes beyond the scope of the question, looking to find an extreme exception to what the question is testing or the "trick" suspected to be somewhere in the phrasing. The student should read the question carefully and judge what the question is saying.

- Finally, review your errors after the exam has been corrected. Students should make time to meet with the instructor to gain an understanding of any questions or concepts that remain unclear. Many of the exams taken in the curriculum are concepts that will be repeated later and ultimately must be understood for success within the clinical portion of the program and the NPTE/NPTAE.

# Lifelong Learning

While it may be difficult for a student to think about lifelong learning activities at the beginning of their career, they must appreciate that learning does not end at graduation. Because of the ever-changing nature of healthcare, conscientious professionals will always be interested in learning new developments. In beginning the process, students should consider all aspects of this textbook that have suggested resources, introduced learning topics, or piqued their interest. Making a list of topics that you find interesting and locating resources for learning can help you create a lifelong learning plan. As your career develops, physical therapy practice changes, and healthcare evolves, so will your lifelong learning plan.

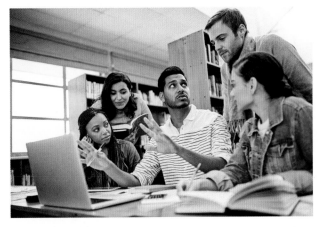

© PeopleImages/E+/Getty Images

## Discussion Questions

1. With your classmates, discuss learning strategies that have helped you in the past. Explain whether this varies by the type of learning task.
2. Complete an online learning inventory using the sources below. Share your results with your classmates.
   a. Personality Max (https://personalitymax.com /personality-test/)
   b. Multiple Intelligences Assessment (www .literacynet.org/mi/assessment/findyourstrengths .html)
   c. The VARK Questionnaire (http://vark-learn .com/the-vark-questionnaire/)
3. Discuss learning services available on your campus.

## Learning Opportunities

1. Utilizing your course syllabi and schedule, create a daily/monthly calendar that includes school, work, and family/social obligations. Identify when completing homework and studying will fit into the schedule.

2. Utilize the SQ3R strategy to read a chapter in a textbook.
3. List activities that will be part of a lifelong learning plan.

## References

1. Dreeben O: Patient Education in Rehabilitation. Sudbury, MA, Jones & Bartlett Learning, 2010

2. American Physical Therapy Association: Guide to Physical Therapist Practice 4.0. Alexandria, VA, American Physical Therapy Association, 2023

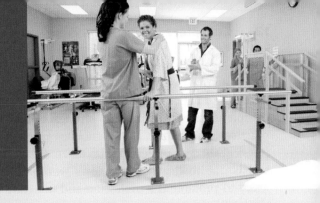

# CHAPTER 2

# The Physical Therapy Profession

## OBJECTIVES

- Discuss the history of rehabilitation treatments from ancient times through the 1900s.
- Describe the history of the physical therapy profession and its six cycles of growth and development.
- Identify the values and culture of the physical therapy profession.
- Describe the American Physical Therapy Association's (APTA) mission and its goals for physical therapists (PTs) and physical therapist assistants (PTAs).
- Explain the organizational structure of the APTA.
- Discuss the benefits of belonging to a professional organization.
- Name organizations involved in the physical therapy profession.

## KEY TERMS

American Physical Therapy
  Association (APTA)
assembly
autonomous practice
board of directors (BOD)
client
combined sections meeting (CSM)
Commission on Accreditation in
  Physical Therapy Education
  (CAPTE)

disability
evidence-based practice
functional limitations
House of Delegates (HOD)
physiatrist
physical therapist assistant (PTA)
  Caucus
Physical Therapy Political Action
  Committee (PT-PAC)
physiotherapists

physiotherapy
poliomyelitis ("polio")
reconstruction aides
Special Interest Group (SIG)
Vision 2020
World Confederation for Physical
  Therapy (WCPT)

## Overview

Physical therapy is delivered by healthcare professionals who help individuals maintain, restore, and improve movement, activity, and functioning, thereby enabling optimal performance in enhancing health, well-being, and quality of life [1]. The physical therapy profession continues to evolve based on societal needs and is driven by medical advancements. While evolving, the profession has strived to provide a unique service while preventing encroachment from other professions, including athletic trainers and chiropractors. Each state regulates the physical therapy profession using legislation known as practice acts, which provide guidelines about practice requirements and help to provide consistency. The physical therapy profession is also managed by the American Physical Therapy Association's (APTA) Guide to Physical Therapist Practice 4.0 ("the Guide"), which provides a comprehensive description of physical therapist (PT) practice (see Chapter 3) [1]. The development of the physical therapy profession has taken over a century and is due to the many pioneers who worked tirelessly to promote the profession and integrate it into the healthcare system.

# The APTA

The APTA is the principal membership organization that stands for and promotes the profession of physical therapy and is a strong voice in Washington, DC, politics for physical therapy services and patient advocacy. In addition, the APTA has worked for payment reform and insurance provider education. The APTA's mission is: "Building a community that advances the profession of physical therapy to improve the health of society."[1]

The APTA has also been involved in several societal issues, including the following:

- Working with other organizations on initiatives of mutual interest in proposed care and payment models, ensuring the inclusion of physical therapy where appropriate
- Supporting the Alliance of Wound Care Stakeholders, a nonprofit multidisciplinary trade association of medical specialty societies and clinical associations that promotes quality care and access to products and services for people with wounds through advocacy and educational outreach in the regulatory, legislative, and public arenas
- CDC recommendations for age-related vaccinations
- Support for public health policies to reduce and prevent firearms-related injuries and death
- Supports the Consortium for Citizens with Disabilities (CCD), an organization that works through federal legislation and regulations to ensure that the 54 million children and adults with physical and mental disabilities are fully integrated into the mainstream of society
- Supports the proposed provision of resources on the use of cannabis or cannabis-based products for health-related conditions
- Working with other organizations on mutually beneficial legislation and regulations for the betterment of the healthcare system

- Supporting the Alliance for Balanced Pain Management (AfBPM), a diverse collection of healthcare advocacy groups, patient organizations, industry representatives, and other stakeholders who ensure people with or affected by pain have appropriate access to integrated, effective, and safe care across the continuum of care, and raise awareness of the need for individualized treatment options
- Is a founding member of the Coalition for Patients' Rights and continues to work with its member organizations to oppose efforts by the American Medical Association and other physician organizations to limit nonphysician scopes of practice
- Advocates the Coalition to Preserve Rehabilitation (CPR), a national coalition of consumer, clinician, and membership organizations to preserve access to rehabilitation services for individuals with disabilities, injuries, or chronic conditions

## The House of Delegates and the Board of Directors

The **House of Delegates (HOD)** is the highest policy-making body of the APTA. It comprises delegates from all chapters, sections, and assemblies, as well as members of the **board of directors (BOD)**. The HOD comprises chapter voting delegates; section, **assembly**, physical therapist assistant (PTA) Caucus nonvoting delegates; and consultants. The voting chapter delegates' number is determined yearly based on membership numbers as of June 30. The annual session of the APTA is the meeting of the HOD. It occurs yearly at the Association's NEXT Conference and Exposition in June.

The role of the BOD is to carry out the mandates and policies established by the HOD and to communicate issues to internal and external personnel, committees, and agencies. The APTA's BOD comprises 15 members—6 officers and 9 directors. Board members assume office at the close of the HOD at which they were elected. A complete term for a board member is 3 years. Only active members of the APTA in good standing for at least 5 years can serve on the BOD. No member can serve more than three consecutive terms on the board or more than two consecutive terms in the same office. The board meets at least once a year, and the executive committee meets at least twice yearly.

The six officers of the APTA are the president, vice president, secretary, treasurer, speaker of the HOD,

---

1 https://www.apta.org/apta-and-you/leadership-and-governance/policies/apta-mission-statement.

and vice speaker of the HOD. The president of the APTA presides at all BOD and executive committee meetings and serves as the official spokesperson of the Association. The president is also an ex officio member of all committees appointed by the BOD except the ethics and judicial committees. The APTA's vice president assumes the president's duties in the absence or incapacitation of the president. In the event of a vacancy in the office of president, the vice president will be the president for the unexpired portion of the term. In this situation, the office of the vice president will be vacant. The secretary of the APTA is responsible for keeping the minutes of the proceedings of the HOD, the BOD, and the executive committee; for making a report in writing to the HOD at each annual session and the BOD on request; and for preparing a summary of the proceedings of the HOD for publication. The treasurer of the APTA is responsible for reporting in writing on the financial status of the Association to the HOD and the BOD on request. The treasurer also serves as the chair of the finance and audit committees. The speaker of the HOD presides at sessions of the HOD, serves as an officer of the HOD, and is an ex officio member of the reference committee. The vice speaker of the HOD serves as an officer of the HOD and assumes the duties of the speaker of the HOD in the absence or incapacitation of the speaker. In the event of a vacancy in the office of the speaker of the HOD, the vice speaker succeeds to the office of the speaker for the unexpired term. In this situation, the office of the vice speaker will be vacant.

## APTA's Headquarters

The Association's headquarters are currently located in Alexandria, Virginia. The Association's personnel are available online at www.apta.org and the toll-free number (800) 999-2782. The address of the Association is 1111 North Fairfax Street, Alexandria, VA,

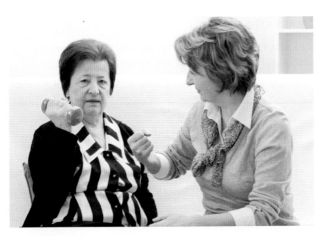

22314-1488. The APTA Centennial Center opened on January 15, 2021.

## APTA Components

Membership in the APTA is voluntary. The components of the APTA are districts (local level), chapters (state level), sections (national level), and assemblies (national level) (**Figure 2-1**):

- Districts: The most local organizational component of the APTA is the district. Not all jurisdictions have a membership at the district level. When present, districts hold educational and networking events for their members throughout the year and serve as a means of representation at the chapter level.
- Chapters: The Association has 51 chapters in the 50 states and the District of Columbia. Membership in a chapter is automatic. Members must belong to the chapter of the state in which they live, work, or attend school (or of an adjacent state if more active participation is possible). Chapters are significant for governance at the state level and contributing to the national integration of members in the Association.
- Sections: The APTA has 19 sections (see **Table 2-1**). They are organized at the national level, allowing

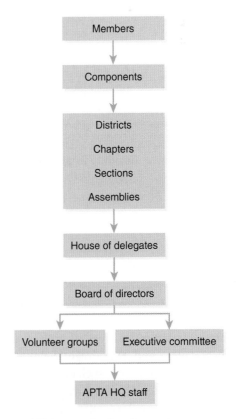

**Figure 2-1** APTA organizational structure.

**Table 2-1** Sections of the APTA

| Section | Mission |
|---|---|
| Acute Care | To foster excellence in acute care practice in all settings, to enhance the health and functioning of patients and clients |
| Aquatics | To champion aquatic physical therapy to optimize lifelong movement, function, and wellness |
| Cardiovascular and Pulmonary | To serve its members and the physical therapy profession by promoting the development, application, and advancement of cardiovascular and pulmonary physical therapy practice, education, and research |
| Clinical Electrophysiology and Wound Management | To optimize patient outcomes by advancing through physical therapy, the practice of clinical electrophysiology, biophysical agents, and integumentary/wound management |
| Education | To inspire all PTs and PTAs in their roles as educators and to enhance the development and implementation of evidence-based education practices |
| Federal | To promote quality health care across the continuum of care for those served by physical therapists in the Federal government |
| Geriatrics | To support those therapists, assistants, and students who work with an aging population in roles of advocacy, direct patient care, consultation, supervision, and education |
| Hand and Upper Extremity | To promote education and research in hand and upper extremity physical therapy while advocating for the ever-changing needs of the communities it serves |
| Home Health | To provide a means by which Association members having a common interest in delivering physical therapy in the home and other alternative settings within the community may meet, confer, and promote these interests |
| Leadership and Innovation | To transform the culture of physical therapy through initiatives that enhance professionalism, leadership, management, and advocacy to foster excellence in autonomous practice for the benefit of members and society |
| Neurology | To empower our members to optimize movement system performance for those impacted by neurologic conditions |
| Oncology | Maximizing movement and wellness across the life span for persons affected by cancer and chronic illness through advocacy, engagement, education, and collaboration |
| Orthopedics | To empower members to excel in orthopedic physical therapy |
| Pediatrics | Bringing people together to advance excellence in pediatric physical therapy |
| Pelvic Health | To advance global excellence in abdominal and pelvic health through evidence-based practice, innovative education, research, and social responsibility |
| Private Practice | To champion the success of the PT in business |
| Research | Optimizing movement through discovery and innovation |
| Sports | To specialize and excel in sports physical therapy by facilitating education, research, networking, and mentoring through our community of established and emerging leaders |

Reproduced from APTA  American Physical Therapy Association

members with similar areas of interest to meet, discuss issues, and encourage the interests of the respective sections. An elected BOD governs each section, all of whom are available to discuss issues affecting the Association and the physical therapy profession. The section president is responsible for governing and directing all section activities. The sections usually have an annual **combined sections meeting (CSM)**, which usually occurs in early February. The purpose of the CSM, which has become the APTA's most popular national education meeting, is to provide educational and business sessions for all sections and product demonstrations.

## Box 2-1 Special Interest Groups

**Special Interest Groups (SIGs)** can be formed within chapters, sections, or assemblies. Each SIG has its own governance, activities, and annual programming. Each SIG provides a forum where members can organize themselves into areas of common interest. Most sections have their own SIGs. For example, the oncology section has the following SIGs: balance and falls, human immunodeficiency virus (HIV) disease, hospice and palliative care, lymphatic diseases, pediatric, and residency.

- Assemblies: The Association has two assemblies: the **physical therapy assistant (PTA) Caucus** and the Student Assembly. The assemblies are composed of members from the same category and provide means for members to communicate and contribute at the national level to their future governance. One of the important positions expressed in 2004 by the National Assembly for the Physical Therapist Assistants was that the PTA is the only educated individual whom the PT may direct and supervise for providing selected interventions in the delivery of physical therapy services. The PTA Caucus is benefiting from and reinforcing the PTA's role in the APTA. A 2014 meeting identified the need for the APTA to develop a membership value plan specifically for the PTA member.

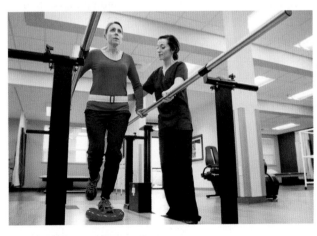

© Andersen Ross Photography Inc/DigitalVision/Getty Images

# History of Rehabilitation Treatments

A historical perspective of rehabilitative techniques dates back to 400 BC. Some of the same interventions we use nowadays, such as therapeutic massage, hydrotherapy, and therapeutic exercises, have helped us recover from injury and illness for centuries. For example, historical figures, such as the father of medicine, Hippocrates, recognized the value of muscle strengthening using exercises (**Figure 2-2**). Hippocrates was the first physician to recommend therapeutic exercises to his patients because he understood the principle of muscle, ligament, and bone atrophy (wasting) due to inactivity. The Greek philosopher Aristotle recommended rubbing massage using oil and water to remedy tiredness. The Romans introduced therapeutic exercises known as gymnastics, and renowned physician Galen described the kinetic principles of human movement. It has long been recognized that exercise gives the body agility and vigor and can cleanse the muscles and ligaments of waste.

Most of what we call physical therapy originated in Europe. During the early 1900s, major theories and techniques were developed due to an increased understanding of human anatomy and physiology. During World War I, many therapeutic techniques were utilized by "reconstruction aides" to rehabilitate disabled soldiers. Through the work of Herman Kabat, Margaret Knott, and Dorothy Voss, proprioceptive neuromuscular facilitation (PNF) was created to assist patients with neurologic dysfunction. Paralysis due to polio inspired Professor Robert Lovett and his senior assistant, Wilhelmine G. Wright [2], to develop training in crutch ambulation. In 1928, Wright

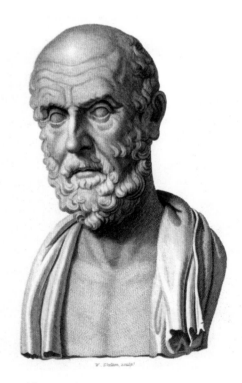

**Figure 2-2** Hippocrates.
Courtesy of National Library of Medicine.

**Box 2-2**

**Reconstruction aides** were civilian women and served an influential role in developing physical therapy by providing treatment to enable service members suffering from wounds or battle neurosis to return to the battlefront.

[2] authored the book Muscle Function (which she started with Dr. Lovett), describing the systematic method of manual muscle testing using palpation, gravity, external manual resistance, and the arc of active movement. Wright believed in the importance of muscle testing on polio patients and using stronger muscles to compensate for the weakness of muscles affected by polio. Between 1917 and the early 1950s, several PTs and rehabilitation clinicians modified Wright's muscle testing method, considering variables such as a patient's fatigue, body position, and incoordination [2]. These clinicians included Florence Kendall, Signe Brunnstrom, Marjorie Dennen, and Catherine Worthingham (**Figure 2-3**). Advances in hydrotherapy led to the creation of the Georgia Warm Springs Foundation, which has become an international polio treatment facility. In 1928, U.S. President Franklin D. Roosevelt, who had polio, used the "hydrogymnastics" therapy at Warm Springs Institute for rehabilitation.

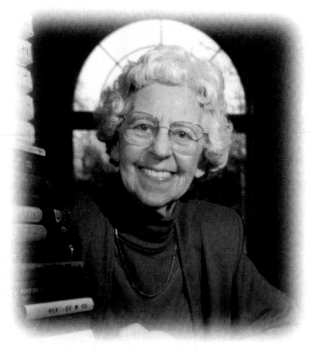

**Figure 2-3** Florence Kendall.
Photo courtesy of Stephen Barrett

The early to mid-1900s were rich in understanding and developing orthopedic surgery and rehabilitation techniques, including the development of Codman pendulum exercises for shoulder rehabilitation by Dr. Ernest A. Codman and postural exercises for back pain by Dr. Paul C. Williams. Following his knee surgery, an Alabama physician, Thomas DeLorme, discovered that he could rapidly restore his quadriceps muscles to full strength by increasing the resistance applied to the exercising muscles. DeLorme's method [3] first introduced the technique of progressive resistive exercise (PRE), which is still used today.

During the second half of the 1900s, therapeutic exercises in the United States advanced tremendously with the arrival of isokinetic and biofeedback exercises. For example, in 1967, the Cybex I Dynamometer was introduced based on Helen Hislop and James Perrine's concept of isokinetic exercise. Hislop and Perrine found that muscular performance can be reduced to the physical parameters of force, work, power, and endurance and that the specificity of exercise should be determined by an exercise system designed to control each training need. Another type of exercise called biofeedback was introduced in the second half of the 1900s due to advances in scientific behavioral psychology and clinical electromyography. Regarding back pain and exercises, in 1953, Paul C. Williams proposed a series of postural exercises known today as the Williams exercises. These helped to strengthen the spine flexors and extensors and relieve back pain. Furthermore, Williams's back flexion exercises were complemented in the 1960s by Robin McKenzie's back extension exercises that relieved pressure posteriorly on the spinal disk. Swiss ball exercises, developed by physiotherapists in Switzerland in the 1960s, found their way to the United States in the 1970s and became popular in physical therapy rehabilitation in the 1980s.

### KNOWLEDGE CHECK

Which two historical events developed the profession?

# History of the Physical Therapy Profession

The creation of the physical therapy profession centered around two major events in U.S. history: the poliomyelitis epidemics and the negative effects of

World Wars I and II. The profession can be compared with a living entity, changing from an undeveloped, young occupation in its formative years (1914–1920) to a firm, growing establishment in its development years (1920–1940). As a mature profession, during its fundamental accomplishment years (1940–1970), physical therapy achieved significant organizational, executive, and educational skills. In the mastery years (1970–1996), the profession acquired greater control, proficiency, and respect within the healthcare arena, expanding education, licensure, specialization, research, and direct access. From 1996 to 2005, in its adaptation years, physical therapy had to adapt, review, and change its objectives and goals due to political, social, and economic changes in the United States. Additionally, the profession underwent rapid educational expansion and research growth, and significant developmental and scientific goals were achieved. From 2006 to the present, in its vision and scientific pursuit years, physical therapy has emerged as a vigorous participant in U.S. healthcare reform, having large responsibilities in research, education, and sociopolitical transformations.

## Formative Years: 1914 to 1920

### *Division of Special Hospitals and Physical Reconstruction*

In the United States, physical therapy began between 1914 and 1919, in a time known as the Reconstruction Era. Before the "Great War" (World War I), most Americans regarded **disability** as irreversible, requiring little or no medical intervention. The war changed this concept of irreversibility because of the many young U.S. service members returning home as disabled veterans. As previously mentioned, physical therapy was created because of World War I and the poliomyelitis epidemics. These two devastating events in U.S. history brought a devastating disease and subsequent disability to U.S. society. The first major outbreak of poliomyelitis occurred in New York State in 1916 [4]. The treatment methods at that time were bed rest, isolation, splinting, and casting of the person's legs [4]. Unfortunately, these forms of healing increased the individual's weakness in the legs and back, so the person required some exercise and physiotherapy.

Before and during World War I, support for people with disabilities grew gradually. For example, the Medical Department of the U.S. Army had two divisions that influenced the growth of physical rehabilitation in the United States: the Division of Orthopedic Surgery and the Division of Physical

Reconstruction [4]. The newly created Division of Physical Reconstruction was needed to apply physiotherapy treatments such as massage and mechanical hydrotherapy to wounded soldiers. The Division of Physical Reconstruction drew its "training corps" personnel from allied health therapies and physical training schools [4]. The Division of Physical Reconstruction had four sections: surgery (including general, orthopedic, and head surgery), neuropsychiatry, education, and physiotherapy (including gymnasiums and equipment) [4].

In April 1917, the United States entered World War I. The U.S. Congress authorized the military draft and passed legislation to rehabilitate all service members permanently disabled from war-related injuries. In August 1917, the Surgeon General of the United States, William Gorgas, authorized the creation of the Division of Special Hospitals and Physical Reconstruction [5]. The role of the division was to give soldiers who were disabled "reconstruction therapy." The people involved in the reconstruction therapy were newly trained physical reconstruction aides. They consisted of a handful of physicians called orthopedists and 1,200 young women called reconstruction aides. These physical and occupational therapy pioneers treated the injured soldiers from World War I. The division included two different groups of reconstruction aides. One group that assisted physicians was to become today's PTs. They provided exercise programs, massage, hydrotherapy, and other therapeutic modalities, including patient education (**Figure 2-4**). The other group of reconstruction aides

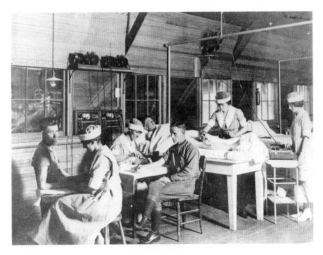

**Figure 2-4** Reconstruction aides treat soldiers at Fort Sam Houston, Texas, in 1919 (World War I Era).

Courtesy of the American Physical Therapy Association.

was to become today's occupational therapists. They provided vocational skills training to help wounded soldiers return to work.

These forms of rehabilitation enabled soldiers to return to combat or their prewar civilian lives. The division had almost a dozen small facilities in Europe and more extensive centers and hospitals in New York Harbor; Lakewood, New Jersey; Tacoma Park, Maryland (a suburb of Washington, DC); Fort McPherson, Georgia; and San Francisco, California [5]. Each hospital had a physical therapy unit containing a gymnasium, a whirlpool room, a massage room, a hot/cold pack room, and other rooms for mechanotherapy and "electricity" (electrotherapy) [5]. The mechanotherapy room was an exercise room equipped with various apparatuses, such as pulley-and-weight systems, trolleys, and ball-bearing wheels.

From its creation, the division recruited unmarried women between the ages of 25 and 40 to be trained as reconstruction aides. Applicants receiving certificates showing practical and theoretical training in any treatment performed, such as hydrotherapy, electrotherapy, mechanotherapy, or massage, received priority and were accepted first. Nevertheless, they were still given additional preparation in all other necessary treatments.

## First PTs: Marguerite Sanderson and Mary McMillan

Marguerite Sanderson and Mary McMillan were the first reconstruction aides who significantly contributed to the physical therapy profession during the Reconstruction Era. Marguerite Sanderson was a physiotherapist who graduated from the Boston Normal School of Gymnastics and used to work with Dr. Joel Goldthwait, an orthopedic surgeon who later became the chairman of the War Reconstruction Committee of the American Orthopedic Association. Because of her prior physiotherapy experience, in 1917, Dr. Goldthwait appointed Sanderson as the first supervisor of reconstruction aides. Her role was to recruit and arrange for the training of reconstruction aides and send them to Europe to help the wounded soldiers. In 1922, Sanderson married and withdrew from active participation in the school.

The training program for the reconstruction aides took place at Walter Reed General Hospital. The program at Walter Reed was assigned to a reconstruction aide named Mary Livingston McMillan (**Figure 2-5**). Mary McMillan was a mature, educated woman born in the United States of Scottish ancestry. When she was 5, her mother and sister died of consumption

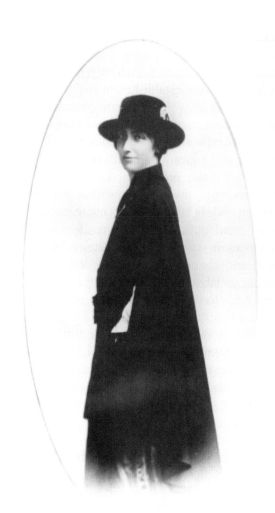

**Figure 2-5** Mary McMillan, one of the founders and the first president of the APTA (World War I Era—1918/1919).
Courtesy of the American Physical Therapy Association.

(tuberculosis). Mary was sent to live with relatives in Liverpool, England. Although acquiring a higher education was unusual at that time for a young woman, as an avid and eager learner, Mary received a college degree in physical education and a postgraduate degree in her chosen career, the science of physical therapy. McMillan's physical therapy degree included corrective exercises, massage, electrotherapy, aftercare of fractures, dynamics of scoliosis, psychology, neurology, and neuroanatomy [5]. In 1910, McMillan took her first professional position in Liverpool, England, working with Sir Robert Jones, nephew and professional heir of the great orthopedist Hugh Owen Thomas. Jones, an orthopedic physician, was renowned for using the Thomas splint (invented by his famous uncle) and performing progressive massage and orthopedic manipulations (invented by the French orthopedist Lucas-Championniere and British surgeon James B. Mennell). Lucas-Championniere and Mennell were pioneers of the principle that following an injury, early movement can enhance healing and prevent disability.

In 1916, McMillan returned home to her family in Massachusetts. Because of her education and experience, she was hired immediately at the Children's Hospital in Portland, Maine. For 2 years, she was director of massage and medical gymnastics, treating children with scoliosis, congenital hip dislocations, and other conditions in pediatric orthopedic bone and joint abnormalities [5]. In 1918, at the recommendation of Sir Robert Jones, Elliott Bracket, a Boston orthopedist and one of the organizers of the Army's Reconstruction Program, asked McMillan to consider serving with the U.S. Army. In February 1918, McMillan was sworn in as a U.S. Army Medical Corps member. She was assigned to Walter Reed General Hospital in Tacoma Park, Maryland, as a reconstruction aide. Shortly after, in June 1918, due to her experience and education in England, McMillan was asked to go to Reed College in Portland, Oregon, to train reconstruction aide applicants in the practical, hands-on segment of the War Emergency Training Program. With her contribution, Reed College's physical therapy curriculum became the standard by which other emergency war training programs were measured. In January 1919, McMillan was awarded the position of Chief Reconstruction Aide in the physiotherapy department at Walter Reed General Hospital [5].

Between 1919 and 1920, the number of physical therapy reconstruction aides was reduced primarily because of a major postwar decrease in military hospitals (at home and overseas). The number of hospitals shrank from 748 to 49. Despite this cutback, the army's commitment to maintaining physical therapy as an important part of its medical services was established. In 1920, McMillan resigned from her duties in the army because she felt her work was essentially completed. She returned to civilian life in Boston as a staff therapist in an orthopedic office. In 1921, McMillan published her book, Massage and Therapeutic Exercise.

## Development Years: 1920 to 1940

### The Development of Professional Organization

While working as a reconstruction aide, Mary McMillan was convinced that physical therapy had a vital future role in America's health care. Before resigning her duties in the army, McMillan wanted to maintain a nucleus of trained people capable of carrying out such a role. She contacted 800 former reconstruction aides and civilian therapists and received 120 enthusiastic responses. On January 15, 1921, at Keene's Chop House, an eatery in Manhattan, New York, McMillan and 30 former reconstruction aides organized themselves into the first association of PTs [5]. The organization was the American Women's Physical Therapeutic Association (AWPTA). McMillan was elected president. The role of the AWPTA was to establish and maintain professional and scientific standards for individuals involved with the profession of physical therapeutics [4]. The members of the AWPTA were graduates of recognized schools of physiotherapy and physical education programs trained in massage, therapeutic exercises, electrotherapy, and hydrotherapy [4]. The executive committee of the AWPTA represented geographically diverse reconstruction aides; in the first year, 274 members came from 32 states.

### The PT Review and Constitution

The official publication of the Association, which first appeared in March 1921, was called the PT Review [5]. It was published quarterly and included the Association's constitution and bylaws, professional interest articles, and a column called "SOS" for job classified advertisements. Also, in 1921, the first textbook written by a physiotherapist (Mary McMillan) was published.

The first edition of the PT Review reported the full text of the constitution and bylaws of the Association. The basic reasons for the Association's existence, as described in its constitution, were to have professional and scientific standards for its members, to increase competency among members by encouraging advanced studies, to promulgate medical literature and articles of professional interest, to make available efficiently trained members, and to sustain professional socialization [5]. The Association's bylaws specified three categories of membership in the Association: charter members, who were the reconstruction aides in **physiotherapy**; active members, who were graduates of recognized schools of physiotherapy or physical education; and honorary members, who were graduates of medical schools.

### American Physiotherapy Association

At its first conference in Boston in 1922, the Association changed its name to the American Physiotherapy Association because although its members were all women, they recognized that men also practiced physiotherapy. At that time, a few male reconstruction aides provided physiotherapy services during World War I.

In 1922, new physiotherapy schools opened at Harvard Medical School and New York City. The graduates of these schools were called **physiotherapists**. By 1923, the membership in the Association had risen appreciably, and McMillan stepped down as president, giving way to a new president, one of the former reconstruction aides, Inga Lohne [5].

In 1926, the Committee on Education and Publicity was formed to draft the minimum standard curriculum for schools offering a complete course in physical therapy. The committee's report, published in 1928, recommended a 9-month course with 33 hours of physical therapy–related instruction per week, for 1,200 hours [5]. The entrance requirement was graduation from a recognized school of physical education or nursing (**Figure 2-6**). In 1930, 11 schools met or exceeded the minimum standards set by the committee, and by 1934, there were 14 approved physiotherapy schools, including higher standard educational institutions, such as Harvard Medical School in Boston, Massachusetts; Stanford University Hospital in Stanford, California; and the College of William and Mary in Williamsburg, Virginia [5].

The American Physiotherapy Association tried to stay alongside the medical profession in the early years. During the 1920s and 1930s, physical therapy physicians formed the American Medical Association (AMA). The AMA recognized their efforts and educated other physicians about the value of physical therapy in rehabilitating World War I veterans. As a result, in 1925, a group of physical therapy physicians founded the American College of Physical Therapy (ACPT). Later that year, the ACPT joined the AMA and changed its name to the American Congress of Physical Therapy. Physical therapy physicians decided to call themselves "physiatrists." Although their name was not officially changed until 1946, the physiatrists established the American Registry of Physical Therapy

Technicians to separate physiotherapists from the medical profession.

In 1930, the American Physiotherapy Association was incorporated and decided to work with the AMA to create standards of education for physiotherapists; to encourage the regulation of physical therapy practice by law; and to cooperate with or under the direction of the medical profession to provide a central registry for physiotherapists [6].

Consequently, by the 1930s, due to pressure from the AMA, registered physiotherapists were called technicians and settled to work under the referral of physical therapy physicians. It seems, however, that members of the AMA were concerned the public might consider physiotherapists to be physicians because their designation as physiotherapists ended in "ists," the same as radiologists, orthopedists, and so on. The AMA wanted no confusion concerning the medical school education of physiatrists compared to physiotherapists. Finally, in the 1940s, the name physiotherapists changed to PTs.

## Poliomyelitis and the Great Depression

By the 1930s, members of the American Physiotherapy Association were confronted with two catastrophes—the growing severity of **poliomyelitis** and its resulting infantile paralysis (which began in the summer of 1916) and the Great Depression of 1929 (**Figure 2-7**). The poliomyelitis epidemics started in 1916 and continued into the 1930s and

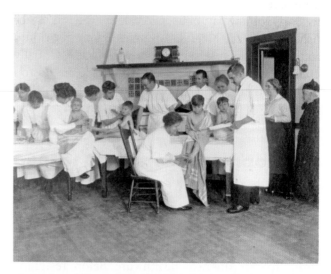

**Figure 2-7** PTs and physicians work together to treat children at a New York poliomyelitis clinic in 1916 (World War I Era).

Courtesy of the American Physical Therapy Association.

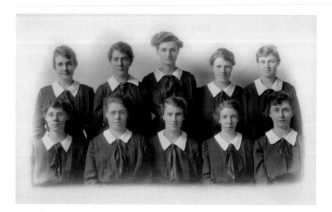

**Figure 2-6** First class at Northeastern University.

Photo courtesy of Champlain Studios, Northeastern University.

1940s. As an example of this disease's high incidence and magnitude, between May and November 1934, approximately 2,500 cases of poliomyelitis were treated at just one hospital, the Los Angeles County General Hospital [4]. The fact that the president of the United States, Franklin Delano Roosevelt, was treated for poliomyelitis by physiotherapists generated large public recognition of the physical therapy profession. At that time, physical therapy for poliomyelitis consisted of hydrotherapy, exercises, massage, heat and light modalities, and assistive and adaptive equipment [4]. The physiotherapists provided "homemade" braces and splints in the home care setting, especially in rural areas.

In 1929, the Depression closed many hospitals and private medical practices, substantially reducing the number of physical therapy services.

Because the country was looking for a cure for poliomyelitis, in 1937, the National Foundation for Infantile Paralysis was founded. Using federal funding and money from charitable organizations, such as the March of Dimes, the foundation opened new facilities and lent equipment to families and hospitals for polio aftercare. The National Foundation for Infantile Paralysis also financially contributed to the development of physical therapy education and the growth of physical therapy schools. PTs without work during the Great Depression could pick and choose positions. They were needed to work in diagnostic clinics, outpatient centers, orthopedic hospitals, convalescent homes, schools for children with disabilities, and therapeutic services.

In 1937, although the physiotherapists were still dominated by their technician mindsets, their plans were progressive and included unity, research, and provision of educational standards. For example, the aims of the American Physiotherapy Association in 1937 were as follows [4]:

- To form a nationwide organization that would establish and maintain professional and scientific standards for its members
- To promote the science of physical therapy
- To aid in the establishment of educational standards and scientific research in physical therapy
- To cooperate with and to work only under the prescription of members of the medical profession
- To provide available information to those interested in physical therapy
- To unite several chapters
- To create a central registry (available for the medical profession) that will make physiotherapists the only "trained assistants" in physical therapy

# Fundamental Accomplishment Years: 1940 to 1970

## The Professional and Educational Developments of Physical Therapy

During World War II, the American Physiotherapy Association continued to grow under its president, Catherine Worthingham. She was the first PT to hold a doctoral degree in anatomy and served as president of the Association from 1940 to 1945. The governance of the American Physiotherapy Association changed substantially to accommodate increased growth and responsibilities and a more national approach. In the summer of 1941, 6 months before the bombing of Pearl Harbor, the first War Emergency Training Course of World War II was initiated at Walter Reed General Hospital. Emma Vogel directed the Walter Reed General Hospital program to train PTs (**Figure 2-8**) [7]. The course at Walter Reed consisted of 6 months of concentrated didactic instruction followed by 6 months of supervised practice at a military hospital.

The physiotherapists graduating from the Emergency Training Course were no longer called reconstruction aides but were referred to as physiotherapy aides. In 1943, the U.S. Congress passed a bill stating that graduates of the Emergency Training Course should be called PTs. Inadvertently, with the change of their titles, PTs started to have increased recognition and wide-ranging responsibilities. These new tasks were related to treating wounded veterans, including rehabilitation for amputations, burns, cold injuries, wounds, fractures, and nerve and spinal cord injuries. Additionally, the U.S. government immediately allocated $1 million to enhance prosthetic services after the war, allowing PTs to participate in the teaching and training programs of the 25-year-old Artificial Limb Program at the University of California at Berkeley, New York University, and the University of California at Los Angeles. Furthermore, in 1946, because of the passing of the Hill–Burton Act and the founding of a nationwide hospital-building program, PTs increased their hospital-based practice. The work

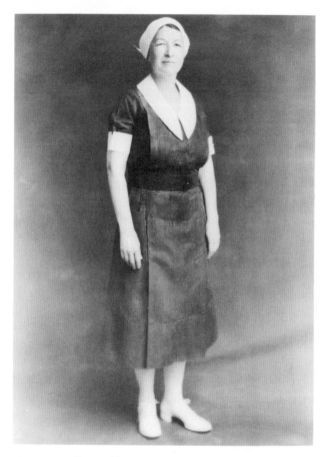

**Figure 2-8** Emma Vogel directed the Walter Reed General Hospital program for PTs. After the outbreak of World War II, Vogel was deployed to direct the War Emergency Training Courses at 10 Army hospitals (Post-World War I through World War II Era).

Courtesy of the American Physical Therapy Association

of PTs expanded even more in the 1950s with the outbreak of the Korean War [7].

In 1944, the American Physiotherapy Association membership voted for a separate internal legislative branch called the HOD [7]. The HOD had the same legislative powers as it does today—to amend or repeal the bylaws of the Association. In 1946, physical therapy physicians practicing physical medicine officially changed their specialty name to **physiatrists**. The same year, the American Physiotherapy Association changed its name to its current one, the American Physical Therapy Association. By 1959, membership in the APTA had increased to 8,028 PTs.

In 1947, the length of physical therapy schools' curricula increased from 9 to 12 months. By the 1950s, 31 accredited schools existed in the United States, 19 of which offered 4-year integrated bachelor's degree programs. By 1959, most states had licensure laws adopting the Physical Therapy Practice Act. In 1951, the Joint Commission on Accreditation

of Hospitals was formed, raising institutional staffing and healthcare standards.

## The Polio Vaccine and the Journal of the American Physical Therapy Association

Because new polio cases were seen every year, PTs from all over the country were called upon to help part-time or full-time as volunteers dealing with polio epidemics. In 1952, there were 58,000 cases of poliomyelitis in the United States. Between 1948 and 1960, nearly 1,000 PTs participated in the polio volunteer program. In 1954, 63 PTs were dispatched to 44 states to help with clinical studies of the polio vaccine developed by Jonas Salk. After successful clinical trial inoculations of 650,000 children, the Salk vaccine was determined to be safe and was approved for commercial production in 1955 by the Food and Drug Administration. Finally, in 1955, a massive national vaccination program started using the Salk vaccine. As a result, poliomyelitis cases were virtually eradicated.

Jessie Wright, PT, MD, was one of the PTs who helped with polio clinical studies by evaluating patient strength. In 1954, Wright and her staff introduced the abridged muscle grading system. Wright, who specialized in physical medicine and rehabilitation at the University of Pittsburgh, Pennsylvania, was a visionary in helping patients achieve function. Wright believed that "the first goal of physical therapy was to relax tight muscles," allowing a complete range of motion in the joints and giving the patient "functional use of residual power, helpful body mechanics, and assistive devices" [8].

The role of the PT in the 1950s expanded from a technical position to that of a professional practitioner [4]. Private practices expanded, and in 1957, the Physical Therapy Fund was established to foster scientific, literary, and educational programs [7]. PTs' licensure started in 1913 in Pennsylvania and in 1926 in New York; it expanded during the 1950s, and by 1959, 45 states and the territory of Hawaii offered licensure [7].

In 1964, the **APTA** formed a research committee to improve the development of scientific inquiry. Regarding dissemination of information (including scientific discovery) among the members of the physical therapy profession, just 2 years earlier (1962), the APTA changed the name of the official journal, the *PT Review*, to the *Journal of the American Physical Therapy Association*. In 1963, the journal modified its format and expanded its content with the help of its editor, Helen Hislop [7]. In 1964, the journal changed to the *Journal of Physical Therapy*. Later, the name was changed to *Physical Therapy*.

### The Beginning of Physical Therapy Assistants

In the 1960s, the U.S. population was changing, primarily because of the doubling of older adults and because people were becoming more health conscious. As with other health professions, physical therapy expanded rapidly with a high demand for physical therapy services. In 1964, the APTA HOD developed a task force to investigate the role of support personnel and the criteria for creating educational programs for the physical therapy assistant (the title was later changed to physical *therapist* assistant) [9]. This investigation was bolstered by a change in physical therapy insurance reimbursement (through diagnostic-related groups introduced by Medicare) and the enactment in 1965 and 1966 of Medicare and Medicaid programs, respectively, which created an even greater demand for PTs. As a result, in 1967, the APTA adopted a policy establishing the physical therapy assistant position in health care. The policy statement adopted by the HOD recommended the following [7]:

- The APTA had to establish the standards for physical therapy assistant education programs, including accreditation of 2-year associate degree education programs by the **Commission on Accreditation in Physical Therapy Education (CAPTE)**.
- A supervisory relationship existed between the PT and the physical therapy assistant.
- The functions of assistants were to be identified.
- Mandatory licensure or registration was encouraged.
- Membership eligibility in the APTA was to be established for the assistants.

At that time, two colleges in the country had already enrolled students in their programs: Miami Dade Community College in Miami, Florida, and St. Mary's Campus of the College of St. Catherine in Minneapolis, Minnesota.

## Mastery Years: 1970 to 1996

### The Societal Developments of Physical Therapy

In 1969, the first 15 PTAs graduated with associate degrees from Miami Dade College and College of St. Catherine. By 1970, there were nine PTA education programs, mostly due to federal financial assistance to

---

**Box 2-3**

- PT (formerly called physiotherapist in the United States): An allied healthcare professional who helps individuals maintain, restore, and improve movement, activity, and functioning, enabling optimal performance in enhancing health, well-being, and quality of life [1]
- PTA: A PTA, who a PT supervises, is the only individual permitted to assist the PT in practice.
- Physical therapy aide (rehabilitation technicians): Under the direction and supervision of PTs and PTAs (in some states), physical therapy aides are support personnel who perform assigned tasks that do not require clinical decision-making or clinical problem-solving. These tasks include helping patients with proper positioning, patient transfers, common exercises, basic modalities, and clinical maintenance. To date, the APTA has opposed the certification or credentialing of physical therapy aides, although many educational institutions offer such programs.
- PT services (practice): Refers to providing physical therapy
- Physical therapy service: Refers to a facility or department in which PT services are provided

---

junior colleges. In the same year, the APTA offered temporary affiliate membership to PTAs. By 1973, eligible PTAs were admitted as affiliate members in the national association, having the right to speak and make motions, hold committee appointments, and have chapter representation in the HOD. In 1983, PTAs formed the Affiliate SIG, and in 1989, the HOD approved the creation of the Affiliate Assembly, which gave PTAs a formal voice in the Association. The first president of the Affiliate Assembly was Cheryl Carpenter-Davis, PTA, MEd. In 2014, the HOD urged the APTA BOD to create a plan to increase the value of a PTA membership for PTAs, to represent the needs and interests of its entire membership better, and to increase inclusiveness [10]. This inclusiveness included the issue of voting strength at the chapter and section level, which, to this point, the APTA bylaws afforded PT members a full vote but PTA members a half vote. However, in 2015, the APTA changed its bylaws to allow chapters and sections to increase voting representation for PTAs to a full vote.

### The Expansion of the Physical Therapy Profession

During the 1970s and 1980s, the physical therapy profession continued to grow and expand. Because of the Occupational Safety and Health Administration (OSHA) establishment by the Department of Labor, physical therapy practices related to prevention, work management, and job injuries and compensation were also developed, contributing to PTs' practice advancement from hospital based to private. In 1972, Congress added physical therapy services to the Social Security Act to be reimbursed [7] when an individual PT furnished them in their office or the patient's home. In 1975, the Individuals with Disabilities Education Act (IDEA) was passed, helping physical therapy expand into treating children with disabilities in public schools.

In 1971, the AMA dissolved the American Registry, and by 1976, all states had physical therapy licensure laws in place. In 1981 and 1982, the HOD adopted the policy that PT practice independent of practitioner referral was ethical [4] (if it was legal in that specific state). This policy separated PTs from the physician's control, giving them the right to practice without a physician's referral (**Figure 2-9**).

During the early 1970s, the APTA formed sections for state licensure and regulations, sports physical therapy, pediatrics, clinical electrophysiology, and orthopedics. The state licensure and regulations section later became the health policy, legislation, and regulation section. In 1976, the first CSM was in Washington, DC. In 1977, the APTA became the sole accrediting agency for all educational programs for PTs and PTAs in the United States, Canada, and Europe through CAPTE.

In 1978, the APTA created the American Board of Physical Therapy Specialties to allow members to receive certification and recognition as clinical specialists in a certain specialty area. During the late 1970s, sections on obstetrics and gynecology (now called women's health) and geriatrics were created. By 1985, the American Board for Physical Therapy Specialties—Certified Cardiopulmonary Specialists was formed, giving cardiopulmonary specialist certifications. Other specialty certifications, such as orthopedic, pediatric, electrophysiology, neurology, and sports, followed. In 1983, the APTA purchased its first four-story building in Alexandria, Virginia.

In 1990, the Americans with Disabilities Act ensured the involvement of PTs as consultants to guarantee every individual with disabilities rightful access to all aspects of life. Many major changes occurred during the 1990s: managed care, point-of-service plans, and other alternative organizational structures, such as health economics resources, also impacted physical therapy delivery. Nevertheless, physical therapy practice developed work conditioning, women's health, and work hardening [4].

During the last two decades of the twentieth century, the following major developments occurred in the physical therapy profession:

- In 1980, the HOD established its goal to raise the minimum entry-level education in physical therapy to a postbaccalaureate degree.
- During the early 1980s, veterans' affairs, hand rehabilitation, and oncology sections were established.
- The PT Bulletin was initiated in 1986. That same year, setting goals and objectives became part of the APTA's annual self-review process.
- In 1989, the HOD approved the formation of the Affiliate Assembly, composed entirely of PTA members. This way, PTAs had a formal avenue to come together and discuss issues that directly concerned them.

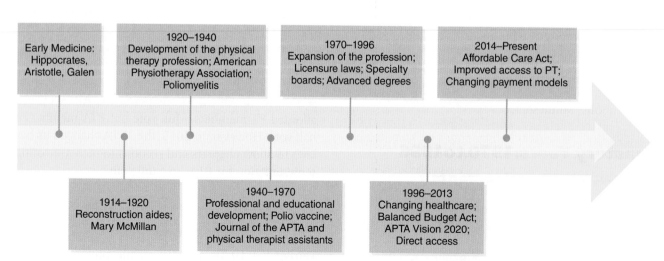

**Figure 2-9** Timeline.

- By 1988, direct access was legal in 20 states, allowing patients and clients to seek direct physical therapy services without first seeing a physician.
- The academic preparation of PTs changed from a bachelor's degree to a postbaccalaureate degree. By January 1994, 55% of physical therapy education programs were at the master's level.
- In 1995, the American Board of Physical Therapy Specialties inaugurated nationwide electronic testing, and the APTA celebrated the 75th anniversary of the Association and the physical therapy profession.
- Also, in 1995, the APTA hosted the 12th **World Confederation for Physical Therapy** Congress in Washington, DC. The Congress had record-breaking crowds [4].

In 1995, the APTA received representation on the AMA Coding Panel, facilitating a better development of PT practice codes.

### KNOWLEDGE CHECK

Which events changed the PT from a technician to a professional?
What caused the development of PTA education?
What is direct access, and how did it change physical therapy practice?

## Adaptation Years: 1996 to 2010

In August 1997, President Clinton signed the Balanced Budget Act to eliminate the Medicare deficit.

### *The Balanced Budget Act*

The Balanced Budget Act, which took effect in January 1999, applied an annual cap of $1,500 (for both physical and speech therapy services) per beneficiary for all outpatient rehabilitation services. Due to the Balanced Budget Act and its resultant reduction in rehabilitation services to Medicare patients, many new graduate PTs and PTAs could not find jobs. Also, some experienced PTs and PTAs suffered an appreciable decrease in income and the number of working hours. Due to pressure from the Association, its members, patients, and the general public, in November 1999, President Clinton signed the Refinement Act, which suspended the $1,500 cap for 2 years in all rehabilitation settings starting on January 3, 2000.

Nonetheless, the Balanced Budget Act was detrimental to the treatment of many Medicare patients and created hardship for PTs and PTAs for at least 3 years. An APTA survey in October 2000 [11] found that PTAs were hurt the most due to the Balanced Budget Act, with an unemployment rate of 6.5%. The PTs also reported that their hours of employment had been involuntarily reduced. In March 2001, the same survey discovered that the unemployment rate among PTAs had improved, going down to 4.2%. PTs also reported an improvement, with a reduction in working hours of only 10.8%. The reduction in the number of working hours for PTAs was even greater, at 24.5% in October 2000; in March 2001, it went down to 19.8%.

In 2000, the Association adopted the new "Evaluative Criteria for the Accreditation of Education for Physical Therapist Assistants," launched the PT Bulletin online, and published the Normative Model for Physical Therapist Professional Education: Version 2000. In 2001, the Association introduced the second edition of the Guide to Physical Therapist Practice (see Chapter 3) and worked hard to maintain the rights of physical therapy in certain states to perform manipulations and provide orthotics and prosthetics within the scope of physical therapy practice. The Association launched Hooked on Evidence on the Web in 2002 to help clinicians review the research literature and utilize the information to enhance their clinical decision-making and practice. In January 2002, all physical therapy educational programs were changed to the master's level. The same year, Pennsylvania became the 35th state to achieve direct access, and the APTA released the Interactive Guide to Physical Therapist Practice. In 2003, the Association built support in Congress for the Medicare Patient Access to Physical Therapists Act to allow licensed PTs to evaluate and treat Medicare patients without a physician's referral.

In 2005, the effects of the Balanced Budget Act of 1997 still influenced the future of rehabilitation services. Rehabilitation providers and patients urged Congress to pass the Medicare Access to Rehabilitation Services Act of 2005 to eliminate the threat that seniors and individuals with disabilities would have to pay out of pocket for rehabilitation or to alter the course of their rehabilitation care. This Act was considered significant to repeal the cap originally instituted through the Balanced Budget Act of 1997. From 1997 to the beginning of 2005, Congress enforced a moratorium three times that delayed the implementation of the cap. On December 31, 2005, the moratorium expired. As a result, on January 1, 2006, the Centers for Medicare and Medicaid Services (CMS) reinstated the

Medicare cap. From January 1, 2006, to December 31, 2006, the dollar amount of the therapy cap was $1,740 for physical therapy and speech-language pathology combined and $1,740 for occupational therapy.

The APTA worked diligently during each Congressional session to reduce the Balanced Budget Act's drastic impact on patient care. Although the therapy cap went into effect in 2006, because of the pressure from the APTA, clinicians, and consumer groups, Congress authorized Medicare to allow exceptions for beneficiaries who needed additional rehabilitation services based on diagnosis and clinicians' evaluations and judgments. Consequently, Congress acted to extend these exceptions through December 31, 2009. On January 1, 2010, without Congressional action, authorization for exceptions to the therapy caps expired. In March 2010, the Patient Protection and Affordable Care Act became law. This Act included a healthcare reform package that extended the therapy cap exception process until December 31, 2010.

The scope of practice for PTs/PTAs has three components:[i]

1. Professional: This scope, grounded in basic, behavioral, and clinical sciences, focuses on the profession's unique body of knowledge, supported by educational preparation, based on a body of evidence, and linked to existing or emerging practice frameworks. This component evolves in response to innovation, research, collaboration, and changes in societal needs. The professional scope of practice consists of patient/client management, which includes diagnosis and prognosis, to optimize physical function, movement, performance, health, quality of life, and well-being across the life span. In addition, the professional scope of practice includes contributions to public health services aimed at improving population health and the human experience.
2. Jurisdictional: This scope is established by a state's practice act governing the specific PT/PTA license and the rules adopted according to that act. All 50 states and the District of Columbia require PTs to be licensed and PTAs to be certified or licensed.
3. Personal: This scope consists of activities for which an individual PT/PTA is educated and trained and their competence to perform.

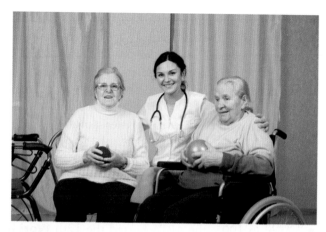
© GBZero/Shutterstock

## The Expansion Years: 2010 to 2022

Since 2010, the APTA has continued to expand and represents more than 100,000 PTs, PTAs, and students in the United States. It works tirelessly to advance the physical therapy profession by promoting evidence-based practice, research, and education, and advocating for policies that support the needs of both patients and practitioners.

The HOD of the APTA has been diligent about providing vision and focus for the profession through mission and vision statements. The HOD and the BOD of the APTA have consistently pushed the profession to move PTs to become a doctoring profession. **Vision 2020** was created in 2000. The APTA vision statement was updated in 2013 and 2019 and currently states that "movement is a key to optimal living and quality of life for all people that extends beyond health to every person's ability to participate in and contribute to society."

Vision 2020 stated:

By 2020, physical therapy will be provided by physical therapists who are doctors of physical therapy, recognized by consumers and other health care professionals as the practitioners of choice to whom consumers have direct access for the diagnosis of, interventions for, and prevention of impairments, functional limitations, and disabilities related to movement, function, and health [12].

The first class of PTs with the designation DPT graduated in 1996, but by 2010, almost all professional-level PT education programs were at the doctoral level.

APTA Vision Statement for Physical Therapy 2020 included the following [12]:

- Physical therapy will be provided by PTs who are doctors of physical therapy and may be board-certified specialists.
- Consumers will have direct access to PTs for patient/client management, prevention, and wellness services in all environments.

A patient is an individual who has conditions that require physical therapy services to improve their function.

A **client** is an individual who seeks physical therapy services to maintain health or a business that hires a PT for consultation.

- PTs will be practitioners of choice in a patient's/client's health network and will hold all privileges of autonomous practice.
- PTs may be assisted by PTAs who are educated and licensed to provide PT-directed and -supervised components of interventions.
- Guided by integrity, lifelong learning, and a commitment to comprehensive and accessible health programs for all people, PTs and PTAs will render evidence-based services throughout the continuum of care and improve the quality of life for society.
- PTs and PTAs will provide culturally sensitive care distinguished by trust, respect, and an appreciation for individual differences.
- While fully availing themselves of new technologies and clinical research, PTs will continue to provide direct patient/client care.
- PTs and PTAs will maintain active responsibility for the growth of the physical therapy profession and the health of the people it serves.

Data from American Physical Therapy Association. Physical therapists scope of practice HOD P06-17-09-16/HOD P06-17-08-07. https://www.apta.org/apta-and-you/leadership-and-governance/policies/position-scope-of-practice. Accessed January 23 2023

The vision sentence/statement terminology relates to the following [12]:

- Autonomous physical therapy practice environments include all physical therapy settings where PTs are responsible for practicing autonomously and collaboratively to provide best practice to the patient/client. Independent, self-determined, professional judgments and actions characterize such PT practices.
- Direct access means that throughout their lifetime, every consumer has the legal right to directly access a PT for the diagnosis of; interventions for; and prevention of impairments, **functional limitations**, and disabilities related to movement, function, and health.

- The Doctor of Physical Therapy (DPT) is a clinical doctorate (entry-level) that reflects the growth in the body of knowledge and the expected responsibilities that a professional PT must master to provide best practices to the consumer. All PTs and PTAs must continually acquire knowledge, skills, and abilities to advance the science of physical therapy and its role in healthcare delivery.
- Practitioner of choice means PTs who personify the elements of Vision 2020 and are recognized among consumers and other healthcare professionals as the preferred providers for the diagnosis of; interventions for; and prevention of impairments, functional limitations, and disabilities related to movement, function, and health.
- **Evidence-based practice** means accessing, applying, and integrating evidence to guide clinical decision-making to provide best practice for the patient/client. Evidence-based practice includes integrating the best available research, clinical expertise, patient/client values and circumstances related to patient/client management, practice management, and healthcare policy decision-making. Plans for evidence-based practice include enhancing patient/client management and reducing unwarranted variation in physical therapy services.
- Professionalism means that PTs and PTAs consistently demonstrate core values by aspiring to and wisely applying principles of altruism, excellence, caring, ethics, respect, communication, accountability, and working with other professionals to achieve optimal health and wellness in individuals and communities.

The vision also includes these guiding principles:

- Identity: The physical therapy profession promotes the movement system as the foundation for optimizing movement to improve the health of society and as the core of PT practice, education, and research.
- Quality: The physical therapy profession will identify, adopt, and utilize evidence-based principles in practice, education, and research.
- Innovation: The physical therapy profession will develop inventive practices in research, education, and practice to lead health care.
- Consumer-centricity: The physical therapy profession will value patient needs as core to all interactions and will create a culture that values the cultures of all people.

The core values for PTs and PTAs guide behavior and include the following:

- Accountability: The active acceptance of the responsibility for the diverse roles, obligations, and actions of the PT and PTA, including self-regulation and other behaviors that positively influence patient and client outcomes, the profession, and the health needs of society
- Altruism: The primary regard for or devotion to the interest of patients and clients, thus assuming the responsibility of placing the needs of patients and clients ahead of the PT's or PTA's self-interest
- Collaboration: Working with patients and clients, families, communities, and professionals in health and other fields to achieve shared goals. Collaboration within the PT–PTA team is working together, within each partner's respective role, to achieve optimal PT services and outcomes for patients and clients.
- Compassion and caring: The desire to identify with or sense something of another's experience, a precursor of caring. Caring is the concern, empathy, and consideration for the needs and values of others.
- Duty: The commitment to meeting one's obligations to provide effective physical therapy services to patients and clients, to serve the profession, and to positively influence society's health
- Excellence: The provision of PT services occurs when the PT and PTA consistently use current knowledge and skills while understanding personal limits, integrate the patient or client perspective, embrace advancement, and challenge mediocrity.
- Inclusion: Occurs when the PT and PTA create a welcoming and equitable environment for all. PTs and PTAs are inclusive when they commit to providing a safe space, elevating diverse and minority voices, acknowledging personal biases that may impact patient care, and taking a position of antidiscrimination.
- Integrity: Steadfast adherence to high ethical principles or standards, being truthful, ensuring fairness, following through on commitments, and verbalizing to others the rationale for actions
- Social responsibility: The promotion of mutual trust between the profession and the larger public that necessitates responding to societal needs for health and wellness

Data from The American Physical Therapy Association. Core values for the physical therapist and physical therapist assistant HOD P09-21-21-09 [Amended: HOD P06-19-48-55; HOD P06-18-25-33; Initial HOD P05-07-19-19] [Previously Titled: Core Values: for the Physical Therapist] [Position]. https://www.apta.org/apta-and-you/leadership-and-governance/policies/core-values-for-the-physical-therapist-and-physical-therapist-assistant. Accessed January 22, 2023.

- Access/equity: The physical therapy profession will identify and develop creative avenues for all who need physical therapy care and education.
- Advocacy: The physical therapy profession will advocate for consumers in research, education, and practice.

### Achieving Direct Access

Direct access means the ability of the public to directly access physical therapy services, such as physical therapy evaluation, examination, and intervention. Direct access eliminates the patient's need to visit their physician to request a physician's referral. Licensed PTs are qualified to provide physical therapy services without referrals from physicians. Direct access decreases the cost of health care and does not promote overutilization. The APTA prioritized direct access to PTs in the Association's federal government affairs activities. In 2005, the Medicare Patient Access to Physical Therapists Act was introduced in the House of Representatives and its companion bill in the Senate. The Act and the bill recognized the ability of licensed PTs to evaluate, diagnose, and treat Medicare beneficiaries requiring outpatient physical therapy services under Part B of the Medicare program without a physician referral. In 2014, all 50 states and the District of Columbia passed legislation that allows PTs to evaluate and treat patients without a physician's referral.

### PTA Caucus

In June 2005, the National Assembly of Physical Therapist Assistants was dissolved, and the PTA Caucus was formed. The National Assembly of PTAs was formed in 1998 as the Affiliate Assembly. The PTA Caucus's purpose was to more fully integrate PTA members into the APTA's governance structure and increase PTAs' influence in the Association. The PTA Caucus represents the PTAs' interests, needs, and issues in the APTA governance. The caucus includes a chief delegate and four delegates representing five regions. Additionally, 51 PTA Caucus members represent 51 chapters. Each PTA Caucus representative is elected or selected by their state chapter. The PTA Caucus also elects one chief delegate and four delegates (representing five regions) to the APTA's HOD. The PTA Caucus representatives work with their chapter delegates and provide input to the delegates to the HOD and the advisory panel of PTAs. Each delegate can speak, debate, and make (and second) motions providing representation in the HOD for a particular region of the country. A major achievement of the PTA Caucus has been the development of *PTA* SIGs, which work to promote PTA membership, provide an outlet for PTA member involvement in chapter and section activities, and provide leadership development opportunities for PTAs. As of January 2023, 39 chapters had PTA SIGs, and the APTA has a SIG for PTA educators that serves as the advocate and expert resource for the education and role of the PTA.

### Physical Therapy Promotion

MoveForwardPT.com was designed to show physical therapy's benefits and make more people aware of APTA's #ChoosePT campaign, an initiative designed to encourage awareness of physical therapy as a safe and effective alternative to opioids to treat chronic pain conditions.

## APTA Strategic Plan 2022–2025

The APTA's 2022–2025 strategic plan (see Appendix A) outlines the Association's purpose based on its goals, outcomes, and connected operational plans with specific reference to the following [13]:

- Member value: Increase member value by ensuring that APTA's community delivers unmatched opportunities to belong, engage, and contribute.
- Sustainable profession: Improve the long-term sustainability of the profession by leading efforts to increase payment, reduce the cost of education, and strengthen provider health and well-being.
- Quality of care: Elevate the quality of care provided by PTs and PTAs to improve health outcomes for populations, communities, and individuals.
- Demand and access: Drive demand for and access to physical therapy as a proven pathway to improve the human experience.

### KNOWLEDGE CHECK

What was the impact of the Balanced Budget Act on physical therapy services?
How did the APTA's Vision 2020 change physical therapy education and practice?
What do the following terms mean: autonomous practice, direct access, a practitioner of choice, evidence-based practice, and professionalism?
What are the seven guiding principles of the current APTA vision?

### Membership in the APTA

The APTA is the national organization that represents the profession of physical therapy. As stated earlier, membership in the APTA is voluntary. Active members of the Association are PTs, PTAs (also called affiliate members), and PT and PTA students. Other Association members are retired members, honorary members (people who are not PTs or PTAs but have made remarkable contributions to the Association or public health), and Fellow members (Catherine Worthingham Fellows of the American Physical Therapy Association). The Fellow member has been an active member for 15 years and has made notable contributions to the profession. As of 2017, the APTA membership comprised over 100,000 PTs, PTAs, and student members. The APTA includes 51 chapters operating in the United States and its territories. Each chapter offers a variety of events, professional development activities, and other opportunities for member interaction.

The requirement for membership in the APTA is graduation from or enrollment in an accredited PT or PTA program. PT or PTA students are welcome as student members of the Association.

The benefits of APTA membership include the following:

1. The Rehabilitation Reference Center at PTNow provides a resource for studying diseases and interventions.
2. The Financial Solutions Center can assist PT/PTA students in creating a school debt management plan.
3. APTA in Action supports physical therapy legislative and payment advocacy, clinical education, clinical practice, and public awareness through membership dues revenue.
4. Career Development and Networking opportunities are available through national, chapter, and section meetings and continuing education courses. Advanced Proficiency Pathway is available for PTAs who want recognition for advanced skills in acute care, cardiovascular/pulmonary, geriatrics, oncology, orthopedics, pediatrics, and wound management.
5. Evidence-Based Practice Tools, including the Clinical Toolbox, Guide to Physical Therapist Practice 3.0, Physical Therapy (PTJ), and the Physical Therapy Outcomes Registry are available to enhance efficient and effective patient care.
6. Current physical therapy news is accessed through PT in Motion magazine, weekly Friday Focus electronic newsletters, PTeam legislative advocacy emails, and the student member blog Pulse.
7. Payment Resources to improve understanding of current and updated policies.
8. Discount and value programs, including insurance, car rentals, hotel, and retail discounts.

# Other Organizations Involved with Physical Therapy

## Commission on Accreditation in Physical Therapy Education

CAPTE grants specialized accreditation to qualified entry-level education programs for PTs and PTAs. The commission is a national accrediting agency recognized by the U.S. Department of Education and the Council for Higher Education Accreditation. Accreditation of physical therapy education programs is a voluntary, nongovernmental, peer-reviewed process that ensures quality education to meet the profession's current needs and promotes graduation outcomes, passing the National Physical Therapy Examination, and employment.

CAPTE's mission is to nurture quality educational experiences taught by qualified faculty that produce acceptable student outcomes. CAPTE consists of three panels: Physical Therapist Review Panel, Physical Therapist Assistant Review Panel, and Central Panel. Appointment to CAPTE is done through the APTA staff members, who provide the APTA BOD with a list of all qualified individuals for open positions who consent to serve. CAPTE reviews the list and recommends individuals who best meet CAPTE's needs. The BOD considers the recommendations of CAPTE and makes final decisions for appointments to CAPTE. The term of appointment is 4 years. Accreditation by CAPTE requires the college and program to submit data to ensure that all required components of a program are in place. Programs must file annual information and complete an in-depth self-study of the program periodically. CAPTE determines the frequency of the self-study process based on the characteristics of the program and the need for oversight by CAPTE to ensure quality.

## American Board of Physical Therapy Specialties

The American Board of Physical Therapy Specialties (ABPTS) is the governing body for the certification and recertification of clinical specialists by coordinating and supervising the specialist certification process.

The ABPTS comprises 11 individuals: 8 individuals appointed by the ABPTS for 4-year terms, 1 member of the APTA BOD appointed by the APTA BOD for a 1-year term, 1 consumer representative appointed by the BOD for a 2-year term, and 1 test and measurement expert appointed by the ABPTS for a 2-year term.

The specialist certification program was established in 1978 by the APTA to provide formal recognition for PTs with advanced clinical knowledge, experience, and skills in a special area of practice and to assist consumers and the healthcare community in identifying these PTs. The APTA describes specialization as a process by which a PT increases their professional education and practice and develops greater knowledge and skills related to a particular practice area. Specialist recertification is when a PT verifies current competence as an advanced practitioner in a specialty area by increasing their education and professional growth.

The Specialty Council on Cardiopulmonary Physical Therapy was the first to complete the process, and the cardiopulmonary specialist certification examination was first administered in 1985. Since then, eight other specialty areas have been established: clinical electrophysiology, geriatrics, neurology, oncology, orthopedics, pediatrics, sports, and women's health physical therapy.

The purposes of APTA's Clinical Specialization Program are as follows:

- To contribute to identifying and developing appropriate areas of specialty practice in physical therapy
- To promote the highest possible level of care for individuals seeking physical therapy services in each specialty area
- To promote the development of the science and the art underlying each specialty area of practice
- To provide a reliable and valid method for certifying and recertifying individuals with advanced knowledge and skill levels in each specialty area
- To help consumers, the healthcare community, and others identify certified clinical specialists in each specialty area
- To serve as a resource in specialty practice for APTA, the physical therapy profession, and the healthcare community

## Federation of State Boards of Physical Therapy

The Federation of State Boards of Physical Therapy (FSBPT) develops and administers the national examination for PTs (NPTE) and PTAs (NPTAE) in 53 jurisdictions: the 50 states, the District of Columbia, Puerto Rico, and the Virgin Islands. The FSBPT aims to protect the public by providing leadership and service encouraging competent and safe physical therapy practice. The exams assess the basic entry-level competence for first-time licensure or registration as a PT or PTA within the 53 jurisdictions. FSBPT's vision is that the organization will achieve a high level of public protection through a strong foundation of laws and regulatory standards in physical therapy, effective tools/systems to assess entry-level and continuing competence, and public and professional awareness of resources for public protection.

For PT and PTA graduates from an accredited education program who are candidates to sit for the national examination, the federation offers a Candidate Handbook that includes all the necessary information about the exam and exam administration. The handbook can be viewed or downloaded online at www.fsbpt.org. The federation has been working with the state boards within its jurisdiction toward licensure uniformity, supporting one passing score. This uniformity in scores assists PTs and PTAs in working across states.

In 2004, the FSBPT developed for purchase an online Practice Exam and Assessment Tool (PEAT) to help PT and PTA candidates prepare for the national examination. The online PEAT allows the candidates to take a timed, multiple-choice exam similar to the national examination and receive feedback. When receiving feedback, the candidates can access the correct answer rationale and the references used for each question. The NPTE PT test content outline is shown in **Table 2-2**, and the PTA test outline is in **Table 2-3**.

**Table 2-2** **The NPTE PT Test Content Outline**

| Body System | Physical Therapy Examination | Foundations for Evaluation, Differential Diagnosis, and Prognosis | Interventions | Total per System |
|---|---|---|---|---|
| Cardiovascular and pulmonary | 7–9 | 8–9 | 8–10 | 23–28 |
| Musculoskeletal | 18–21 | 17–20 | 16–19 | 51–60 |
| Neuromuscular and nervous | 15–17 | 14–16 | 15–17 | 44–50 |
| Integumentary | 3–4 | 3–4 | 3–4 | 9–12 |
| Metabolic and endocrine | — | 3–4 | 2–3 | 5–7 |
| Gastrointestinal | 0–2 | 2–3 | 1–2 | 3–7 |
| Genitourinary | 1–2 | 2–3 | 1–2 | 4–7 |
| Lymphatic | 0–2 | 1–3 | 2–3 | 3–8 |
| System interactions | — | 8–12 | — | 8–12 |
| **Total across systems** | 44–57 | 58–74 | 48–60 | — |
| **Nonsystem** | | | | **Total per Nonsystem** |
| Equipment, devices, and technologies | | | | 5–6 |
| Therapeutic modalities | | | | 6–8 |
| Safety and protection | | | | 5–6 |
| Professional responsibilities | | | | 4–5 |
| Research and evidence-based practice | | | | 3–5 |
| Total | | | | 200 |

**Table 2-3** The NPTE PTA Test Content Outline

| Body System | Data Collection | Diseases/Conditions | Interventions | Total per System |
|---|---|---|---|---|
| Cardiovascular and pulmonary | 6–8 | 6–7 | 9–11 | 21–26 |
| Musculoskeletal | 12–14 | 9–11 | 15–16 | 36–41 |
| Neuromuscular and nervous | 8–10 | 8–10 | 12–14 | 28–34 |
| Integumentary | 2–3 | 1–3 | 2–4 | 5–10 |
| Metabolic and endocrine | — | 3–4 | 2–3 | 5–7 |
| Gastrointestinal | — | 0–2 | 0–2 | 0–4 |
| Genitourinary | — | 0–2 | 0–2 | 0–4 |
| Lymphatic | 1–2 | 1–2 | 1–2 | 3–6 |
| System interactions | — | 5–7 | — | 5–7 |
| **Total across systems** | 29–37 | 33–48 | 41–54 | — |
| **Nonsystem** | | | | **Total per Nonsystem** |
| Equipment, devices, and technologies | | | | 7–9 |
| Therapeutic modalities | | | | 9–11 |
| Safety and protection | | | | 4–6 |
| Professional responsibilities | | | | 3–4 |
| Research and evidence-based practice | | | | 2–3 |
| Total | | | | 150 |

Reproduced from Federation of State Boards of Physical Therapy. NPTE-PTA Test Content Outline. January 2018. https://www.fsbpt.org/Portals/0/documents/free-resources/ContentOutline_2018PTA_20170126 .pdf?ver=JHEpTkOiWP39AlgeOJPZtg%3D%3D

## Political Action Committee

The APTA's **Physical Therapy Political Action Committee (PT-PAC)** is vital to the Association's success on Capitol Hill in Washington, DC. The PT-PAC ensures that future legislative actions on Capitol Hill are helpful to physical therapy practice. PT and PTA members make donations to the political action committee. The PT-PAC committee uses membership donations to influence legislative and policy issues through lobbying efforts directed toward policy decision-makers. The vision of PT-PAC is "to become the #1 health professions PAC providing the resources to create a network of Congressional champions on physical therapy issues." The 2019 Priority Issues of the PT-PAC are Barriers to Care, Public Health Epidemics, New Models of Care, Shortage of Health Care Providers, and Health Care Delivery Obstacles.

## APTA's Position Regarding Licensure

Regarding licensure, the APTA desires that all PTs and PTAs be licensed or otherwise regulated in all U.S. jurisdictions. State regulation of PTs and PTAs should require, at a minimum, graduation from an accredited physical therapy education program (or, in the case of an internationally educated PT, an equivalent education) and passing an entry-level competency exam; should provide title protection; and should allow for disciplinary action. In addition, PTs' licensure should include a defined scope of practice. Relative to temporary jurisdictional licensure, the APTA supports the elimination of temporary jurisdictional licensure of PTs or temporary credentialing of PTAs for previously non–U.S.-licensed or non–U.S.-credentialed applicants in all jurisdictions.

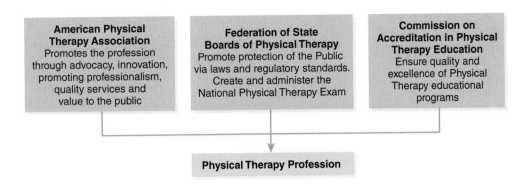

## Discussion Questions

1. List the values and culture of the physical therapy profession.
2. A second-year student member of the APTA is developing a presentation for incoming students. What should the student highlight as the purpose and value of becoming a member of the APTA?
3. List contributions that PTAs can make to the profession.
4. Identify the role and benefits of being a PTA.

## Learning Opportunities

1. Go online at www.apta.org and research information about becoming a PTA.
2. Create a brochure identifying the vision, mission, and function of the APTA and the benefits of belonging to the APTA.
3. Participate in a district or chapter/subchapter meeting of the APTA.

## References

1. American Physical Therapy Association: Guide to Physical Therapist Practice 3.0. Alexandria, VA, American Physical Therapy Association, 2014
2. Neumann DA: Polio: its impact on the people of the United States and the emerging profession of physical therapy. J Orthop Sports Phys Ther 34(8):479–492, 2004
3. DeLorme T, Watkins A: Techniques of Progressive Resistance Exercise. New York, Appleton-Century, 1951
4. Moffat M: The history of physical therapy practice in the United States. J Phys Ther Educ 17(3):15–25, 2003
5. Moffat M: Three quarters of a century of healing the generations. Phys Ther 76(11):1242–1252, 1996
6. Vogel EE: The beginning of "modern physiotherapy." Phys Ther 56(1):15–21, 1976
7. Murphy W: Healing the Generations: A History of Physical Therapy and the American Physical Therapy Association. Alexandria, VA, American Physical Therapy Association, 1995
8. Wright J: Physical and occupational therapy in poliomyelitis. Pediatr Clin North Am 1(1A):26–34, 1953
9. Woods EN: PTAs their history and development. PT Mag Phys Ther 4(1):34–39, 1993
10. American Physical Therapy Association: RC 11-14 Membership Value for the Physical Therapist Assistant, in House of Delegates Minutes. Alexandria, VA, American Physical Therapy Association, 2014
11. Goldstein M: Positive employment trends in physical therapy. PT Mag Phys Ther 9, 2001
12. American Physical Therapy Association House of Delegates: Vision 2020, in HOD P06-13-18-22. Alexandria, VA, American Physical Therapy Association, 2014
13. American Physical Therapy Association: APTA Strategic Plan 2022–2025 [Internet]. [cited 2023 Jan 31]. Available from: https://www.apta.org/apta-and-you/leadership-and-governance/vision-mission-and-strategic-plan/strategic-plan

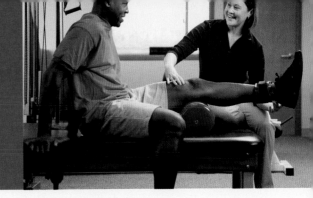

# CHAPTER 3

# Physical Therapist Clinical Practice

## OBJECTIVES

- Describe the significance of the Guide to Physical Therapy Practice.
- Discuss the six elements of patient/client management.
- Compare and contrast physical therapy and medical diagnosis.
- List examples of procedural interventions.
- Describe the International Classification of Functioning, Disability, and Health.
- List employment settings for physical therapists and physical therapist assistants.
- Compare and contrast the three types of skilled nursing facilities.
- Discuss physical therapy clinical practice issues such as policy and procedure manuals, meetings, budgets, quality assurance, and risk management.
- Describe contemporary clinical trends regarding wellness, health promotion, and disease prevention.

## KEY TERMS

diagnosis
direct access
evaluation
examination
goals
history
intervention

medical diagnosis
outcomes
physical therapy diagnosis
plan of care (POC)
policy
primary care
procedure

prognosis
secondary care
systems review
tertiary care
tests and measures

## Overview

Throughout a career in physical therapy, the American Physical Therapy Association's (APTA) scope of practice (see Chapter 2) evolves based on considerations including, but not limited to, societal needs; progressive professional development activities of the physical therapist (PT); modifications to jurisdictional laws and regulations; advancements in knowledge, research, clinical skills, and technology; and the evolving health delivery system [1]. For the PT, the doctor of physical therapy (DPT) degree is the entry-level (professional) degree; currently, an associate degree is required for the physical therapist assistant (PTA). Although becoming a PTA is not a stepping stone to becoming a PT, 10% of PTAs pursue PT careers through bridge programs or Bachelor of Science completion degrees [1].

# General Terminology Used in Physical Therapy

- A patient is an individual who receives healthcare services, including direct physical therapy intervention.

- A client is an individual who is not necessarily sick or injured but who can benefit from a PT's consultation, professional advice, or services. Examples of a client can be a student in a school system or an employee in a business.

- The **examination** gathers subjective and objective data about the patient/client. It is also a comprehensive screening and specific testing process leading to diagnostic classification or, as appropriate, a referral to another practitioner. Physical therapy examination has three components: the patient/client history, the systems review, and tests and measures.

- The **evaluation** is a dynamic process in which the PT makes clinical judgments based on data gathered during the examination [1]. The evaluation results in the determination of the **diagnosis**, **prognosis**, and interventions. The evaluation reflects the severity of the current problem, the presence of preexisting conditions, the possibility of more than one site involvement, and the condition's stability.

- **Interventions** are skilled techniques and activities that make up the treatment plan [1].

- Discharge is defined as the process of discontinuing interventions in a single episode of care [1].

- **Goals** are functional activities that are the intended response to the physical therapy intervention and are set by the PT, the patient, and the patient's family/caregivers. Written goals must be Specific, Measurable, Achievable, Relevant, and Time-Bound (SMART).

- An **outcome** is a functional activity achieved by the physical therapy episode of care. The value of physical therapy can be documented by measuring preintervention and postintervention outcomes [1].

- Coordination. In addition to the collaboration between the PT and PTA, the physical therapy team must interact efficiently and effectively with other healthcare team members, including but not limited to occupational therapists (OTs), speech and language pathologists (SLPs), orthotists/prosthetists, physicians, nurses, dentists, and social workers.

- Communication. Communication is crucial for providing a constant exchange of information (see Chapter 8).

- Documentation. Written communication is used extensively in health care (see Chapter 10).

# Clinical Practice Settings

PTs/PTAs practice in a broad range of inpatient, outpatient, and community-based settings (see Physical Therapy Clinical Settings). Health care is generally divided into primary, secondary, and tertiary levels.

- Primary care: This level of care, which accounts for 80–90% of physician or other caregiver visits, is the entry level of health care. It includes diagnostic, therapeutic (e.g., hypertension, diabetes, or arthritis), or preventive services (e.g., mammograms or vaccinations) for common health issues. The care is provided on an outpatient basis by primary care physicians (PCPs), including family practice physicians, internists, and pediatricians who have traditionally served as gatekeepers to other subspecialists, such as physical therapy. However, with **direct access**, an individual seeking physical therapy can do so without obtaining a referral from another healthcare provider in all 50 states and the District of Columbia.

- **Secondary care**: Medical specialists (e.g., orthopedists, cardiologists, urologists, or dermatologists) provide this level of care for problems requiring more specialized clinical expertise. This level of care may require inpatient hospitalization or ambulatory same-day surgery. The degree of physical therapy involvement at this level varies according to how much the patient's condition impacts their function.

- **Tertiary care**: This level of care involves the management of complex or rare disorders (e.g., major surgical procedures, congenital malformations, or organ transplants) that require high-level care. Physical therapy may be prescribed as needed at this level of care and is often provided in specialized units, such as wound care or burn care.

# Elements of PT Practice

In 1992, the APTA's board of directors (BOD) began determining practice parameters to delineate the physical therapy profession. The BOD initiated the development of a document describing PT practice—content and processes—for members of the physical therapy profession, healthcare policymakers, and third-party payers. The deliberations resulted in the BOD's development of A Guide to Physical Therapist Practice, Volume I: A Description of Patient Management, published in the August 1995 issue of Physical Therapy. Volume II contained descriptions of preferred PT practice for patient groupings defined by common PT management.

In early 1997, volumes I and II became part one and part two of a single document ("the Guide"), the first edition of which was published in the November 1997 issue of Physical Therapy (PTJ). Then, in 1998, the APTA began developing part three to catalog the tests and measures used by PTs.

Over the years, the Guide has been revised based on research evidence and the suggestions of the APTA's members and produced in various formats, including a CD-ROM. Indeed, the APTA is currently working on the fourth revision of the Guide.

In 2014, the Guide to Physical Therapist Practice 3.0 was published online, and several significant changes occurred. For example, the language of the Guide became more consistent with the International Classification of Functioning, Disability, and Health (ICF) language and removed the preferred practice patterns. The preferred practice patterns are still available online as an educational tool but no longer serve to inform the public or payer sources.

A further revision, 4.0, was posted as a web resource in February 2023.

The Guide, as the result of collaboration among hundreds of PTs, continues to be a resource for physical therapy practice and the professional education of PTs and PTAs. Clinicians can use the Guide to help organize their management process and choose the most helpful data to collect and analyze during the examination process. The Guide effectively defines PT practice, including the roles of the PT and the PTA. It describes the setting and practices; defines terminology; and creates a road map for PT examination, evaluation, diagnosis, prognosis, and intervention.

### The ICF

The ICF is a biopsychosocial classification system developed by the World Health Organization (WHO) based on the concept of health as a state of complete physical, mental, and social well-being and not merely the absence of disease or infirmity. Thus, the ICF provides a framework to help recognize the complex interplay between an individual's health condition, environmental factors, and personal factors that may influence their functioning and participation in society.

The ICF consists of two parts:

- Functioning and disability: This part describes the person's health condition and its impact on their body functions, structures, activities, and participation. It is organized into four domains:
  - Body functions
  - Body structures
  - Activities and participation
  - Environmental factors
- Contextual factors: This part includes personal and environmental factors affecting the person's functioning and participation.
  - Personal factors include factors such as age, gender, race, and education.
  - Environmental factors include factors such as social support, access to health care, and physical barriers.

The APTA's House of Delegates has also chosen to use this model and its definitions to describe physical therapy for this exact reason. In addition, current physical therapy practice emphasizes prevention services programs for promoting health, wellness, and fitness and programs for maintaining function.

## Patient and Client Management Model

The Patient and Client Management Model (PCMM) is a framework that provides a structured approach to clinical decision-making and patient management in healthcare settings. It was developed by the WHO as part of its efforts to improve the quality of care provided by health professionals. The PCMM is based on a patient-centered approach that considers the patient's specific needs, preferences, and circumstances when making clinical decisions. It emphasizes the importance of communication and collaboration between healthcare professionals and patients, and it recognizes that effective patient management requires a coordinated, multidisciplinary approach. The PCMM consists of six steps:

1. Engagement: This step involves establishing a relationship with the patient and assessing their needs, preferences, and expectations.
2. Assessment: This step involves gathering information about the patient's health status, including their medical history, physical examination, and diagnostic tests.
3. Diagnosis: This step involves identifying the patient's health problem and determining the underlying cause or causes.
4. Planning: This step involves developing a **plan of care (POC)** tailored to the patient's needs and circumstances.
5. Implementation: This step involves putting the POC into action, including providing treatment,

The ICF is a medical and social model that allows medical intervention to correct a patient's health problem and demands social change to prevent or right an injustice due to societal attitudes or lack of environmental accessibility.

A person's ability to complete an activity is affected by various factors, including body functions, structures, and personal and environmental traits.

An example:

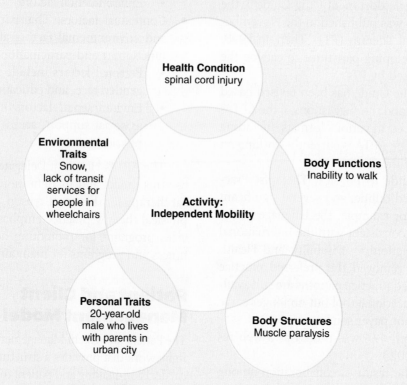

Suppose a person with a spinal cord injury was placed into the ICF model. In that case, their mobility impairment might cause an activity limitation (inability to use public transportation) and a participation restriction (inability to attend the local college sporting activities).

monitoring the patient's progress, and adjusting the plan as needed.

6. Evaluation: This step involves evaluating the effectiveness of the POC and making any necessary changes to improve the patient's outcomes.

The Guide describes the PCMM to help inform and guide the PT [1]. The PCMM in physical therapy is a modification of the one designed by the WHO. It is a patient-centered approach that emphasizes communication, collaboration, and the coordination of care among healthcare professionals, patients, and their families. Like the WHO model, the PCMM in physical therapy includes the following six steps (see Chapters 5 and 12):

1. Examination: This step involves collecting relevant data about the patient's health status, including their medical history, physical examination, and diagnostic tests.

2. Evaluation: This step involves analyzing the data collected during the examination and identifying impairments, activity limitations, and participation restrictions that affect the patient's functional status.

3. Diagnosis: This step involves identifying the underlying cause or causes of the patient's impairments and functional limitations.

4. Prognosis: This step involves predicting the expected outcomes of physical therapy interventions, including the anticipated improvement level in the patient's functional status.

5. Intervention: This step involves implementing a POC that includes physical therapy interventions designed to improve the patient's functional status, reduce impairments, and increase participation.

6. Outcomes: This step involves evaluating the effectiveness of the interventions and determining

whether the patient's goals have been met. If the goals have not been met, the POC is revised, and additional interventions are implemented as needed.

Using these elements, the PT gathers information, analyzes the information, establishes a POC that identifies goals and outcomes, and describes the proposed intervention, including frequency and duration.

Patient and client management requires an ongoing process that includes working with others managing the patient, consultation services, direction and supervision of personnel, and referrals for other services. The PCMM helps PTs maintain and improve a person's health, well-being, and function to optimize independence.

# Clinical Practice

The PT and PTA work together (and, when appropriate, with other individuals) using various physical therapy techniques and procedures to produce changes in the patient's/client's condition. This collaborative relationship between the PT and the PTA occurs through all patient/client management phases (see Chapter 5).

## Examination

As indicated previously, the PT performs the initial examination, which involves gathering information about the individual's past and current status, termed the **history**. The patient/client history accounts for the patient's/client's past and current health status [1]. The history is obtained by gathering data from the patient/client, immediate family, caregivers, other members of the patient's/client's family, and other interested persons, such as an employer or a rehabilitation counselor. This data includes the medical and surgical history, functional status, living environment, social and employment history, and general health.

The **systems review** is a part of the history that provides additional information about the anatomic and physiological status of the individual's musculoskeletal, genitourinary, cardiovascular/pulmonary, neuromuscular, and integumentary systems and the patient's communication, affect, cognition, learning style, and education needs.

The **tests and measures** component of the examination is the procedures selected by the PT to acquire additional information about the patient's condition, the physical therapy diagnosis, and the necessary therapeutic interventions [1]. Sometimes tests and measures are unnecessary; at other times, they are extensively required. **Table 3-1** includes examples of tests and measures that PTs use.

## Evaluation

The evaluation, a clinical judgment based on the findings from the clinical presentation, history, systems review, and tests and measures, is the clinical decision-making component of the PCMM. This clinical decision-making may also require additional guiding factors, such as coordination, consultation, and collaboration of care consistent with the nature of the problem and the patient's needs [1].

## Diagnosis

The diagnosis or physical therapy diagnostic process includes the following: obtaining relevant patient/

**Table 3-1** Tests and Measures

| Aerobic Capacity/Endurance | Anthropometric Characteristics | Assistive Technology |
|---|---|---|
| Balance | Circulation (arterial, venous, lymphatic) | Community, social, and civic life |
| Cranial and peripheral nerve integrity | Education life | Environmental factors |
| Gait | Integumentary integrity | Joint integrity and mobility |
| Mental functions | Mobility (including locomotion) | Motor function |
| Muscle performance (including strength, power, endurance, and length) | Neuromotor development and sensory processing | Pain |
| Posture | Range of motion | Reflex integrity |
| Self-care and domestic life | Sensory integrity | Skeletal integrity |
| Ventilation and respiration | Work life | |

**Box 3-1 Diagnosis by PTs**

PTs shall establish a diagnosis for each patient/client.

Before making a patient/client management decision, PTs shall utilize the diagnostic process to establish a diagnosis for the specific conditions needing the PT's attention.

A diagnosis is a label encompassing a cluster of signs and symptoms commonly associated with a disorder or syndrome or category of impairments in body structures and function, activity limitations, or participation restrictions. It is the decision reached due to the diagnostic process, which evaluates information obtained from the patient/client examination. The purpose of the diagnosis is to guide the PT in determining the most appropriate intervention strategy for each patient/client. If the diagnostic process does not yield an identifiable cluster, disorder, syndrome, or category, intervention may be directed toward alleviating symptoms and remedying impairments in body structures and function, activity limitations, or participation restrictions.

The PT's responsibility in the diagnostic process is to organize and interpret all relevant information collected. The diagnostic process includes obtaining the relevant history, performing a systems review, and selecting and administering specific tests and measures.

When indicated, PTs order appropriate tests, including but not limited to imaging and other studies, that are performed and interpreted by other health professionals. PTs may also perform or interpret selected imaging or other studies.

PTs may need additional information (including diagnostic labels) from other health professionals when performing the diagnostic process. In addition, as the diagnostic process continues, PTs may identify findings that should be shared with other health professionals, including referral sources, to ensure optimal patient/client care. When the patient/client is referred with a previously established diagnosis, the PT should determine that the clinical findings are consistent with that diagnosis. If the diagnostic process reveals findings outside the scope of the PT's knowledge, experience, or expertise, the therapist should refer the patient/client to an appropriate practitioner.

Modified from American Physical Therapy Association: Diagnosis by Physical Therapists HOD P06-12-10-09 [Amended HOD P06-08-06-07; HOD P06-97-06-19; HOD 06-95-12-07; HOD 06-94-22-35; Initial HOD 06-84-19-78] [Internet] [cited 2023 Jan 24]. Available from: https://www.apta.org/apta-and-you/leadership-and-governance/policies/diagnosis-by-physical-therapist

client history, performing systems review, selecting and administering specific tests and measures, and organizing and interpreting all data [1]. A **physical therapy diagnosis** describes the system(s) affected by the alteration in function and identifies the specific patient complaint and the overall effect on the person [1].

- Impairments are abnormalities or dysfunctions of body structure or function. Examples of impairments include muscle weakness, tendon or ligament inflammation, muscle spasms, or edema.
- Activity limitations are the inability of a patient/client to function adequately in their environment. Activity limitations include an inability to ambulate or perform activities of daily living (ADLs), such as brushing the hair, washing the face, or dressing.
- Participation restriction refers to a person's challenges in interacting with the world around them. An example of a participation restriction would be a person's inability to work, attend community activities, or access healthcare resources.
- Disability is the inability to perform or participate in activities or tasks related to a person's work, home, or community. Disability affects individual and societal functioning and changes the person's

social roles. Examples of disability are the inability to perform occupational tasks, school-related tasks, home management (that can be a disability for a homemaker), caring for dependents, community responsibilities, or service.

## Prognosis

The prognosis is the PT's judgment about the optimal improvement the patient/client may achieve and the time needed to reach that level [1]. The prognosis is often subjective as many factors, including an individual's unique characteristics, attitude, and motivation, can influence it. During this phase, the PT designs a POC comprising measurable and achievable goals, outcomes (intended level of function), and interventions based on the examination findings; patient/client input; and determined diagnosis and prognosis. It is important to remember that the goals (short-term and long-term) are written in terms that are oriented to function and are time-sensitive. For example, a short-term goal might be: In 10 days, the patient will be able to walk from the bed to the bathroom unassisted, while a long-term goal might be: The patient will walk 30 feet from the family room to the kitchen with one hand held at dinner time 5/7 days per week.

# Intervention

Interventions are purposeful and skilled interactions of the PT with the patient/client and, when appropriate, with other individuals involved in patient/client care to produce changes in the condition consistent with the diagnosis and prognosis [1]. The interventions are altered following changes in response or status of the patient/client. The interventions are provided at a level consistent with current physical therapy practice. The APTA's intervention categories used in the provision of PT services include the following [1]:

- Therapeutic exercise: Physical movements or activities that improve physical function and health status
- Manual therapy techniques: Skilled techniques to increase motion and reduce pain in soft tissues and joints
- Motor functioning training: Physical movements, postures, or activities that require planning
- Functional training: Activities to improve function in the home, work, community, and education environments
- Airway clearance techniques: Activities or techniques to create or maintain clear airways
- Assistive technology: The selection, fitting, and training in the use of devices and equipment that improve function, prevent further impairments, and reduce pain
- Biophysical agents: The use of thermal, electrical, mechanical, acoustic, or radiant energy equipment to improve neuromuscular performance, improve skin condition, increase joint motion, and decrease pain and swelling
- Patient/client education: Informing the patient/client, family, or caregiver about a condition and the available services to optimize outcomes.

# Outcomes

**Outcomes**, the result of the interventions and the entire POC, are important in patient care as they provide the opportunity to compare care collectively and determine effectiveness [1]. It is not uncommon to modify goals and outcomes based on a patient reexamination during an episode of care if the POC does not appear to be achieving the desired results. In addition, the patient may require a referral to another practitioner to achieve the desired outcomes.

The PT concludes an episode of care when the goals and outcomes for the patient or client have been achieved, when the patient or client cannot further

## Box 3-2 PT Responsibilities

Regardless of the setting in which the physical therapy service is provided, the following responsibilities must be borne solely by the PT: (1) interpretation of referrals when available; (2) initial examination, evaluation, diagnosis, and prognosis; (3) development or modification of a POC based on the initial examination or reexamination, which includes the physical therapy goals and outcomes; and (4) determination of when the expertise and decision-making capability of the PT require the PT to render physical therapy interventions personally and when it may be appropriate to utilize the PTA. The PT shall also determine the most appropriate utilization of the PTA to provide safe, effective, and efficient service delivery. For example, the interventions are provided to make the directed and supervised responsibilities commensurate with the PTA's qualifications and legal limitations.

progress toward goals, or when the PT determines that the patient or client will no longer benefit from physical therapy [1].

## *Physical Therapy Diagnosis versus Medical Diagnosis*

The physical therapy diagnosis is different from the medical diagnosis.

### Definition of Medical Diagnosis

A **medical diagnosis** is determined by a physician (medical doctor [MD] or doctor of osteopathy [DO]) who identifies an illness or disorder in a patient through an interview, physical examination, medical tests, and other procedures. Consequently, the medical diagnosis recognizes a disease and finds the pathology's cause and nature.

Data from American Physical Therapy Association. Guide to Physical Therapist Practice 3.0. Alexandria, VA: APTA; 2014.

### Definition of Physical Therapy Diagnosis

The PT determines a physical therapy diagnosis. Consequently, the physical therapy diagnosis is defined as the end result of evaluating information obtained from the examination, which the PT organizes to determine the functional losses and to help determine the most appropriate intervention strategies [1].

Data from American Physical Therapy Association. Guide to Physical Therapist Practice 3.0. Alexandria, VA: APTA; 2014.

## The Importance of Physical Therapy Diagnosis.

Diagnosis is essential to PT practice to provide proper physical therapy interventions. PTs diagnose based on PT practice as authorized by state law. In diagnosing a patient's condition under such law, PTs do not conflict with the diagnosis provisions of state laws governing the practice of medicine. No states prohibit a PT from performing a diagnosis.

As indicated in the definition of physical therapy diagnosis, PTs utilize the diagnostic process before making a patient/client management decision. They establish a diagnosis for the specific conditions needing the PT's attention. The purpose of the physical therapy diagnosis is to guide the PT in determining the most appropriate intervention strategy for each patient/client. Suppose the diagnostic process does not generate an identifiable cluster, disorder, syndrome, or category. In that case, physical therapy intervention may alleviate symptoms and remedy impairment, functional limitation, or disability.

During the diagnostic process, PTs can obtain additional information, including diagnostic labels, from other health professionals. As the diagnostic process continues, PTs may identify findings that should be shared with other health professionals (including referral sources) to ensure optimal patient/client care. When the patient/client is referred with a previously established diagnosis, the PT should determine that the clinical findings are consistent with that diagnosis. If the diagnostic process reveals findings outside the guide of the PT's knowledge, experience, or expertise, the PT should refer the patient/client to an appropriate practitioner.

### KNOWLEDGE CHECK

What portions of the PCMM can the PTA perform?
What are the differences among an impairment, an activity limitation, a participation restriction, and a disability?
How are a medical diagnosis and a physical therapy diagnosis different?

## *Physical Therapy Intervention*

Physical therapy intervention has three components: coordination, communication, and documentation; patient/client-related instruction; and direct interventions. Coordination, communication, documentation, and patient/client-related instruction are provided for all patients/clients and may include the following:

- Case management
- Coordination of care with the patient/client, family, or other healthcare professionals

- Computer-assisted instruction
- Periodic reexamination and reassessment of the home program
- Demonstration and modeling for teaching, verbal instruction, and written or pictorial instruction

Direct interventions are based on the following elements:

- Examination and evaluation of data
- The diagnosis and the prognosis (including the POC)
- The anticipated goals and expected outcomes for a particular patient in a specific patient/client diagnostic group [1]

Through coordination, communication, documentation, and patient/client-related instruction, the PT ensures appropriate, coordinated, comprehensive, and cost-effective physical therapy services and patient/client integration in the home, community, and workplace.

Some examples of PT interventions include:

1. Patient or client instruction (used with every patient and client)
   The PT provides instruction to patients with some portions provided by the PTA. Patient/client-related instruction may include direction, education, and training of patients/clients and caregivers regarding current condition (pathology, pathophysiology, impairments, functional limitations, or disabilities); enhancement of performance; health, wellness, and fitness; POC; risk factors (for pathology, pathophysiology, disease, disorder or condition, impairments, functional limitations, or disabilities); patient's/client's transitions across settings; and patient's/client's transitions to new roles.

2. Airway clearance techniques (such as breathing, positioning, and/or manual/mechanical techniques)
   Examples of breathing exercises include paced breathing and pursed-lip breathing. Examples of positioning include techniques to maximize ventilation and pulmonary drainage (of specific lobes). Examples of manual/mechanical techniques include chest percussion, vibration, and mechanical suctioning.

3. Assistive technology
   The assistive technology category includes the prescription, application, and fabrication/modification of assistive devices. This category can be divided into locomotion aids (wheelchairs, walkers, canes, etc.), orthoses (braces and splints), prostheses, wheelchair seating systems,

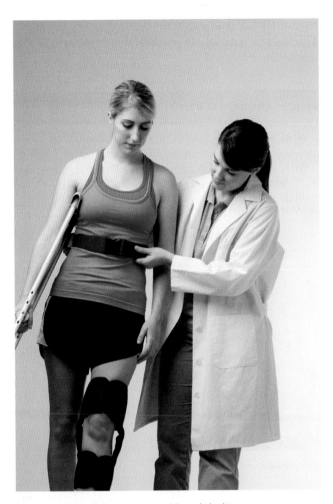

**Figure 3-1** Crutch training with gait belt.
© DNY59/E+/Getty Images

positioning devices (prone and supine standers or upper extremity supportive wheelchair trays), and other technologies that improve safety (home modification devices, slide boards, and mechanical transfer assists) (**Figure 3-1**).

4. Biophysical agents that include electrotherapeutic modalities

    Examples of electrotherapeutic modalities include utilizing electrical stimulation, such as high-voltage pulsed current (HVPC), transcutaneous electrical nerve stimulation (TENS), and neuromuscular electrical stimulation (NMES). Physical agents and mechanical modalities also fit under this heading. Examples of physical agents include cold packs, ice massages, hot packs, paraffin baths, and hydrotherapy (whirlpool tanks or pools). Examples of mechanical modalities include standing frames or tilt tables.

5. Functional training in self-care, domestic, work, community, social, and civic life

    Functional training in self-care and home management includes ADLs and instrumental activities

of daily living (IADLs). ADLs include bathing, bed mobility and/or transfer training, developmental activities, dressing, eating, grooming, and toileting. Examples of IADLs include caring for dependents, household chores, shopping, yard work, structured play for children, and home maintenance. Functional training in work (job/school/play), community, and leisure integration or reintegration includes IADLs, work hardening, and work conditioning. Examples of functional training in work (which can take place as back schools, job coaching, or simulated work environments) include injury prevention or reduction, education during work, safety awareness training, or use of devices and equipment.

6. Integumentary repair and protection techniques

    An example of integumentary repair would be wound or burn care. Protection techniques include aseptic and isolation procedures.

7. Manual therapy techniques

    Manual therapy techniques include mobilization and/or manipulation (such as of soft tissue or spinal and peripheral joints).

8. Motor function training

    Motor function training involves interventions to improve balance, motor control, perceptual awareness, gait training with or without using an assistive device, postural awareness, strength and control, and vestibular training.

9. Therapeutic exercise

    Therapeutic exercise includes aerobic conditioning and endurance training, flexibility, coordination, strength and power training, and relaxation strategies [1].

The PT's POC identifies a plan for discharge of the patient/client, considering the achievement of anticipated goals and expected outcomes, and provides for appropriate follow-up or referral.

## Discharge from Physical Therapy and Discontinuation of Physical Therapy Services

Discharge is "the process of ending physical therapy services that have been provided during a single episode of care when the anticipated goals and expected outcomes have been achieved" [1]. Discharge does not occur with a transfer (when the patient is moved from one site to another within the same setting or across settings during a single episode of care). Discharge is based on the PT's analysis of the achievement of anticipated goals and expected outcomes.

Discontinuation is described as the process of discontinuing interventions that have been provided during a single episode of care when: (1) the patient/client, caregiver, or legal guardian declines to continue interventions; (2) the patient/client is unable to continue to progress toward anticipated goals and expected outcomes because of medical/psychosocial complications or financial/insurance resources have been expended; or (3) the PT determines that patient/client will no longer benefit from physical therapy [1]. When physical therapy services are terminated before achieving anticipated goals and expected outcomes, patient/client status and the rationale for discontinuation should be documented.

> Indications for patient's/client's discharge include the following:
>
> - The patient's/client's desire to stop treatment
> - The patient's/client's inability to progress toward goals due to medical or psychosocial complications
> - The PT's decision that the patient/client will no longer benefit from physical therapy [1]

Data from American Physical Therapy Association. Guide to Physical Therapist Practice 3.0. Alexandria, VA: APTA; 2014.

The PT reexamines the patient/client as necessary during an episode of care to evaluate progress or change in patient/client status and modifies the POC accordingly or discontinues physical therapy services. In consultation with appropriate individuals and considering the anticipated goals and expected outcomes, the PT plans for discharge or discontinuation and provides the appropriate follow-up or referral.

## Preferred Practice Patterns

The original Guide included preferred practice patterns in musculoskeletal, neuromuscular, cardiovascular/pulmonary, and integumentary systems. The most recent edition does not include these patterns; however, they are available on the APTA website for educational purposes. To guide professionals to provide effective, efficient, and evidence-based practice, an APTA initiative supports the development of clinical practice guidelines (CPGs). The APTA sections develop the CPGs for specific diagnoses and interventions. A list of currently developing CPGs is available on the APTA website in PTNow.[1] PTs may also consider utilizing clinical prediction rules (CPRs) to assist in the

examination, diagnosis, and development of a POC. Throughout a variety of physical therapy journals, PTs can access CPRs.

**KNOWLEDGE CHECK**

What are some examples of interventions within a POC?

What conditions indicate that a patient should be discharged from physical therapy?

What are CPGs?

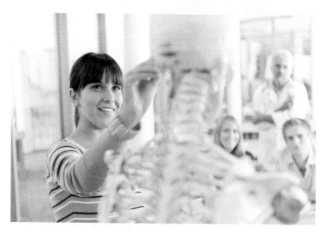

© CandyBox Images/Shutterstock

# Physical Therapy Clinical Settings

Typically, PTs and PTAs work together in the same clinical facilities. These facilities range from acute care to extended care in skilled nursing facilities (SNFs) and private practices.

## Acute Care Facilities

Acute care physical therapy is practiced in hospitals, where patients usually remain for a short period. The average length of stay for a patient is less than 30 days. Acute care physical therapy practices are very demanding for PTs and PTAs because of the variety of patients having diverse and sometimes critical pathophysiological impairments and functional limitations. For example, in acute care hospitals, after the physical therapy examination and evaluation, PTAs may need to provide physical therapy treatments for patients after major surgical procedures, such as heart or liver transplants. Additionally, other major surgeries are performed by highly specialized physicians and surgeons in technologically equipped hospitals. These hospitals increasingly rely on information technology solutions to help deliver better quality patient care while containing costs.

Consequently, PTs and PTAs should learn to use the technology while applying expert and focused physical therapy. Furthermore, due to the fast and demanding pace of acute care hospitals, the rapid discharge of patients increases the role of the PT and the PTA as patient/family/caregiver educators. The healthcare providers functioning in acute care clinical settings (in addition to PTs and PTAs) include physicians (MDs or DOs), physician assistants (PAs), nurses (registered nurses, licensed practical nurses), OTs, social workers, and SLPs.

Due to the fast-paced, ever-changing environment in acute care, the Academy of Acute Care, a section of the APTA, created the Core Competencies for Entry-Level Physical Therapist Assistants in the Acute Care Setting document. The document describes the necessary clinical and decision-making skills to make a PTA successful in this practice area.

## Primary Care Facilities

**Primary care** is a type of healthcare practice provided by a PCP, where PTs and PTAs work on an outpatient physical therapy basis. PCPs can be family practice physicians or specialists, such as pediatricians, internists, or obstetricians/gynecologists. These physicians provide basic or first-level health care. The PTs support the physicians as part of the primary care team supplying the patient's examination, evaluation, physical therapy diagnosis, and prognosis. PTAs support the PTs on the primary care team by implementing the treatment plan. The treatment plan is usually implemented after the PT has established a POC.

## Subacute Care Facilities

Subacute care is an intermediate level of care for medically fragile patients too ill to be cared for at home. Subacute care is offered within a subacute hospital or an SNF. Typically, SNFs offer rehabilitation services daily. There are three types of SNFs:

- SNFs provide subacute care (a higher level of care than extended care).
- SNFs provide transitional care (hospital-based SNFs).
- SNFs provide extended care.

Patients who receive health care in a transitional care SNF often are discharged to home, assisted living

facilities, or extended-care SNFs. Extended-care SNFs are freestanding or may be part of a hospital. They provide healthcare services daily, 7 days per week. In these facilities, rehabilitation services are offered 5 days per week. In extended-care SNFs, patients are not in an acute phase of illness but require skilled interventions on an inpatient basis. Extended-care SNFs need to be certified by Medicare. Extended-care SNFs must offer 24-hour nursing care coverage and physical, occupational, and speech therapy to comply with Medicare certification. PTs/PTAs work with the rehabilitation team in these facilities, including OTs, SLPs, certified occupational therapy assistants (COTAs), social workers, and nurses. PTAs deliver skilled interventions to patients after the supervising PT establishes the POC. PTAs also may be involved in delegation and supervision (when allowed by the individual facility or state practice) of non-skilled tasks performed by the rehabilitation aides.

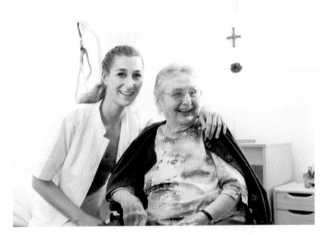

© Kzenon/Shutterstock

## Outpatient Care Facilities

A large area of employment for PTs and PTAs includes outpatient care centers (or ambulatory care). These facilities provide outpatient preventive services, diagnostic services, and treatment services. Outpatient care centers are situated in medical offices, surgery centers, and outpatient clinics. The healthcare providers are MDs, PAs, nurse practitioners, PTs, OTs, PTAs, and other rehabilitation personnel. The services in outpatient centers are less costly than in inpatient centers and are favored by managed care insurance companies. The PTAs implement the treatment programs after the PTs complete the POC.

## Rehabilitation Hospitals

Rehabilitation hospitals provide rehabilitation, social, and vocational services to patients with a disability, facilitating their return to maximal functional capacity. PTAs implement all or part of the physical therapy POC delegated by the PTs. PTAs work with other healthcare providers, participating in team meetings and performing patient and family education when necessary.

## Chronic Care Facilities

Chronic care or long-term care facilities provide services to patients who must stay 60 days or longer. Medical services are offered to patients with permanent or residual disabilities caused by a nonreversible pathological health condition. The rehabilitation services in these facilities may need to be specialized based on the patient's pathology. PTs/PTAs deliver skilled physical therapy interventions to meet a patient's daily living needs. The interventions needed are not necessarily only to maintain the patient's function but also to improve the patient's function.

## Hospice Care Facilities

A hospice care facility is a healthcare facility that offers care for patients who are terminally ill and dying. The care is offered in an inpatient setting or at home. The healthcare team includes nurses, social workers, chaplains, physicians, and volunteers. Rehabilitation services are optional. Medicare and Medicaid insurance companies require that most health care (80%) be provided in the patient's home.

## Home Health Care

Home health care is typically provided to patients and their families in a home environment. The government, private insurance, volunteer organizations, or nonprofit or for-profit organizations can financially sponsor home health care. The patient must be homebound to be eligible, meaning they require physical assistance to leave home. Also, eligibility for home health care requires skilled interventions from at least one of the following disciplines: nursing, physical therapy, occupational therapy, or speech therapy. In addition, a physician has to certify that skilled interventions are necessary. If physical therapy is needed, the PT has to reevaluate the patient every 3–6 weeks or periodically, depending on the patient's rehabilitation needs. The PT or the PTA must document every visit and reevaluation.

The patient's safety is the main concern for home healthcare physical therapy. An ongoing patient's environmental assessment occurs during the PT's or the PTA's visits. The PT or the PTA must report any

information regarding substance abuse by the patient or physical abuse of the patient. The PTA provides skilled interventions in bed mobility training, transfer training, gait training, and implementation of a home exercise program. State regulations differ in the use of the PTA in home health care. Some states require 1 year of experience as a PTA, and some do not allow a PTA to practice in home healthcare environments. If the PTA can practice home health care, the PT needs to examine and evaluate the patient, develop a POC, establish treatment goals, and discuss the patient's program with the PTA before the PTA's first visit. The PT should always be accessible to the PTA by way of telecommunications. Ongoing conferences between the PT and the PTA must occur weekly or biweekly, and the PT's supervisory visits must be made every 4–6 weeks or sooner at the PTA's request.

## School System

School system physical therapy takes place in school settings. The PTA collaborates with the PT, teachers, and teacher aides to improve the student's function in school. The child's team and parents develop an individual education plan (IEP) for the student who has a disability. The IEP focuses on increasing the student's school and classroom function. The PTA provides the necessary interventions for achieving goals delegated by the PT. Examples of physical therapy recommendations for a student would be to help the student's functional mobility by having the student use a computer or improving a student's mobility in the school building by use of an assistive device (such as a walker).

## Private Practice Facilities

Private practice physical therapy is provided in a privately owned physical therapy facility. The private practice can offer outpatient or contract services for SNFs, schools, or homecare agencies. Insurance reimbursement is allowed with a provider number, and the provider needs to be a PT. The PTA works with

### KNOWLEDGE CHECK

Where would patients receive physical therapy services if they are too ill to be cared for at home but do not need hospitalization?

Which settings utilize healthcare teams to treat patients/clients?

What condition must exist for a patient to be eligible for home health services?

the PT to provide physical therapy services under the PT's supervision (as allowed by the state practice acts). The PT needs to examine and evaluate the patient and provide a POC. Documentation describing the treatment must take place for every visit, and a complete reevaluation by the PT is necessary every 30 days.

# Practice Areas

Upon entering a physical therapy educational program, students are instructed in all practice areas to become competent healthcare workforce members (see Chapter 5).

# Physical Therapy Employment Practices

## Policy and Procedure Manual

The general purpose of a policy and procedure manual is to familiarize the employees with the practice's specific mission, culture, expectations, and benefits. Although the manual is not a contract, it provides a clear, common understanding of the practice's goals, benefits, and policies and what is expected concerning the employee's performance and conduct. The manual also contributes to the employee's comfort level because it spells out what is expected of them to comply with practice guidelines and fit in with the practice culture.

> The purposes of the policy and procedure manual include the following:
>
> - It provides extensive information on what should be done and how it should be done in a physical therapy department.
> - The Joint Commission, Commission on Accreditation of Rehabilitation Facilities, and other physical therapy accrediting agencies require it.

A **policy** is defined as a broad statement that guides the decision-making process. A policy represents a principle, a law, or a decision that guides actions. Examples of policies in a physical therapy department include the following:

- Time off, leave of absence, sabbaticals for military service, maternity leave, medical issues, and jury duty
- Vacation according to the length of employment and seniority; vacation is paid time off from work

- Dress code required by the facility
- Probationary period

**Procedures** are defined as specific guides to job functions for all departmental personnel, visitors, and patients to standardize activities with a high level of risk. Procedures represent the sequence of steps to perform an action typically described in a policy. Procedures are also criteria for how things are done. Procedures can assist employees in dealing with situations that may arise during the daily operations of a practice. Examples of procedures in a physical therapy department include the following:

- Equipment management, cleaning, and maintenance; safety inspections; and training requirements
- Safety and emergency procedures
- Hazardous waste management
- Disciplinary procedures for actions such as violation of the dress code or a patient's confidentiality

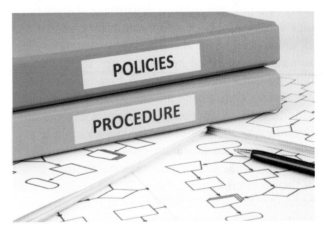

© vinnstock/Shutterstock

### Content of the Policy and Procedure Manual

The policy and procedure manual has an introduction that may include the employee welcome message, an introductory statement, and an employee acknowledgment form. This section is written in a friendly, conversational style designed to make the employee welcome and comfortable and provides basic information about the practice and its operating philosophy. The remaining sections of the manual contain very detailed and precise language regarding the rights and obligations of both the employee and the employer and should be reviewed by a legal counsel to ensure compliance with federal and state laws.

The policy and procedure manual must be guided by various state and federal laws and organizations, such as the Equal Employment Opportunity Commission (EEOC), the Americans with Disabilities Act

(ADA), the Family and Medical Leave Act (FMLA), the Fair Labor Standards Act (FLSA), the Occupational Safety and Health Administration (OSHA), the Health Insurance Portability and Accountability Act (HIPAA) (see Chapter 7), and the Centers for Medicare and Medicaid Services (CMS). The FMLA is an example of federal legislation included in the policy and procedure manual. The FMLA requires employers with 50 or more employees to allow up to 12 workweeks of unpaid leave in any 12 months for the birth, adoption, or foster care placement of a child, or serious health condition of the employee, spouse, parent, or child, provided the leave is taken within 12 months of such an event. The policy and procedure manual must include all the information related to the FMLA.

## Emergency Preparedness

Preparation for emergencies will be part of the policy and procedure manual and part of the daily operations of a physical therapy department. Larger facilities usually have a communication process that lets all employees know about facility emergencies. Examples of this would be code words such as "code blue" to call assigned caregivers to a person in cardiac arrest, "code red" to indicate a fire, or "code gray" to indicate a weather emergency, such as a tornado. Regardless of the size of the facility, all facilities will have standardized procedures to help deal with such situations, and each staff member needs to be aware of their role in the procedures. To this end, staff may be required to practice procedures or maintain certification for cardiopulmonary resuscitation and first aid. All employees will be expected to be alert to safety issues throughout their workday, whether noticing spilled water on a tile floor that may pose a fall hazard or identifying symptoms of cardiac instability in their exercising patient.

## Departmental Meetings

PTAs participate in facility and departmental meetings. The following types of meetings occur in the physical therapy department:

- Staff/departmental meetings: These are held regularly to discuss departmental (or hospital or management) business.
- Team meetings: Scheduled weekly and involving the interdisciplinary team members, such as the physician, nurse, PT, PTA, OT, COTA, SLP, social services, and other team members, the purpose of team meetings is to discuss and coordinate patient care services, set patients' goals, discuss goal achievement necessary for a patient's discharge, and discuss discharge plans and continuum of care, including equipment needs or home health services.
- Supervisory meetings: These take place regularly between the supervisor and the staff. The supervisory meeting's purpose is to discuss patient care issues. Sometimes, a supervisory meeting can be a one-on-one meeting between a staff member (such as the PTA) and the supervisor (such as the PT) to discuss the immediate needs of the staff member concerning patient care. The goal of the supervisory meetings is to achieve positive outcomes.
- Strategic planning meetings provide an organizational/departmental planning process for the future. These meetings discuss the results of the strategic planning process included in the strategic plan. They also make a statement about the mission and the philosophy of values of the organization/department before implementing the strategic plan. Strategic planning meetings also can reveal the organizational/departmental strengths and weaknesses and the course of action for achieving future goals. In addition, strategic planning meetings can provide the following:
  - Directions on how to achieve the organization's/department's goals
  - Identification of the people responsible for developing and carrying out the strategic plan (such as staff members and/or the supervisor)
  - Information to external parties (such as the accrediting agencies) about the organization/department
  - Analysis of the progress toward the strategic plan goals

The strategic plan goals are time-related and can be for 1, 2, or 5 years. Analysis of progress toward the goals is generally done quarterly by the supervisor (or director/manager) of the organization/department.

# Fiscal Management of a Physical Therapy Service

## Budgets

A budget fiscally manages physical therapy services. A budget is a financial projection for the allocated funds to cover specific aspects of operating a physical therapy department or a private practice over a specific period.

Budget periods vary from 1 year for personnel and supplies to 5 years (or longer) for capital expenses (purchase expenses). Budgets need to be revised when conditions in the organization/department change.

The purposes of a budget include the following:

- Explains in detail the anticipated income and expenditures (expenses) for personnel, buildings, equipment, supplies, and/or space
- Represents an integral aspect of the planning process
- Provides a mechanism for assessing the success of the practice, programs, or projects

The various types of budgets include the following:

- Operating expense budget: A financial projection of daily organizational/departmental operations. Examples include salaries, benefits (such as sick days or vacation days), utilities (such as electricity, gas, or telephone), supplies (such as ultrasound gel, changing gowns, or gloves), linen, housekeeping, maintenance, and continuing education.
- Capital expense budget: A financial projection related to the purchase of large items for future use. An example is physical therapy equipment to be utilized for more than a year (such as an ultrasound machine).
- Accounts receivable budget: A financial projection assessing expected benefits from future operations; includes money owed to a company, such as a physical therapy private practice for providing physical therapy services. An example could be money to be received from Medicare for physical therapy services provided to Medicare patients.
- Accounts payable budget: A financial projection assessing money owed to a creditor that provided services or equipment to the company; it is the part of the budget where debts are listed. An example could be money paid to a company that regularly services physical therapy equipment.

## Costs

In physical therapy, there are four different costs associated with providing physical therapy services:

- Direct costs: Costs directly related to the provision of physical therapy services. Examples include salaries, equipment, treatment supplies, or continuing education.
- Indirect costs: Costs related to the provision of physical therapy services in an indirect way. Examples include housekeeping, utilities, laundry, and marketing.

- Variable costs: Costs related to the provision of physical therapy services that are not fixed and can vary depending on the volume of services. Examples include linen or utility costs, which will increase with an increase in the number of patient visits.
- Fixed costs: Costs related to the provision of fixed physical therapy services regardless of the changes in the volume of services. An example is rent, which will not increase regardless of the number of patient visits.

Every employee of a physical therapy department should be aware of appropriate billing practices and cost containment measures to maintain a fiscally sound operation. Employees should review the department's billing practices to ensure that payer rules are followed and that billing is consistent and accurate. To ensure a successful business model, all staff should consider their productivity, equipment, supply use, and awareness of cost-saving measures, such as the appropriate use of theraband, kinesio tape, electrodes, paper, water, and electricity. Many employers have specific productivity goals for their employees to meet. The productivity model needs to be balanced with an appropriate value of patient care to provide quality care. Understanding the department's mission and value statements can assist the PT or PTA in adhering to the department's standards.

### KNOWLEDGE CHECK

What kinds of topics are part of a policy and procedure manual?
What are the purposes of departmental meetings in a physical therapy department?
What is the role of all department members in fiscal responsibility?

## Quality Assurance

Quality assurance (QA) is defined as activities and programs designed and implemented in a clinical facility to achieve high-quality levels of care. QA activities are intended to identify areas of success in outcomes and patient satisfaction and to improve in areas of weakness. In physical therapy, QA is responsible for the following:

- Monitoring the quality of physical therapy services
- Monitoring the appropriateness of patient care
- Resolving any identified problems related to the quality of service and patient care

## Utilization Review

QA can be implemented in a clinical facility using a utilization review, which evaluates the necessity, quality, effectiveness, or efficiency of medical services, procedures, and facilities. For example, a hospital's utilization review includes the appropriateness of admission, services ordered, services provided, length of stay, and discharge practices. In physical therapy, utilization review can be implemented through a written plan to review the use of resources and determine their medical necessity and cost efficiency. For example, a utilization review can analyze the cost and the outcome of interferential electrical stimulation for patients diagnosed with posterior disk impingement. If the patients' outcomes were positive, it means the use of interferential electrical stimulation was appropriate, and the cost of the treatment was efficient.

## Peer Review

Utilization review can be applied in clinics by using peer review. As a general definition, peer review means the evaluation of the quality of the work effort of an individual by their peers. In addition to the clinical quality of medical care administered by an individual, group, or hospital, peer review is also used to evaluate articles submitted for publication in different scientific journals.

In physical therapy peer review, PTAs can review the work of other PTAs, and PTs can review the work of other PTs. In general, peer review is not punitive but educational. The goal of peer review is to improve the quality of care and to evaluate how well physical therapy services are performed when delivering care.

Types of peer review in physical therapy clinical settings include the following:

- Retrospective peer reviews are conducted after physical therapy services are rendered. They are used to determine whether physical therapy services were necessary, appropriate, and comprehensive based on patient needs.
- Concurrent peer reviews are conducted during physical therapy treatments. They are used to immediately improve the quality of physical therapy treatments and determine current patient outcomes and satisfaction.

Peer review can also be performed in physical therapy clinical facilities by different accrediting agencies or third-party payers, such as Medicare, Medicaid, or managed care plans. In these situations, a peer review is done by professional review organizations. An example of such an organization is the Professional Standards Review Organization (PSRO), which performs peer review at the local level as required by Public Law 92-603 (started in 1973) of the United States for the services provided under Medicare, Medicaid, and Maternal and Child Health programs funded by the federal government.

The major goals of the PSRO are the following:

- To ensure that healthcare services are of acceptable professional quality
- To ensure the appropriate use of healthcare facilities at the most economical level consistent with professional standards
- To identify lack of quality and overuse problems in health care and improve those conditions
- To attempt to obtain voluntary correction of inappropriate or unnecessary practitioner and facility practices, and if unable to do so, recommend sanctions against violators

## Risk Management

QA can be implemented in a clinical facility by using risk management. As a general definition, risk management is the methods healthcare organizations use to defend their assets against the threats posed by legal liability. Accurate self-assessment of implementing policies, procedures, and matters of practice can identify issues that can be rectified before significant damage or errors occur. Risk management includes the following:

- Identification of healthcare delivery problems in an institution (as evidenced by previous lawsuits and patient or staff complaints)
- Development of standards and guidelines to enhance the quality of care
- Anticipation of problems that may arise in the future

For example, risk management issues found in a hospital could include breaches of patients' privacy, failure to disclose risks and alternatives to treatment, intubation errors during anesthesia, or infant trauma or death during childbirth. In physical therapy, risk management can identify, evaluate, and prevent risk to staff or patients. Examples of risk management in physical therapy could include delegating issues, such as PTs delegating to PTAs or PTAs delegating to physical therapy aides. In such situations, the PTs and the PTAs must consult their state practice acts. Another risk management issue in physical therapy could be providing quality care for managed care patients or

Medicaid patients. For example, if a managed care company does not provide enough visits, and the patient needs additional visits, the PT may need to ask the managed care company for more visits or to ask the owner of the facility to allow free-of-charge services to the patient.

The general purposes of physical therapy risk management include the following:

- To decrease risks in physical therapy practice by maintaining equipment safety and providing ongoing staff safety education in the use of equipment
- To identify potential patient or employee injuries
- To identify potential property loss or damage
- To implement procedures to clean the equipment properly and prevent contamination
- To increase patient and staff safety by reporting all incidents, documenting incidents by making reports, reviewing incident reports by a supervisor, identifying all risk factors concerning patient care and safety, and having all staff certified (and recertified annually) in cardiopulmonary resuscitation

## Patient Satisfaction Surveys

A common QA strategy that healthcare practices employ is a patient satisfaction survey. It is important to survey discharged patients soon after completing their care as the survey return rate is higher. Some facilities offer electronic surveys that are taken after the last treatment to ensure feedback from all patients.

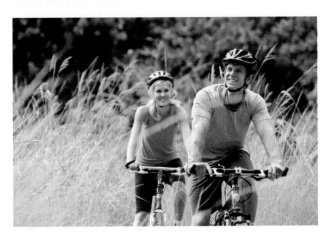

© Warren Goldswain/Shutterstock

---

### KNOWLEDGE CHECK

Which of the QA activities is the evaluation of the necessity, quality, effectiveness, or efficiency of physical therapy services?

What is an example of risk management?

# Nonclinical Roles

Wellness, disease prevention, and health promotion were physical therapy goals included in the 2020 Vision Statement. The APTA took the initiative to promote health by participating in the Healthy People Consortium, assisting with Healthy People 2010 and Healthy People 2020. Both Healthy People programs are leading the way to eliminate health disparities and attain years of healthy life. PTs' educational and practice guidelines emphasize health promotion, wellness, and disease prevention in schools' curricula and physical therapy practice. The Guide also stresses the importance of prevention and promoting health, wellness, and fitness for patients/clients. Physical therapy goals for the twenty-first century include preventing diabetes (and prediabetes), obesity, arthritis, stroke, and falls in older adults [2]. In addition, the goals incorporate the promotion of regular physical activity. Encouraging children and adults to adopt a healthy lifestyle using exercises and activities is crucial. It is well established that regular physical activity can enhance health and prevent disease [2]. One way to promote physical activity is for PTs to provide individualized assessments and exercise programs for patients/clients who are overweight and need to lose weight. PTAs can assist PTs in promoting a healthy lifestyle through physical activity.

## Wellness and Health Promotion

The concept of wellness is the patient's/client's capacity to be in good physical and emotional health and appreciate and enjoy high-quality health. This notion of wellness also means having a harmonious relationship between a patient's/client's internal and external environments. Health promotion is the science and art of helping patients/clients change their lifestyles and attain optimal health. Both wellness and health promotion can guide a patient/client toward a healthy lifestyle. In clinical practice, PTs can use patient education to increase a patient's/client's health awareness and ability to maintain good health. Examples of health promotion could be the PT's assessments of the following elements of a patient's/client's situation:

- Physical activity and exercise: Physical activity is any movement that requires energy expenditure and can include everything from daily tasks such as housework to gardening. Exercise refers to a planned, structured, and repetitive movement, including aerobics, strength training, and stretching.
- Behavioral health risks: Behavioral health risks refer to negative health outcomes from individual

behavior, such as substance abuse, physical inactivity, and poor nutrition, which can lead to physical and mental health problems, such as addiction, heart disease, diabetes, obesity, and depression.

- Sleep patterns: Adequate sleep is important for maintaining good health and well-being, as a lack of it may lead to various physical and mental health problems, such as decreased immune function, obesity, cardiovascular disease, depression, and cognitive impairment. PTs/PTAs can help by discussing strategies for good sleep hygiene, including the recommended amount of sleep by age, establishing a consistent sleep schedule, creating a sleep-conducive environment, avoiding stimulants such as caffeine and nicotine, and engaging in relaxing activities before bedtime.

- Level of physical fitness: Physical fitness has several components: cardiovascular endurance, muscular strength and endurance, flexibility, and body composition. Fitness needs vary with each individual's work and lifestyle, but maintaining a high level of physical fitness by engaging in regular physical activity and eating a balanced diet can improve overall health and reduce the risk of chronic diseases, such as heart disease, stroke, and diabetes.

- Psychological function: Psychological function refers to an individual's mental and emotional well-being, including their ability to cope with stress, form and maintain relationships, think and reason, and experience pleasure and happiness. Factors that can affect psychological function include genetic predisposition, life experiences, and behavior. Depression, anxiety, and schizophrenia can impair psychological function and require treatment. Stress management is the process of

identifying, understanding, and managing the factors that contribute to stress. Effective strategies for managing stress include regular physical activity, relaxation techniques, time management, a healthy, well-balanced diet, social support, sufficient sleep, hobbies and interests, and mindfulness.

- Nutrition advice: Although a specific diet prescription is not within the scope of physical therapy practice, PTs/PTAs must encourage patients to follow the national nutrition guidelines and refer patients to a dietitian when a specific diet might be indicated [3]. PTs/PTAs are also expected to provide suggestions to educate and support patients to eat healthily and manage their weight.

Many variables are involved in a patient's/client's wellness and health promotion, including the patient's/client's own health beliefs and values, personal expectations, and/or physical and social environments.

## Assessing Health and Wellness

There is increased recognition of the importance of the patient's perception of health and functional outcomes. Numerous tools are available to assess health and wellness (**Table 3-2**). At the basic level, health can be assessed by measuring blood pressure, body fat, cholesterol, and aerobic capacity. The number of cognitive factors involved makes wellness more difficult to determine.

Several biological, psychological, and social factors can influence how health and wellness are experienced, expressed, and interpreted. Disease-specific instruments determine the impact a disease/dysfunction has on the patient producing a higher degree of increased responsiveness. Examples of the primary focus of these instruments include symptoms (back

**Table 3-2  Health and Wellness Tools**

| | |
|---|---|
| International Classification of Functioning, Disability, and Health (ICF) | A standard framework using a biopsychosocial model with the following categories: body functions and structures, activity and participation restriction, environmental factors, and personal factors |
| Medical Outcomes Short Form Health Survey (SF-36) | A generic set of coherent and easily administered quality-of-life measures that relies upon the self-reporting of patients of all types |
| Patient-Specific Function Scale (PSFS) | A self-reported valid, reliable, and responsive outcome measure for patients with back, neck, knee, and upper extremity problems that allows goal setting and monitoring of progress at an individual level, making it more sensitive to change than conventional measures |
| Perceived Wellness Survey (PWS) | A 36-item measure designed to assess an individual's perceptions of their wellness through physical, spiritual, intellectual, psychological, social, and emotional dimensions |

pain), populations (rheumatoid arthritis), and function (ADLs) [4]. Complicating health and wellness assessments are maladaptive cognitions, which are illogical or incorrect beliefs related to the symptoms that produce behavioral changes (e.g., fear of pain, injury, physical activity, and movement).

### Changing Behaviors

Several theories have been proposed to explain why and how people adopt new behaviors and change existing behaviors. Understanding the underlying motivations and factors that influence behavior can help the PT/PTA assist a patient in developing effective strategies for behavior change. Some common theories include the following:

- Social cognitive theory: Suggests that personal, behavioral, and environmental factors influence behavior. For example, it is important to determine a patient's home and work environments when advising a patient on activities to avoid.
- The transtheoretical model (Stages of Change): Outlines the stages individuals go through as they move from precontemplation to action in changing a behavior. For example, a patient with low back pain may contemplate going to physical therapy before hearing about the advantages.
- The health belief model: Explains how an individual's beliefs about a specific behavior and its consequences and perceived barriers to change impact their behavior. For example, a patient may have read on the internet that chiropractic care is better than physical therapy care.
- Self-determination theory: Emphasizes the importance of psychological needs for autonomy, competence, and relatedness in motivating behavior change. For example, some patients benefit from receiving input and feedback when trying to master a particular task.
- Social influence theory: Suggests that the attitudes and behaviors of others, including family, friends, and media, shape behavior. The three areas of social influence are conformity, compliance, and obedience. For example, a patient may attend physical therapy because their uncle told them it would benefit them.

Much literature has conceptualized or reported poor motivation and slower progress in rehabilitation secondary to patient-related factors, including apathy, low self-efficacy (e.g., low confidence in one's ability to rehabilitate successfully), depression, cognitive impairment, fatigue, and personality factors [5]. Thus, motivation is critical to maintaining behavior and increasing compliance in a rehabilitation program. Several considerations should be made to increase compliance:

- The patient's age: Older individuals tend to adhere to exercise programs more than younger individuals.
- The patient's education: Individuals with high levels of education show more compliance to exercise programs than uneducated individuals [6].
- The patient's marital status: Singles tend to have lower adherence rates to physical activity/exercise than their married counterparts [6].
- The patient's gender: Males report greater total and vigorous activity levels than females.
- The patient's biomedical status: Poorer health tends to lead to decreased adherence [7].
- The patient's socioeconomic status: An individual's income bracket tends to influence the ability to access medical care, exercise equipment, and venues [8].
- The patient's ethnicity: Caucasians appear to participate in more physical activities than other racial or ethnic groups, regardless of age [6].

Several factors have been outlined to improve motivation and compliance, including:

- Involving the patient in intervention planning and goal setting
- Setting realistic and challenging short- and long-term goals
- Promoting high prospects regarding the outcome
- Promoting the benefits
- Projecting a positive attitude
- Providing clear instructions/demonstrations with appropriate feedback
- Pain-free or low-level pain exercises
- Encouraging patient problem-solving

## Disease Prevention

Disease prevention involves avoiding exposure to pathogens or reducing infection risk factors when exposure is unavoidable. Some common strategies for disease prevention in health care include:

- Vaccination: Getting immunized against specific diseases
- Hand hygiene: Washing hands frequently with soap and water can help to remove pathogens and prevent the spread of disease.
- Avoiding close contact with individuals who are ill or showing symptoms of a disease
- Maintaining a clean and healthy work environment

In physical therapy clinical practice, PTs can educate patients/clients to identify their risk factors and provide protective measures. Typically, the prevention of risk factors is implemented at three levels: primary, secondary, and tertiary.

- Primary: Primary prevention is the most cost-effective because it occurs before the onset of the disease/disorder. For example, in clinical settings, PTs/PTAs can provide primary prevention to patients/clients by educating patients about guarding against accidents while performing basic ADLs.
- Secondary: Secondary prevention refers to activities and measures taken to detect (e.g., screening) and treat a disease in its early stages to reduce the progression and severity of the disease, prevent complications, and improve outcomes.
- Tertiary: Tertiary prevention refers to activities and measures taken to manage and treat a disease's complications that have already been established to minimize its impact and improve the quality of life for affected individuals.

## Community Education

Health promotion can also include community education and providing educational programs for schools, colleges, businesses, industries, third-party payers, families, and caregivers. PTs/PTAs find that civic groups, wellness centers, senior citizen centers, and other community health groups welcome the addition of PTs and PTAs as educators. Physical therapy professionals may be able to offer education on topics such as disease awareness and prevention, fall prevention strategies, and chronic disease management. Many hospitals have implemented preoperative educational sessions for people receiving total joint arthroplasty to teach patients about the exercises and activities they will experience as part of their rehabilitation process. The opportunity to improve community health and promote physical therapy to assist in health and wellness efforts has become important for all physical therapy professionals.

Finally, PTs/PTAs may assume additional clinical and nonclinical roles, including consultation, research, education, and health facility administration.

# Clinical Trends in Physical Therapy

Several clinical trends in physical therapy are shaping the future of the profession. In addition to health and wellness and evidence-based practice, these trends include:

- Telehealth: Telehealth delivers healthcare services using technology, such as videoconferencing, to connect patients and providers remotely. This trend has become increasingly popular in physical therapy due to its convenience, accessibility, and cost-effectiveness.
- Personalized medicine: Personalized medicine involves tailoring treatment plans to an individual's unique needs, including their genetic makeup, lifestyle factors, and medical history. This trend is becoming more prevalent in physical therapy as new research emerges on the effectiveness of personalized treatment plans.
- Interprofessional collaboration: Interprofessional collaboration involves working with other healthcare professionals, such as physicians, nurses, and OTs, to provide comprehensive care to patients. This trend is becoming more prevalent in physical therapy as healthcare systems shift toward a team-based approach to care.
- Advanced technology: Advanced technology, such as virtual reality, wearable devices, and robotics, is being used to enhance the delivery of physical therapy services. This trend is expected to continue as new technology emerges and becomes more accessible to patients and providers.

## KNOWLEDGE CHECK

What are some topics that would address the goal of physical therapy in promoting wellness and disease prevention?

## Discussion Questions

1. Discuss the terminology related to physical therapy interventions in the Guide to Physical Therapist Practice.
2. List the five elements of patient/client management and identify components in which the PTA may participate.
3. Develop and share with the group a list of healthy lifestyle tips for a patient with a chronic health condition such as diabetes mellitus or heart disease.
4. Describe three recommendations for a patient to prevent falls at home.

## Learning Opportunities

1. Compare and contrast the different types of physical therapy settings.
2. Identify the impairment, functional limitation, and disability of a patient who has a rotator cuff tear pathology.
3. Write one policy and one procedure appropriate for a physical therapy department.

## References

1. American Physical Therapy Association: Guide to Physical Therapist Practice 4.0. Alexandria, VA, American Physical Therapy Association, 2023
2. Dreeben O: Patient Education in Rehabilitation. Sudbury, MA, Jones & Bartlett Learning, 2010
3. Bezner JR: Promoting health and wellness: implications for physical therapist practice. Phys Ther 95(10):1433–1444, 2015
4. Fisher C, Dvorak M: Orthopaedic Research: What an Orthopaedic Surgeon Needs to Know, in Orthopaedic Knowledge Update: Home Study Syllabus. Rosemont, IL, American Academy of Orthopaedic Surgeons, 2005, pp 3–13
5. Lenze EJ, Munin MC, Quear T, et al: The Pittsburgh Rehabilitation Participation Scale: reliability and validity of a clinician-rated measure of participation in acute rehabilitation. Arch Phys Med Rehabil 85(3):380–384, 2004
6. Keele-Smith R, Leon T: Evaluation of individually tailored interventions on exercise adherence. West J Nurs Res 25(6): 623–640, 2003; discussion 641–651
7. Boyette LW, Lloyd A, Boyette JE, et al: Personal characteristics that influence exercise behavior of older adults. J Rehabil Res Dev 39(1):95–103, 2002
8. Cohen B, Vittinghoff E, Whooley M: Association of socioeconomic status and exercise capacity in adults with coronary heart disease (from the Heart and Soul Study). Am J Cardiol 101(4):462–466, 2008

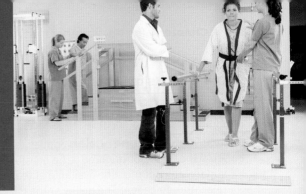

# The Physical Therapist Assistant as a Member of the Healthcare Team

## OBJECTIVES

- Describe the role of the physical therapist assistant in physical therapy.
- Discuss the supervisory role of the physical therapist in the healthcare team.
- Describe the differences in role, function, and supervisory relationships of the physical therapist, physical therapist assistant, and other healthcare personnel.
- List the events in the collaborative path between a physical therapist and a physical therapist assistant.
- Compare and contrast the types of healthcare teams.
- Identify the members of the rehabilitation team and their responsibilities.

## KEY TERMS

Commission on Accreditation in
   Physical Therapy Education
   (CAPTE)
direct personal supervision

direct supervision
general supervision
interprofessional team
intradisciplinary team

multidisciplinary team
occupational therapist
physical therapist assistant (PTA)
plan of care (POC)

## Overview

A **physical therapist assistant (PTA)** is part of a team directed and supervised by a physical therapist (PT) that works with patients of all ages who have difficulties performing everyday tasks and activities. The PTA helps to gather specific data (requested by the PT) and acknowledges the delegated tasks within the limits of their capabilities and any legal, jurisdictional, and ethical guidelines, including examination, evaluation, diagnosis, prognosis, interventions, and outcomes.

## Direction and Supervision of the PTA

The American Physical Therapy Association (APTA) defines a PTA as "a technically educated health care provider who assists the PT in the provision of physical therapy" [1]. The Association considers a PTA to be the only individual who assists the PT in delivering selected physical therapy interventions.

## Box 4-1 Levels of Supervision

The following levels of supervision are the minimum required for safe and effective PT services.

*General*: **General supervision** applies to the PTA. The PT is not required to be on-site for supervision but must be available at least by telecommunication. The ability of the PTA to provide services shall be assessed on an ongoing basis by the supervising PT.

*Direct*: Direct supervision applies to the supervision of the student PT and student PTA. When supervising a student PTA, the PT, or the PTA, is physically present and immediately available for supervision. In both cases, the PT or PTA will be in direct contact with the patient or client on each service date. Contact by telecommunication does not meet the requirement of this level of supervision.

*Direct personal*: **Direct personal supervision** applies to the supervision of a physical therapy aide. The PT, or where allowable by law the PTA, is physically present and immediately available to supervise tasks related to patient/client services. The PT maintains responsibility for patient/client management at all times.

Modified From American Physical Therapy Association: Levels of Supervision P06-19-13-45 [Internet]. [cited 2023 Jan 24]. Available from: https://www.apta.org/apta-and-you/leadership-and-governance/policies/levels-supervision

## Levels of Supervision

When a PTA provides care to a patient, the PT is responsible for the direction and supervision of that care. The APTA currently defines three levels of supervision (see **Box 4-1**).

State statutes and insurance provider requirements also dictate the requirements of supervision. For example, Medicare requires that PTAs who practice in private practice outpatient clinics have direct supervision when working with a Medicare beneficiary. Each state delineates what type of supervision is required and how frequently the PT is required to directly supervise the patient's care. This PT visit is defined by the number of physical therapy visits the patient has had or the number of calendar days. Some states also require this visit to be a co-treat of the PT and the PTA with the patient.

The PTA's performance must be safe and legal in all physical therapy practice settings. The decision by the PT to use a PTA depends on several variables, including the following [2]:

- The type of clinical practice: The type of clinical practice can determine the criticality, security, stability, and complexity of a patient/client. For example, a 14-year-old student-athlete with patellar tendinopathy presents a much more stable clinical picture than a 62-year-old with dementia in an intensive care unit.

- The environmental surroundings of the practice: The level of available medical staff to provide consultation and assistance varies significantly from an outpatient private practice setting to an acute care hospital.

- The type of communication between the PT and the PTA: Typically, the communication levels between a PT and the PTA take time to develop. Verbal communication tends to be more effective than written communication.

- The PTA's education, training, experience, and skill level: As with any occupation, education and training usually determine an individual's competency and skill level. However, if a PTA does not understand something or is being asked to do something they are not trained in or comfortable with, the PTA must feel comfortable raising these issues with the supervising PT.

- The patient's/client's needs: In an outpatient setting, a patient typically has a single diagnosis (e.g., rotator cuff tendinopathy), whereas in an acute care hospital setting, a patient may have multiple comorbidities and less functional ability.

- The needed frequency of reexaminations: Depending on the caseload, frequent reexaminations can be very time-consuming. In other settings, where the drive is to discharge patients as soon as is safely possible, reexaminations occur less frequently.

- The PT's expectations for the patient/client: If the status of a patient is not expected to fluctuate (e.g., a comatose patient requiring passive range of motion exercises), the PT is more likely to feel comfortable delegating patient care responsibilities to the PTA compared to a patient who has poor exercise tolerance and wildly fluctuating vital signs.

- The necessary modification(s) to the **plan of care (POC)**: Some patients require frequent modifications to the POC, so, in the interest of time, it is often more convenient for the PT to see them.

- The accessibility of the PT: The accessibility needs of the PT depend on the required level of supervision, which is a factor of third-party payer regulations and the state practice act.

- Federal and state statutes: A PT must understand their state's practice act delineations regarding services the PTA may not provide as some do not list any restrictions but leave the decision to the PT's judgment, while others are far more explicit. Furthermore, third-party payer regulations at the state or federal level may also influence the decision to use a PTA's services because, in many cases, third-party payers may pay less for their services than a PT.

- Liability and risk management concerns: The APTA delineates four specific interventions not to be performed by a PTA: spinal joint mobilization/manipulation, peripheral joint mobilization/manipulation, dry needling, and sharp debridement. While APTA policies do not have the force of state law, they are a second resource of legal authority, and although a PTA may understand the theoretical background or be trained in the necessary peripheral joint mobilization skills, they are not allowed to perform the required immediate reevaluation following such techniques as the reevaluation of a patient/client is the sole responsibility of the PT. *Note:* While it is not mandated as a minimum skill for PTA graduates, many PTA programs teach the basics of joint mobilization with the understanding that some clinical practice sites expect PTAs to perform these interventions. However, state physical therapy practice acts differ regarding the PTA's responsibilities and may prohibit or allow different skills, including joint mobilization.

## The Role of the PTA in a Clinical Setting

The PT conducts the practice of physical therapy. The PT remains the only individual responsible for the physical therapy services when the PTA provides selected interventions (treatments). The PT must direct and supervise PTAs and other personnel to provide quality physical therapy services. Many considerations are involved to ensure quality in physical therapy clinical settings. These considerations can directly affect clinical practice and may include the PT's and PTA's education, experience, responsibilities, and the organizational structure in which the physical therapy services are provided. The PT is directly responsible for the actions of the PTA regarding patient/client management [1]. The APTA Minimum Required Skills of the PTA Graduate at Entry Level describes specific skills that can be delegated to the PTA.

## APTA Minimum Required Skills of PTA Graduates at Entry Level [3]

A committee developed this document to list the required skills for a graduating PTA. This list includes skills considered essential for any PTA graduate, including musculoskeletal, neurologic, cardiovascular, pulmonary, and integumentary system care skills. The terms used in this list are based on the Guide to Physical Therapist Practice, and an asterisk (*) denotes a skill identified on the PTA (NPTE) Test Content Outline.

| PTA Skill Category | Description of Minimum Skills for PTA |
|---|---|
| POC Review<br>■ Review of physical therapy documents<br>■ Review of medical record<br>■ Identification of pertinent information<br>■ Identification of indications, contraindications, precautions, safety considerations, and expected outcomes<br>■ Access to related literature<br>■ Match patient goals to selected interventions<br>■ Identify their role in patient care<br>■ Identification of items to be communicated to the PT | 1. Read all physical therapy documentation, including initial examination and POC.<br>  A. Note indications, contraindications, precautions, and safety considerations for the patient.<br>  B. Note goals and expected outcomes.<br>  C. Seek clarification from the PT as needed.<br>2. Review the information in the medical record at each visit, including:<br>  A. Monitor the medical record for changes in medical status and/or medical procedures.<br>  B. Collect data on the patient's current condition, compare results to previously collected data and safety parameters established by the PT, and determine if the safety parameters have been met.<br>  C. Seek clarification from appropriate health team members for unfamiliar or ambiguous information.<br>3. Identify when the directed interventions are either beyond the scope of work or the personal scope of work of the PTA.<br>4. Communicate to the PT when there are significant changes in the patient's medical status, physician referral, or when the patient's criticality and complexity are beyond the PTA's knowledge, skills, and abilities.<br>5. Explain the rationale for selected interventions to achieve patient goals as identified in the POC. |

*(continues)*

## APTA Minimum Required Skills of PTA Graduates at Entry Level [3] *(continued)*

| PTA Skill Category | Description of Minimum Skills for PTA |
|---|---|
| Provision of Procedural Interventions<br><br>■ Compliance with policies, procedures, ethical standards, etc.<br>■ Risk management strategies<br>■ Protection of patient privacy, rights, and dignity<br>■ Competent provision of interventions, including:<br>  • Therapeutic exercise<br>  • Functional training<br>  • Manual therapy techniques<br>  • Application and adjustment of devices and equipment*<br>  • Airway clearance techniques<br>  • Integumentary repair and protection techniques<br>  • Electrotherapeutic modalities*<br>  • Physical agents and mechanical modalities*<br>■ Assessment of patient response<br>■ Clinical problem-solving<br>■ Ability to modify techniques | 1. Provide interventions compliant with federal and state licensing requirements, APTA standards documents (e.g., Guide for Conduct for the PTA, Code of Ethics—see Appendix D), and facility policies and procedures.<br>2. Ensure the safety of the patient and self throughout patient care.<br>  A. Identify the need for and take action when the safety of the patient or self may be at risk or is compromised.<br>  B. Utilize risk management strategies (e.g., universal precautions, body mechanics).<br>3. Ensure patient privacy, rights, and dignity.<br>  A. Follow Health Insurance Portability and Accountability Act (HIPAA) requirements and observe the Patient Bill of Rights.<br>  B. Position/drape to protect patient modesty.<br>4. Provide competent provision of physical therapy interventions, including:<br>*Therapeutic exercise*<br>  A. Aerobic capacity/endurance conditioning or reconditioning<br>    1. Increase workload over time.<br>    2. Movement efficiency and energy conservation training<br>    3. Walking/wheelchair propulsion programs<br>  B. Balance, coordination, and agility training<br>    1. Developmental activities training<br>    2. Neuromuscular education or reeducation<br>    3. Postural awareness training<br>    4. Standardized, programmatic, complementary exercise approaches (protocols)<br>    5. Task-specific performance training (e.g., transfer training, mobility exercises, functional reaching)<br>  C. Body mechanics and postural stabilization<br>    1. Body mechanics training<br>    2. Postural stabilization activities<br>    3. Postural awareness training<br>  D. Flexibility exercises<br>    1. Range of motion<br>    2. Stretching (e.g., passive, active, mechanical)<br>  E. Gait and locomotion training<br>    1. Developmental activities training<br>    2. Gait training (with and without devices)<br>    3. Standardized, programmatic, complementary exercise approaches<br>    4. Wheelchair propulsion and safety<br>  F. Neuromotor development training<br>    1. Developmental activities training<br>    2. Movement pattern training<br>    3. Neuromuscular education or reeducation<br>  G. Relaxation<br>    1. Breathing strategies (relative to the delivery of an intervention)<br>    2. Relaxation techniques (relative to the intervention delivery)<br>  H. Strength, power, and endurance training for head, neck, limb, trunk, and ventilatory muscles<br>    1. Active assistive, active, and resistive exercises, including concentric, dynamic/isotonic, eccentric, isometric, diaphragmatic breathing, and low-level plyometrics (e.g., kicking a ball, throwing a ball) |

| PTA Skill Category | Description of Minimum Skills for PTA |
| --- | --- |
| | *Functional training in self-care and home management*<br>I. Activities of daily living (ADL) training<br>   1. Bed mobility and transfer training<br>   2. Activity-specific performance training<br>J. Device and equipment use and training<br>   1. Assistive and adaptive device or equipment training during ADL<br>K. Injury prevention or reduction<br>   1. Injury prevention education during self-care and home management<br>   2. Injury prevention or reduction with the use of devices and equipment<br>   3. Safety awareness training during self-care and home management<br>*Manual therapy techniques*<br>L. Therapeutic massage<br>M. Soft tissue mobilization<br>N. Passive range of motion<br>*Application and adjustment of devices and equipment*<br>O. Adaptive devices<br>   1. Hospital beds<br>   2. Raised toilet seats<br>P. Assistive devices<br>   1. Canes<br>   2. Crutches<br>   3. Long-handled reachers<br>   4. Walkers<br>   5. Wheelchairs<br>Q. Orthotic and prosthetic devices<br>   1. Braces<br>R. Protective devices<br>   1. Braces<br>S. Supportive devices, such as:<br>   1. Compression garments<br>   2. Elastic wraps<br>   3. Soft neck collars<br>   4. Slings<br>   5. Supplemental oxygen<br>*Breathing strategies/oxygenation*<br>   6. Identify a patient in respiratory distress.<br>   7. Reposition the patient to improve respiratory function.<br>   8. Instruct patient in various breathing techniques (pursed lip breathing, paced breathing, etc.).<br>   9. Administration of prescribed oxygen during interventions<br>*Integumentary protection*<br>  10. Recognize interruptions in integumentary integrity.<br>  11. Repositioning<br>  12. Patient education<br>  13. Edema management<br>*Electrotherapeutic modalities, such as:*<br>  14. Electrotherapeutic delivery of medications<br>  15. Electrical muscle stimulation<br>  16. Electrical stimulation for tissue repair<br>  17. Functional electrical stimulation<br>  18. High-voltage pulsed current<br>  19. Neuromuscular electrical stimulation<br>  20. Transcutaneous electrical nerve stimulation<br>*Physical agents*<br>  21. Cryotherapy (e.g., cold pack, ice massage, vapocoolant spray, hydrotherapy) |

*(continues)*

## APTA Minimum Required Skills of PTA Graduates at Entry Level [3] *(continued)*

| PTA Skill Category | Description of Minimum Skills for PTA |
|---|---|
| | 22. Ultrasound<br>23. Thermotherapy (e.g., dry heat, hot packs, paraffin baths, hydrotherapy)<br>*Mechanical modalities*<br>24. Compression therapies<br>25. Mechanical motion devices<br>26. Traction devices<br>5. Determine a patient's response to the intervention:<br>  A. Interview a patient and accurately interpret verbal and nonverbal responses.<br>  B. Identify secondary effects or complications caused by the intervention.<br>  C. Determine the intervention outcome (positive or negative), including data collection and functional measures.<br>6. Use clinical problem-solving skills in patient care.<br>  A. Determine if a patient is safe and comfortable with the intervention, and if not, determine appropriate modifications.<br>  B. Compare the results of an intervention to previously collected data and determine if there is progress toward the expectations established by the PT or if the expectations have been met.<br>  C. Determine if modifications to the interventions are needed to improve patient response.<br>7. Modify interventions to improve patient response.<br>  A. Determine modifications that can be made to the intervention within the POC.<br>  B. Communicate with the PT when modifications are outside the scope of work or the personal scope of work of the PTA.<br>  C. Select and implement the modification.<br>  D. Determine patient outcomes from the modification. |
| Patient Instruction<br>▪ Application of principles of learning<br>▪ Use of a variety of teaching strategies<br>▪ Methods to enhance compliance<br>▪ Clarity in instructions<br>▪ Assessment of patient response | 1. Apply principles of learning using a variety of teaching strategies during patient instruction.<br>2. Provide clear instructions (e.g., verbal, visual).<br>3. Apply methods to enhance compliance (e.g., handouts, reporting forms).<br>4. Determine patient response/understanding of instruction. |
| Patient Progression<br>▪ Competent patient progression<br>▪ Communication of pertinent information<br>▪ Relationship of psychosocial factors to patient's progress<br>▪ Clinical problem-solving | 1. Implement competent patient progression.<br>  A. Identify the need to progress via data collection.<br>  B. Determine what progression can be made within the POC.<br>  C. Identify possible progressions that will continue to advance patient response.<br>  D. Select and implement the progression of the intervention.<br>  E. Determine the outcomes of the intervention.<br>2. Communicate pertinent information.<br>  A. Identify changes in patient response due to intervention.<br>  B. Describe adjustments to an intervention within the POC.<br>  C. Describe the response to a change in the intervention.<br>3. Recognize when other variables (psychological, social, cultural, etc.) affect the patient's progression with the intervention.<br>4. Determine if the patient is progressing toward goals in the POC. If not, determine if modifications to the intervention are required to improve patient response. |

| PTA Skill Category | Description of Minimum Skills for PTA |
|---|---|
| Data Collection<br><br>■ Competent data collection<br>■ Interview skills<br>■ Accurate and timely<br>■ Clinical problem-solving<br>■ Ability to modify techniques<br>■ Documentation and communication | 1. Provide accurate, reproducible, safe, valid, and timely collection and documentation of data to measure the patient's medical status and/or progress within the intervention as indicated in the following categories:<br>*Anthropometric characteristics*<br>  1. Measure body dimensions (e.g., height, weight, girth, limb length).<br>*Arousal, attention, and cognition*<br>  2. Determine the level of orientation to situation, time, place, and person.<br>  3. Determine the patient's ability to process commands.<br>  4. Determine the level of arousal (lethargic, alert, agitated).<br>  5. Test the patient's recall ability (e.g., short-term and long-term memory).<br>*Assistive and adaptive devices*<br>  6. Measure for assistive or adaptive devices and equipment.<br>  7. Determine components, alignments, and fit of devices and equipment.<br>  8. Determine the patient's safety while using the device.<br>  9. Monitor the patient's response to the use of the device.<br> 10. Check the patient's or caregiver's ability to care for devices and equipment (maintenance, adjustment, cleaning).<br>*Body mechanics*<br> 11. Determine the patient's ability to use proper body mechanics during functional activity.<br>*Environmental barriers, self-care, and home management*<br> 12. Identify potential safety barriers.<br> 13. Identify potential environmental barriers.<br> 14. Identify potential physical barriers.<br> 15. Determine the ability to safely perform bed mobility and transfers in self-care home management.<br>*Gait, locomotion, and balance*<br> 16. Determine the patient's safety while engaged in gait, locomotion, balance, and mobility.<br> 17. Measure the patient's progress with gait, locomotion, balance, and mobility, using standardized tests.<br> 18. Describe gait deviations and their effect on gait and locomotion.<br>*Integumentary integrity*<br> 19. Identify activities, positioning, and postures that may produce or relieve trauma to the skin.<br> 20. Identify devices and equipment that may produce or relieve trauma to the skin.<br> 21. Observe and describe skin characteristics (e.g., blistering, continuity of skin color, dermatitis, hair growth, mobility, nail growth, sensation, temperature, texture, and turgor).<br> 22. Observe and describe changes in skin integrity, such as the presence of a wound, blister, incision, and hematoma.<br> 23. Test for skin sensation and describe any absent or altered sensation.<br>*Muscle function*<br> 24. Perform manual muscle testing.<br> 25. Observe the presence or absence of muscle mass.<br> 26. Describe changes in muscle tone.<br>*Neuromotor function*<br> 27. Identify the presence or absence of developmental reflexes, associated reactions, or abnormal tone.<br> 28. Identify the performance of gross and fine motor skills.<br>*Orthotic and prosthetic devices and equipment*<br> 29. Check components and ensure alignment and fit of orthotic devices, braces, and/or splints.<br> 30. Determine the effectiveness of components (Is it working or not?), alignment, and fit of orthotic devices, braces, and splints during functional activities. |

*(continues)*

## APTA Minimum Required Skills of PTA Graduates at Entry Level [3]    *(continued)*

| PTA Skill Category | Description of Minimum Skills for PTA |
|---|---|
| | 31. Determine patient's/caregiver's ability to don/doff orthotic, device, brace, and/or splint. |
| | 32. Determine patient's/caregiver's ability to care for orthotic device, brace, and/or splint (e.g., maintenance, adjustments, and cleaning). |
| | *Pain* |
| | 33. Define the location and intensity of pain. |
| | *Posture* |
| | 34. Determine postural alignment and position (static and dynamic, symmetry, deviation from midline). |
| | *Range of motion* |
| | 35. Perform tests of joint active and passive movement, muscle length, soft tissue extensibility, tone, and flexibility (goniometry, tape measure). |
| | 36. Describe the functional range of motion. |
| | *Sensory response* |
| | 37. Perform tests of superficial sensation (coarse touch, light touch, cold, heat, pain, pressure, and/or vibration). |
| | 38. Check peripheral nerve integrity (sensation, strength). |
| | *Vital signs* |
| | 39. Monitor and determine cardiovascular function (e.g., peripheral pulses, blood pressure, heart rate). |
| | 40. Monitor and determine physiological responses to position change (e.g., orthostatic hypotension, skin color, blood pressure, and heart rate). |
| | 41. Monitor and determine the respiratory status (e.g., pulse oximetry, rate, rhythm, pattern). |
| | 2. Provide timely communication to the PT regarding findings of data collection techniques. |
| | 3. Recognize when intervention should not be provided or modified due to a change in patient status. |
| Documentation<br><br>■ Select relevant information.<br>■ Accuracy<br>■ Ability to adapt | 1. Document in writing/electronic entry in the patient care record using language that is accurate, complete, legible, timely, and consistent with institutional, legal, and billing requirements.<br>2. Use appropriate grammar, syntax, and punctuation in communication.<br>3. Use appropriate terminology and institutionally approved abbreviations.<br>4. Use an organized and logical framework to document care.<br>5. Identify and communicate with the PT when further documentation is required. |
| Safety, Cardiopulmonary Resuscitation (CPR), and Emergency Procedures<br><br>■ Safety<br>■ Initiate emergency response system.<br>■ CPR | 1. Ensure the safety of self and others while providing care in all situations.<br>2. Initiate and/or participate in emergency life support procedures (simulated or actual).<br>3. Initiate and/or participate in an emergency response system (simulated or actual).<br>4. Maintain competency in CPR.<br>5. Prepare and maintain a safe working environment for interventions (e.g., clear walkways, equipment checks). |
| Healthcare Literature | 1. Reads and understands the healthcare literature. |
| Education<br><br>■ Colleagues<br>■ Aides, volunteers, peers, coworkers<br>■ Students<br>■ Community | 1. Instruct other healthcare team members using established techniques, programs, and instructional materials commensurate with the learning characteristics of the audience.<br>2. Educate colleagues and other healthcare professionals about the PTA's role, responsibilities, academic preparation, and scope of work. |

| PTA Skill Category | Description of Minimum Skills for PTA |
|---|---|
| Resource Management<br>■ Human<br>■ Fiscal<br>■ Systems | 1. Follow legal and ethical requirements for the direction and supervision of other support personnel.<br>2. Select appropriate nonpatient care activities to be directed to support personnel.<br>3. Identify and eliminate obstacles to completing patient-related duties.<br>4. Demonstrate efficient time management.<br>5. Provide accurate and timely information for billing and reimbursement purposes.<br>6. Adhere to legal/ethical requirements, including billing.<br>7. Maintain and use physical therapy equipment effectively. |
| Behavioral Expectations<br>■ Accountability<br>■ Altruism<br>■ Compassion and caring<br>■ Cultural competence<br>■ Duty<br>■ Integrity<br>■ Social responsibility | *Accountability*<br>1. Adhere to federal and state legal practice standards and institutional regulations related to patient care and fiscal management.<br>2. Act consistently with the Standards of Ethical Conduct for the Physical Therapist Assistant and Guide for Conduct of the Physical Therapist Assistant.<br>3. Change behavior in response to understanding the consequences (positive and negative) of the PTA's actions.<br>*Altruism*<br>1. Place the patient's/client's needs above the PTA's self-interests.<br>*Compassion and caring*<br>1. Exhibit compassion, caring, and empathy in providing services to patients; promote active patient involvement in their care.<br>*Cultural competence*<br>1. Identify, respect, and act with consideration for the patient's differences, values, preferences, and expressed needs in all physical therapy activities.<br>*Duty*<br>1. Describe and respect the PT's and other team members' expertise, background, knowledge, and values.<br>2. Demonstrate reliability in meeting normal job responsibilities (e.g., attendance, punctuality, following directions).<br>3. Preserve the safety, security, privacy, and confidentiality of individuals.<br>4. Recognize and report when signs of abuse/neglect are present.<br>5. Actively promote physical therapy.<br>*Integrity*<br>1. Demonstrate integrity in all interactions.<br>2. Maintain professional relationships with all persons.<br>*Social responsibility*<br>1. Analyze work performance and behaviors and seek assistance for improvement as needed. |
| Communication | *Interpersonal communication*<br>1. Develop rapport with patients/clients and others to promote confidence.<br>2. Actively listen and display sensitivity to the needs of others.<br>3. Ask questions in a manner that elicits needed responses.<br>4. Modify communication to meet the audience's needs, demonstrating respect for the knowledge and experience of others.<br>5. Demonstrate congruence between verbal and nonverbal messages.<br>6. Recognize when communication with the PT is indicated.<br>7. Initiate and complete verbal and written communication with the PT on time.<br>8. Ensure ongoing communication with the PT for optimal patient care.<br>9. Recognize the role and participate appropriately in communicating patient status and progress within the healthcare team.<br>*Conflict management/negotiation*<br>1. Recognize the potential for conflict.<br>2. Implement strategies to prevent and/or resolve conflict.<br>3. Seek resources to resolve conflict when necessary. |

*(continues)*

**APTA Minimum Required Skills of PTA Graduates at Entry Level [3]** *(continued)*

| PTA Skill Category | Description of Minimum Skills for PTA |
| --- | --- |
| Promotion of Health, Wellness, and Prevention | 1. Demonstrate health-promoting behaviors.<br>2. Recognize opportunities to educate the public or patients about health, wellness, and prevention (e.g., benefits of exercise, prevention of falls) and communicate opportunities to the PT.<br>3. Educate the public or patients about health, wellness, and prevention (e.g., benefits of exercise, prevention of falls).<br>4. Recognize patient indicators of willingness to change health behaviors and communicate with the PT. |
| Career Development | 1. Engage in self-assessment.<br>2. Identify individual learning needs to enhance their role in the profession.<br>3. Identify and obtain resources to increase knowledge and skill.<br>4. Engage in learning activities (e.g., clinical experience, mentoring, skill development).<br>5. Incorporate new knowledge and skill into clinical performance. |

The PTA cannot evaluate, develop, or change the POC or the treatment plan and cannot write a discharge plan or a summary [2]. Furthermore, the APTA has a position that the PTA cannot perform joint mobilization/manipulation techniques and sharp debridement wound therapy because it requires evaluative skills during and after the intervention application. Some PTs allow PTAs with the appropriate knowledge and skills to perform these interventions.

### KNOWLEDGE CHECK

What are the levels of PTA supervision?
What are some of the tasks that a PTA may perform?

## The PT's Responsibilities in the Clinical Setting

The PT integrates the five elements of patient/client management to optimize patient/client outcome(s). These five elements are examination, evaluation, diagnosis, prognosis, and intervention. The PT's POC may involve having the PTA assist with selected interventions. The PT is responsible for directing and supervising the PTA consistent with the APTA's House of Delegates positions (Direction and Supervision of the Physical Therapist Assistant [American Physical Therapy Association: Direction and Supervision of the Physical Therapist Assistant [Internet]. [cited 2019 June]. Available from: http://www.apta.org/uploadedFiles/APTAorg/About_Us/Policies/Practice/DirectionSupervisionPTA.pdf]). All selected interventions are directed and supervised by the PT. Also, there should be ongoing communication regarding the patient's/client's care between the PT and the PTA.

Regardless of the setting where the services are provided while supervising the PTA, the APTA has established that the PT has the following responsibilities[1]:

- Referral interpretation
- Initial examination, evaluation, diagnosis, and prognosis
- Development or modification of a POC based on the initial examination and reexamination; the POC includes the physical therapy goals and outcomes.
- Determination of when the expertise and decision-making capability of the PTA require the PT to administer physical therapy interventions personally and when it may be appropriate to utilize the PTA. A PT must determine the most appropriate use of the PTA to provide safe, effective, and efficient physical therapy services.

---

- Reexamination of the patient/client considering the patient's/client's goals and revision of the POC
- Establishment of the discharge plan and documentation of discharge summary/status
- Oversight of all documentation for physical therapy services rendered to each patient/client

Ultimately, the PT remains responsible for the physical therapy services provided when the PT's POC involves the PTA assisting with selected interventions.

---

The APTA's recommendations for ongoing communication between the supervising PT and the PTA in off-site settings may include the following actions [2]:

- The supervising PT must be accessible by telecommunication to the PTA at all times while the PTA is treating patients/clients. This requirement is dependent on the jurisdiction of the clinical site. Some jurisdictions require general supervision, whereas others require direct, on-site supervision.
- There must be regularly scheduled and documented conferences between the supervising PT and the PTA regarding patients/clients. The needs of the patient/client and the needs of the PTA must determine the frequency of these conferences. In those situations in which a PTA is involved in the care of a patient/client, a supervisory visit by the PT will be made for the following reasons:
  - Upon the PTA's request for a patient's reexamination
  - When a change in the POC is needed
  - Before any planned discharge
  - In response to a change in the patient's/client's medical status
  - At least once a month, or at a higher frequency when established by the supervising PT, in accordance with the needs of the patient/client

  A supervisory visit should include an on-site reexamination of the patient/client, an on-site review of the POC with appropriate revision or termination, and an evaluation of the need and recommendation for using outside resources.

## The Collaboration Path Between the PT and the PTA

A collaborative path between the PT and the PTA allows appropriate communication and patient care. This collaborative path includes the following steps:

1. The PT performs the initial examination of the patient/client. During the examination, the PTA helps the PT by gathering specific data that the PT requested. The PTA accepts the delegated tasks within the limits of their capabilities and considers legal, jurisdictional, and ethical circumstances and principles. Although the PTA cannot perform the initial examination and evaluation, they may take notes and help gather some data as requested by the PT. Taking notes should not compromise the decision-making process of the PT, the integrity of the evaluation, or the establishment of the POC.

2. The PT performs the initial evaluation of the patient/client by comprehensively assessing all the initial examination results. The PT assesses the examination data to judge the data value. This judgment is called evaluating. The PTA is not involved in this process. The PTA does not interpret the results of the initial examination.

3. The PT establishes a diagnosis by organizing the examination data into defined clusters, syndromes, or categories to determine the prognosis, including the POC. The PTA is not involved in this process.

4. The PT determines the patient's/client's prognosis (level of optimal improvement) that may be obtained through specific interventions; the PT also decides the necessary amount of time, frequency, and types of interventions required to reach the patient's/client's optimal level. The PTA is not involved in this process.

5. The PT establishes the goals/outcomes to be accomplished by the POC and the plan for interventions. The PT creates a POC to use various physical therapy procedures and techniques to produce changes in the patient's/client's condition.

6. The PT performs the patient's/client's interventions, delegating selected patient/client interventions to the PTA.

7. The PTA performs the selected patient/client interventions as directed by the PT. There is established ongoing communication between the PT and the PTA.

8. The PTA may collect data during the patient's/client's interventions to record the patient's/client's progress or lack of progress since the initial examination and evaluation. The PTA may ask the PT for a reexamination. The PTA's utilization and understanding of problem-solving are integral to patient care.

9. The PT performs the reexamination and establishes new patient/client outcomes and POC.

10. The PT performs the patient's/client's new interventions. The PT delegates to the PTA selected new patient/client interventions.

11. The PTA performs new patient/client interventions as directed by the PT. There is, again, established, ongoing communication between the PT and the PTA.

12. The PT performs the discharge examination and evaluation of the patient/client when the outcomes are met. As with the initial examination, the PTA can gather examination data that the PT can utilize in the discharge evaluation.

The preferred collaborative relationship between the PT and the PTA is characterized by trust, mutual respect, and value and appreciation for individual and cultural differences. In this relationship, the PTA's role is to offer suggestions, provide feedback, carry out agreed-upon delegated activities, and freely express concerns to the PT about clinical issues or other difficulties. The PT and the PTA modify communication to treat patients effectively; collaborate as team members; ensure a continuum of care in all settings; and educate patients, families, caregivers, other healthcare providers, and payers. The mechanisms for effective communication and feedback between the PT and the PTA relating to patient/client care include:

- Discussion of the goals and expectations for the patient
- Frequent and open communication
- Information on response to patient care
- Recommendations for discharge planning
- Discussion of modifications of a POC established by the PT
- Recommendations from other disciplines
- Considerations of precautions, contraindications, or other special problems included in the interventions

The PT is the administrator and supervisor of the clinical services, and the PTA can assist with delegated clinical services or administrative tasks.

## Differences in Supervision Requirements for PTAs

PTs are licensed providers in all states, and PTAs are licensed or certified providers in most states. PTs and PTAs are governed by their state's specific physical therapy practice act, including specific supervision rules. Some states have more stringent standards of supervision than other states. The state-specific practice act dictates the number of assistive personnel (including PTAs) the PT can supervise. For example, in Arizona, one PT can supervise no more than three assistive personnel (PTAs, PT aides, or PT/PTA students), whereas in Kansas, they can supervise four PTAs, and in Iowa, only two PTAs. The majority of states limit the number of personnel a PT can supervise.

In addition, there are supervision requirements for PTAs that relate to the type of insurance that reimburses physical therapy services, such as Medicare, and the setting type, such as outpatient or inpatient departments, home health agencies (HHAs), private facilities, and others. For example, in certain settings (reimbursed by Medicare), such as HHAs, physical therapy services can be performed safely and effectively under the "general" supervision of a PT. This type of supervision means the PT need not always be present on the premises when the PTA is delivering physical therapy services. However, this Medicare rule for HHAs may be superseded by a specific state physical therapy practice act.

Another example of Medicare supervision for PTAs is the "direct" form of supervision, which takes place in the office of a PT in private practice. **Direct supervision** means that the supervising PT (who owns their physical therapy practice) must always be physically present in the office suite when physical therapy services are provided by PTAs (and other PTs). PTAs must consult the Medicare supervision requirements (at www.apta.org) and their state practice act for more information.

## PTA Practice Influences

| Individual State Practice Acts and Regulatory Standards | Payer Requirements | APTA Standards of Practice |
|---|---|---|
| Requirements for licensure or certification<br>Continuing education requirements<br>PTA's supervision rules<br>Prohibits specific tasks | Supervision requirements<br>Limitations on PTA's provision of care<br>Decrease in reimbursement rates | Ethical Practice Guidelines<br>Practice Position Statements |

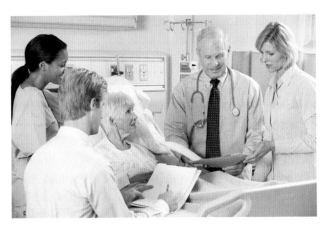

© Monkey Business Images/Shutterstock

# Clinical Decision-Making

Before the initial treatment session, the PTA must thoroughly review the PT's POC, determine the medical and physical therapy diagnosis, the structure(s) involved, the stage of healing, any comorbidities that could adversely impact the patient, and the short- and long-term goals documented by the PT. Before entering the patient's room, the PTA should have a plan for the introductions, what to say to the patient about what is planned for the session, and ensure that all necessary equipment is at hand.

At the beginning of every subsequent treatment session, the PTA must determine whether there has been any change in the patient's status from the prior session, which normally involves obtaining a patient's subjective report.

While carrying out a PT's directions during a treatment session, the PTA must continually monitor the patient/client so that any results from the data collection of impairments and outcomes can be documented or shared directly with the PT. A major part of this monitoring is ensuring the patient/client moves toward their established goals. The PTA should become proficient at recognizing patient changes that may occur during a patient care episode, as some changes should trigger immediate action. For example, changes in levels of consciousness, cognitive status, vital signs, or pain may indicate imminent danger to the patient. Certain conditions, such as myocardial infarction (heart attack), cerebrovascular attack (stroke), or respiratory distress, have their specific characteristic signs and symptoms. Other patient status changes warrant documentation and continued observation in subsequent visits. For example, a patient with patellar tendinopathy is experiencing increased pain and decreased motion following a home exercise program of lower extremity eccentric strengthening exercises. Changes in symptoms from one visit to the next may indicate a progressive nature of a condition or may necessitate a reevaluation by the PT. During the PTA program, students will learn about signs and symptoms of pathology, normal values of vital signs, expected responses to interventions, and possible complications that occur with different diagnoses. These combined concepts and understanding of risks will help the student develop the clinical reasoning necessary to work as a PTA. Perhaps one of the more difficult concepts for a PTA is determining when patients can advance their resisted exercises. For example, determining when a patient can transition from active to resisted exercise or from open-chain to closed-chain activities.

The APTA has developed a Decision-Making Algorithm that can assist the PTA in developing this skill. The Algorithm can be located in Appendix A.

# The Healthcare Team and the Rehabilitation Team

As healthcare professionals and providers, PTs and PTAs always work together with other professionals and providers. Typically, this collaborative effort between disciplines involves the healthcare and rehabilitation teams.

## Healthcare Team

A healthcare team is a group of equally important individuals with a common interest: collaborating to develop common goals and building trusting relationships to achieve these goals. Members of the healthcare team are the patient/client, family member(s), caregiver(s), various healthcare professionals involved in the patient's/client's care, and insurance companies. The patient/client, the patient's/client's family, and the caregiver(s) are extremely important in the team. Healthcare team members must be committed to the team's and the patient's goals to work effectively. They must address all the patient's medical needs. Team members must communicate effectively with each other, sharing a common language of care, respect, dedication, and teamwork. All members must also show leadership skills to effectively work together and help the patient/client in their care.

There are three types of healthcare teams: intradisciplinary, multidisciplinary, and interdisciplinary. **Intradisciplinary team** members work together within the same discipline. Other disciplines are not involved. An example of such a team is the PT and the PTA working in a home healthcare physical therapy practice when other services are unnecessary. Although the members collaborate effectively, this team is not the most efficient because only one discipline is involved, leaving the patient/client with only one type of care.

In a **multidisciplinary team**, members work separately and independently in their different disciplines. They do not meet or try to collaborate. The members' allegiance is mostly geared toward their particular discipline. Sometimes, competition between members may develop. An example of such a team may be different medical specialties trying to evaluate a patient for a specific pathology and having very little communication with each other. The lack of communication and cooperation between the multidisciplinary team members may cause problems for the patient/client. For example, the patient's/client's final diagnosis may be controversial because some team members have a competitive approach and limited consultation. This team approach is not the most effective; however, its success depends on the members of the team.

Unlike the first two teams, **interprofessional team** members work together within all disciplines to set goals relevant to a patient's/client's case. All the members collaborate in decision-making; however, the evaluations and interventions are done independently. An example of such an interprofessional team would be healthcare members working together in a skilled nursing facility. In such a facility, members from different disciplines meet, exchange information, and try to understand each other's discipline to help the patients. The outcomes and the goals are team directed and not bound to a specific discipline. This team is the most efficient and successful regarding patient outcomes.

## Rehabilitation Team

The rehabilitation team may include the PT, the PTA, the occupational therapist (OT), the certified occupational therapist assistant (COTA), the speech-language pathologist (SLP), the certified orthotist and prosthetist, the kinesiologist, the primary care physician (PCP; a medical doctor such as a physiatrist and/or a doctor of osteopathy or other specialty/physician who is concurrently treating the patient), the physician assistant (PA), the registered nurse (RN), the social worker, and the certified athletic trainer (ATC). It may also include the physical therapy aide, the physical therapy volunteer, the PT or the PTA student, and the home health aide.

### *Physical Therapy Director*

The rehabilitation team also includes the physical therapy director (who may also be called the physical therapy manager or supervisor). The physical therapy director may be an experienced PT or PTA (with knowledge and experience beyond entry level) who manages and supervises a physical therapy department. They are in charge of the department's functions, the responsibilities of all department members, and the relationships of all personnel in the department.

The physical therapy director has to ensure that the department's policies and procedures are applied efficiently and that the department's goals and strategic planning are set. The director also has clinical knowledge and skills plus abilities in administration, education, leadership, and other areas. They have the responsibility for the following:

- Motivate subordinates.
- Communicate effectively with supervisors.
- Impartially evaluate staff and give feedback.
- Educate all employees.
- Interview new personnel and help them develop skills.
- Delegate tasks to appropriate staff.

### *Physical Therapist*

As a rehabilitation team member, the PT clinician is a skilled healthcare professional with a postbaccalaureate degree (doctorate—Doctor in Physical Therapy). The APTA considers the attainment of a postbaccalaureate as the minimum professional education qualification for PTs who graduated from a **Commission on Accreditation in Physical Therapy Education (CAPTE)**-accredited program after 2003.

As of 2019, all PT postbaccalaureate degrees were from Doctor of Physical Therapy (DPT) programs. Per the APTA, the DPT is a postbaccalaureate degree conferred upon completing a doctoral-level professional (entry-level) or postprofessional education program. The transition to the regulatory designation of "DPT" was adopted by the 2014 House of Delegates. This transition will require changes in the practice acts of all states by the year 2025. After graduation and following a successful performance on the National Physical Therapy Examination (NPTE), every PT is licensed (or registered) by each state or jurisdiction where they practice. As a member of the rehabilitation team, the PT is responsible for the patient's/client's:

- Screening
- Evaluation
- Diagnosis
- Prognosis
- Intervention
- Education
- Prevention of injury and disease

- Coordination of care
- Referral to other providers

The PT also must prevent or decrease the patient's/client's impairments, functional limitations, and disabilities and achieve cost-effective clinical outcomes.

PTs also educate patients, clients, families of patients/clients, and caregivers on how to do the following:

- Use assistive and adaptive devices, such as crutches, prostheses, and wheelchairs.
- Perform home exercise programs.
- Help facilitate patient independence at home, work, and/or play.
- Prevent disease.
- Promote wellness and healthy behaviors.

According to the U.S. Bureau of Labor Statistics, "employment of physical therapists is expected to grow by 28 percent from 2016 to 2026, much faster than the average for all occupations" [2]. Over the long run, the demand for PTs should continue to rise as the increase in individuals with disabilities or limited function spurs demand for therapy services. The growing elderly population is particularly vulnerable to chronic and debilitating conditions that require therapeutic services. Also, the baby boomer generation is entering the prime age for heart attacks and strokes, increasing the demand for cardiac and physical rehabilitation. Young people will need physical therapy as technological advances save the lives of a larger proportion of newborns with severe congenital disabilities. Future medical developments also should permit more trauma victims to survive, creating additional demand for rehabilitative care. Employment growth in the physical therapy field may also result from advances in medical technology that would permit the treatment of more disabling conditions. In addition, widespread interest in health promotion should increase demand for physical therapy services. Many employers use PTs to evaluate worksites, develop exercise programs, and teach employees safe work habits to reduce injuries.

## *Physical Therapist Assistant*

The PTA is a technically educated healthcare provider who assists the PT in providing physical therapy. A PTA must graduate from a CAPTE-accredited PTA education program earning an associate degree from a technical or community college, college, or university. The PTA program is typically 2 years (five semesters) and includes classes in anatomy, physiology, exercise physiology, biomechanics, kinesiology, neuroscience, clinical pathology, behavioral sciences, communication, and ethics/values.

Following a successful performance on the National Physical Therapist Assistant Examination (NPTAE), administered by the Federation of State Boards of Physical Therapy, every PTA is licensed or certified by each state or jurisdiction where they practice.

As discussed earlier, the PT is directly responsible for the actions of the PTA related to patient/client management. The PTA may perform selected physical therapy interventions under the PT's direction or at least general supervision. The PT can determine the most appropriate use of the PTA to deliver services safely, effectively, and efficiently.

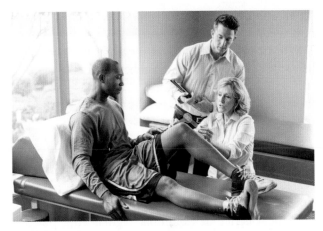

© kali9/E+/Getty Images

PTAs perform a variety of tasks. These treatment procedures, performed under the direction and supervision of PTs, include the following:

- Therapeutic exercises
- Therapeutic massages
- Therapeutic modalities such as electrical stimulation, paraffin baths, hot and cold packs, traction, and ultrasound
- Patient/caregiver/family education

PTAs also record the patient's responses to treatment and report the outcome of each treatment to the PT.

Most PTAs work in hospitals or privately owned physical therapy practices, while others work in home health, schools, and rehab units.

In addition to clinical practice, PTAs may work in PTA educational programs. They act as program directors, instructors, and clinical instructors (CIs). They provide students with an appropriate PT–PTA relationship role model.

According to the U.S. Bureau of Labor Statistics, employment of PTAs is expected to grow "by 24 percent from 2021 to 2031, much faster than the average for all occupations."[2] The reasons for growth are similar to those for PTs: the increase in individuals with disabilities or limited function, the growing elderly population vulnerable to chronic and debilitating conditions that require therapeutic services, and the large baby boomer generation in need of rehabilitation. In addition, future medical developments would also create demand for physical therapy services.

Throughout their careers, PTAs are guided in all aspects of their role by the *Standards of Ethical Conduct of the Physical Therapist Assistant* (Appendix E) and *Core Values for the Physical Therapist and Physical Therapist Assistant* (see Chapter 2).

## KNOWLEDGE CHECK

What components of care can only be performed by the PT?

What are the supervision requirements of the PT working with the PTA?

## Occupational Therapist

The licensed (or registered) **occupational therapist** (OTR/L) is a skilled healthcare professional having a doctorate or master's degree. All states, Puerto Rico, and the District of Columbia regulate the practice of occupational therapy; however, specific eligibility requirements for licensure vary by state. To obtain a license, applicants must graduate from an accredited educational program and pass a national certification examination. OTs who pass the exam are awarded the title occupational therapist registered (OTR) or occupational therapist licensed (OTL).

OTs help people improve their ability to perform tasks in their daily living and working environments. They work with individuals who have conditions that are mentally, physically, developmentally, or emotionally disabling. They also help these individuals to develop, recover, or maintain daily living and work skills. OTs help patients and clients improve their basic motor functions and reasoning abilities and compensate for permanent loss of function. OTs' areas of expertise include the following:

- Patient education and training in ADLs
- Development and fabrication of orthoses (splints)
- Training, recommendation, and selection of adaptive equipment (such as a long-arm shoehorn)

- Therapeutic activities for a patient's/client's functional, cognitive, or perceptual abilities
- Consultation in the adaptation of the environment for a physically challenged patient/client

OTs may work exclusively with individuals in a particular age group or with particular disabilities. In schools, for example, they evaluate children's abilities, recommend and provide therapy, modify classroom equipment, and help children participate in school programs and activities as fully as possible.

Most OTs work in acute hospitals, rehabilitation centers, and orthopedic settings.

Like physical therapy, "employment of occupational therapists is expected to increase by 14 percent from 2021 to 2031, much faster than the average for all occupations."[3] The baby boomer generation's movement into middle age and the growth in the population 75 years or older will increase the demand for occupational therapy services. Hospitals will continue to employ many OTs to provide therapy services to acutely ill inpatients. Hospitals also will need OTs to staff their outpatient rehabilitation programs. Employment growth in schools will result from expanding the school-age population and extending services for disabled students. OTs will be needed to help children with disabilities prepare to enter special education programs.

## Occupational Therapy Assistant

Occupational therapy assistants must complete an associate or bachelor's degree program from an accredited community college or technical school. Occupational therapy assistants are regulated in most states and must pass a national certification examination after they graduate. Those who pass the test are awarded the title of certified occupational therapist assistant. The COTA's duties do not include patient evaluation and establishing or revising a POC. The COTA's areas of practice are in a patient's/client's functional deficits of dressing, grooming, personal hygiene, and housekeeping.

The supervisory relationship of the OTR/L and the COTA follows similar guidelines to the supervisory relationship between the PT and the PTA.

## Speech-Language Pathologist

The SLP or speech therapist is a skilled healthcare professional with a master's degree in speech pathology

---

2 https://www.bls.gov/ooh/healthcare/physical-therapist-assistants-and-aides.htm
3 https://www.bls.gov/ooh/healthcare/occupational-therapists.htm

(including 9 months to 1 year of clinical experience). The SLP needs to pass a national examination to obtain the certification of clinical competence to practice speech and language pathology. The national examination on speech-language pathology is offered through the Praxis Series of the Educational Testing Service.

Medicaid, Medicare, and private health insurers require an SLP practitioner to be licensed to qualify for reimbursement. All states regulate SLPs through licensure or registration. SLPs can also acquire the Certificate of Clinical Competence in Speech-Language Pathology (CCC-SLP) offered by the American Speech-Language-Hearing Association.

SLPs assess, diagnose, treat, and help to prevent speech, language, cognitive, communication, voice, swallowing, fluency, and other related disorders. The SLP's general area of practice is to restore or improve communication of patients with language and speech impairments. In the rehabilitation team, the SLP works closely with the PT, PTA, OTR/L, and COTA to correct a patient's swallowing and cognitive deficits.

As per the U.S. Department of Labor office, "the employment of speech-language pathologists is expected to grow by 21 percent from 2021 to 2031, faster than the average for all occupations."[4] The reasons for this growth may be the baby boomer generation's problems associated with speech, language, swallowing, and hearing impairments and the high survival rate of premature infants and trauma and stroke victims, whose speech or language may need assessment and possible treatment. Many states now require that all newborns be screened for hearing loss and receive appropriate early intervention services. Employment of SLPs in educational services will increase along with growth in elementary and secondary school enrollments, including enrollment of special education students.

### KNOWLEDGE CHECK

What are the roles of OTs and COTAs?
How might the PT and PTA interact with the SLP on the healthcare team?

### Orthotist and Prosthetist

Both orthotists and prosthetists are important members of the rehabilitation team. They work closely with orthopedic surgeons, physicians from many disciplines, and physical and occupational therapy practitioners. As per the U.S. Department of Labor, "orthotists and prosthetists can fit and prepare orthopedic braces and prosthetic devices for patients/clients who have disabilities of limbs or spine" (including partial or total absence of the limb).[5] Regarding educational requirements, orthotists and prosthetists must complete an accredited master's degree program and a residency in prosthetics and orthotics. Certification as an orthotist or prosthetist is available through the American Board for Certification in Orthotics and Prosthetics. The certified orthotist designs, fabricates, and fits patients with orthoses prescribed by the physician. The orthoses can be braces, splints, cervical collars, and corsets. The certified prosthetist designs, fabricates, and fits prostheses for patients with partial or total limb loss(s). Prosthetists and orthotists are responsible for making any modifications and alignments of the prosthetic limbs and orthotic braces, evaluating the patient's progress, keeping accurate records on each patient, and teaching patients how to care for their prosthetic or orthotic devices. Prosthetists and orthotists work in private practice laboratories, hospitals, or government agencies.

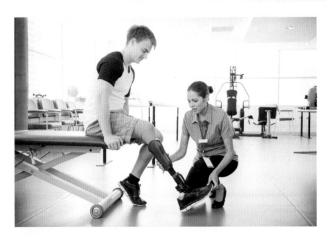

© JohnnyGreig/E+/Getty Images

### Kinesiologist

Kinesiologists are individuals who complete a bachelor's or master's degree in the study of human movement and try to improve the efficiency and performance of the human body in sports, at work, and during ADLs. Kinesiologists work closely with PTs and PTAs to help patients/clients in specific areas of exercise, biomechanics, psychomotor skills, and the workplace environment. Regarding exercise kinesiology, the kinesiologist will work with the PT to assess and monitor a patient's/client's response to exercises.

4  https://www.bls.gov/ooh/healthcare/speech-language-pathologists.htm
5  https://www.bls.gov/ooh/healthcare/orthotists-and-prosthetists.htm

## Primary Care Physician

The PCP is a medical doctor (MD) or an osteopathic doctor (DO). The PCP provides primary care services and manages routine healthcare needs. Although both MDs and DOs may use all accepted treatment methods, including drugs and surgery, DOs emphasize the body's musculoskeletal system, preventive medicine, and holistic patient care. DOs are more likely than MDs to be primary care specialists, although they can be found in all specialties. About half of the DOs practice general or family medicine, internal medicine, or pediatrics. The PCP acts as the "gatekeeper" for patients covered under managed healthcare systems (such as a health maintenance organization), authorizing referrals to other specialties or services, including physical therapy.

It takes many years of education and training to become an MD: 4 years of undergraduate school; 4 years of medical school; and between 3 and 8 years of internship and residency, depending on the specialty selected. A few medical schools offer combined undergraduate and medical school programs that last 6 years rather than the customary 8 years. The minimum educational requirement for entry into a medical school is 3 years of college; most applicants, however, have at least a bachelor's degree and many have advanced degrees. Following medical school, almost all MDs enter a residency. Residency is a graduate medical education in a specialty that takes the form of paid on-the-job training, usually in a hospital. Most DOs serve a 12-month rotating internship after graduation and before entering a residency, which may last 2–6 years, depending on the selected specialization.

All states, the District of Columbia, and U.S. territories license physicians. To be licensed, physicians must graduate from an accredited medical school, pass a licensing examination, and complete 1–7 years of graduate medical education.

The rehabilitation team has five distinct physician specialties that PTs and PTAs may interact with the most: family and general practitioners, physiatrists, orthopedic surgeons, neurologists, and pediatricians.

Family and general practitioners are often the first points of contact for people seeking health care, acting as the traditional family doctor. They assess and treat various conditions, ailments, and injuries, from sinus and respiratory infections to broken bones and scrapes. Family and general practitioners typically have a patient base of regular, long-term visitors. Patients with more serious conditions are referred to specialists or other healthcare facilities for more intensive care.

The physiatrist is a physician specializing in physical medicine and rehabilitation. Physiatrists see patients in all age groups and treat problems that touch upon all the major systems in the body. Physiatrists practice in rehabilitation centers, hospitals, and private offices. They often have broad practices, but some concentrate on one area, such as pediatrics, sports medicine, geriatric medicine, brain injury, or other special interests.

Orthopedic surgeons are highly trained physicians who diagnose, treat, give medical advice, and perform surgery on people with bone and joint disorders. Orthopedic surgeons have one of the longest training periods of all doctors.

Neurologists are physicians skilled in diagnosing and treating nervous system diseases, including the brain. These doctors do not perform surgery; however, neurologists often help determine whether a patient is a surgical candidate. They are known to employ various diagnostic tests, such as nerve conduction studies, and are often called upon to make cognitive assessments and offer medical advice.

Pediatricians are concerned with the health of infants, children, and teenagers. They specialize in diagnosing and treating various ailments specific to young people and track their patients' growth to adulthood. Most of the work of pediatricians involves treating day-to-day illnesses common to children, such as minor injuries, infectious diseases, and immunizations. Some pediatricians specialize in serious medical conditions and pediatric surgery, treating autoimmune disorders or serious chronic ailments.

## Physician Assistant

The PA is a skilled healthcare professional with a master's degree from an accredited program. The PA is required to have 1 year of direct patient contact and to pass a national certification examination. All states and the District of Columbia have legislation governing the qualifications or practice of PAs. All jurisdictions require PAs to pass the Physician Assistant National Certifying Examination, administered by the National Commission on Certification of Physician Assistants and open to accredited PA education program graduates. Only those completing the examination may use the credential "Physician Assistant—Certified."

The PA's responsibilities include therapeutic, preventive, and health maintenance services in settings where physicians practice. The PA works under the supervision and direction of a physician; however, PAs may be the principal care providers in rural or inner-city clinics where a physician may be present for only 1 or 2 days per week. In most states, the PA can prescribe medications and refer patients to medical and rehabilitation services, including physical therapy. The duties of PAs are determined by the supervising physician and by state law. Many PAs work in primary care specialties, such as general internal medicine, pediatrics, and family medicine.

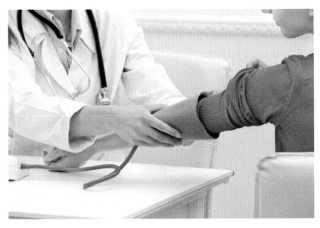

© Monkey Business Images/Shutterstock

### Registered Nurse

The RN is a skilled healthcare professional who has graduated from an accredited program and is licensed by a state board after completing a licensure examination. In all states and the District of Columbia, nursing students must graduate from an approved nursing program and pass a national licensing examination to obtain a nursing license. Nurses may be licensed in more than one state by examination, endorsing a license issued by another state, or through a multistate licensing agreement. All states require periodic renewal of licenses, which may involve continuing education. In the rehabilitation team, the RN is the primary liaison between the patient and the physician. The RN communicates changes in the patient's social and medical status to the physician, makes patient referrals (under the physician's direction) to other services, educates the patient and patient's family, and performs functional training such as ambulation or transfers with patients (after instruction from the PT or PTA). The RN also supervises other levels of nursing care, such as licensed practical nurses, certified nursing assistants, and home health aides.

Registered nursing has three major educational paths: a Bachelor of Science degree in nursing, an associate degree in nursing (ADN), and a diploma program. Most nursing educational programs offer degrees at the bachelor level that take about 4 years to complete. ADN programs, offered by community and junior colleges, take about 2–3 years to complete. Diploma programs, administered in hospitals, last about 3 years. Only a small and declining number of programs offer diplomas. Generally, licensed nursing graduates of any of the three educational programs qualify for entry-level positions as staff nurses. There are several types of nurses: hospital nurses, office nurses, nursing care facility nurses, home health nurses, public health nurses, occupational health nurses (also called industrial nurses), head nurses (or nurse supervisors), nurse practitioners (NPs), clinical nurse specialists, certified registered nurse anesthetists, and certified nurse-midwives. Hospital nurses form the largest group of nurses.

## Nurse Practitioners

An NP is an advanced practice registered nurse (APRN) who has completed additional education and training beyond that of an RN. NPs are licensed to practice medicine and prescribe medication in all 50 states in the United States. NPs provide a wide range of healthcare services, including:

- Conducting physical exams and medical histories
- Diagnosing and treating acute and chronic conditions
- Ordering and interpreting diagnostic tests
- Educating patients about their health and wellness
- Collaborating with physicians and other healthcare professionals
- Managing patients' overall healthcare needs

At the advanced level, NPs provide basic, primary health care. They diagnose and treat common acute illnesses and injuries. NPs also can prescribe medications. However, certification and licensing requirements vary by state. Other advanced practice nurses include clinical nurse specialists, certified registered nurse anesthetists, and certified nurse-midwives. Advanced practice nurses must meet educational and clinical practice requirements beyond the basic nursing education and licensing required of all RNs.

### Social Worker

Generally, a social worker needs a bachelor's degree in social work. Although a bachelor's degree is sufficient for entry into the field, a master's degree in social work (MSW) or a related field has become the standard for many positions. An MSW is typically required for positions in healthcare settings and clinical work. Some social work jobs in public and private agencies also may require an advanced degree, such as a master's degree in social services policy or administration.

All states and the District of Columbia have licensing certification or registration requirements regarding social work practice and the use of professional titles. Some health insurance providers require social workers to have credentials to be reimbursed for services.

Social workers help people function optimally in their environment, deal with relationships, and solve personal and family problems. Social workers often see clients who face a life-threatening disease or a social problem, such as inadequate housing, unemployment, serious illness, disability, or substance abuse. Social workers also assist families with serious domestic conflicts, including child or spousal abuse.

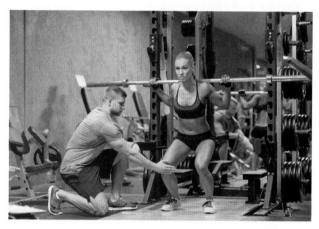

© Syda Productions/Shutterstock

## Certified Athletic Trainer

The ATC is a healthcare professional with a master's degree who works mainly with sports injuries. Athletic trainers can become certified by the National Athletic Trainers' Association Board of Certification (NATABOC). The certification examination administered by NATABOC consists of a written portion with multiple choice questions, an oral/practical section that evaluates the skill components of the domains within athletic training, and a written simulation test consisting of athletic training–related situations designed to approximate real-life decision-making. Athletic trainers can use the designation Certified Athletic Trainer when they pass the certification exam. Usually, the ATC works under the supervision of a physician, providing injury prevention and treatment and rehabilitation to a patient after an injury. The ATC also can work in colleges and universities, secondary schools, private or hospital-based rehabilitation clinics, and professional athletic associations.

## Physical Therapy Aide

The physical therapy aide is a nonlicensed worker who performs assigned tasks related to the operation of the physical therapy service. A physical therapy aide cannot perform tasks that require the PT's clinical decision-making or the PTA's clinical problem-solving. The aide can only function if they are directly and continuously supervised (on-site) by the PT or when permissible by law by the PTA. Direct personal supervision requires that the PT/PTA be physically present and immediately available to direct and supervise patient/client management tasks throughout the time these tasks are performed. The physical therapy aide, typically trained on the job, can perform routine tasks such as patient transportation, equipment cleaning and maintenance, and secretarial or housekeeping duties. The APTA opposes certification or credentialing of physical therapy aides and does not endorse or recognize certification programs for physical therapy aides.

## Physical Therapy Volunteer

The physical therapy volunteer is a community member interested in assisting physical therapy personnel with departmental activities. They may take telephone calls and messages, transport patients from their rooms to the rehabilitation department in acute care hospital settings, and file patients' charts. The volunteer cannot provide direct patient care.

## PT Student and PTA Student

PT and PTA students perform duties commensurate with their level of education. The PT or PTA CI facilitates clinical learning experiences, is responsible for all actions and duties of the PT or PTA student in the clinical setting, and directly instructs, supervises, and assesses students during their clinical learning experiences. The CI must cosign all student documentation. The PTA cannot be a CI for a PT student but can be a CI for a PTA student, although the PT retains responsibility for all services provided by the PTA student. Patients must be informed that they will be treated by a student and have the right to refuse treatment.

## Home Health Aide

The home health aide is a nonlicensed worker who provides personal care and home management services. Some home health aides are certified in their jurisdictions. The home health aide assists the patient in their home setting with bathing, grooming, light housework, shopping, and cooking. After receiving instruction and supervision from the PT or the PTA, the HHA may provide supervision or assistance to a patient performing a home exercise program.

### Community Healthcare Worker

A community healthcare worker is a healthcare-trained person who assists community individuals in accessing healthcare resources, educates on high-risk health concerns, monitors at-risk individuals, and facilitates communication between healthcare providers and patients. This relatively new healthcare team member can help bridge the service gap, recognize compromised situations before they become critical, and assist a community in effectively and efficiently using resources through proactive healthcare work.

## Discussion Questions

1. While working in a skilled nursing facility, the PTA has been asked to attend a care team meeting for a resident. Who will attend the meeting, and what role do they play on the team?

2. Utilizing Appendix A, review the Problem-Solving Algorithm utilized by PTAs in the Patient/Client Intervention document. Discuss the role of the PT and PTA in clinical care.

## Learning Opportunities

1. Utilizing the APTA webpage (www.apta.org), review the Value-Based Behaviors for the PTA. Locate the section PT/PTA Collaboration and create strategies to promote the PT/PTA relationship.

2. Interview a healthcare professional, such as a PT, OT, SLP, or social worker. Create a class presentation about this healthcare professional's function, role, and interactions.

3. Create a class presentation about who PTAs are and what they do.

## References

1. American Physical Therapy Association: A Normative Model of Physical Therapist Professional Education: Version 2007. Alexandria, VA, American Physical Therapy Association, 2007

2. American Physical Therapy Association: Direction and Supervision of the Physical Therapist Assistant, HOD P06-18-18-28-35. House of delegates standards, policies, positions, and guidelines. Alexandria, VA, APTA, 2020

3. American Physical Therapy Association: Minimum Required Skills of Physical Therapist Assistants at Entry-Level, BOD G11-08-09-18. Board of Directors, policies, positions, and guidelines. Alexandria, VA, APTA, 2012

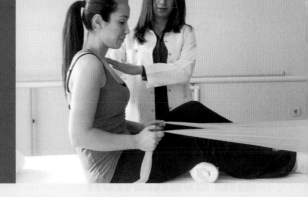

# CHAPTER 5

# Examination, Evaluation, Plan of Care, and Intervention

## OBJECTIVES

- Discuss the elements of a physical therapy examination.
- Compare and contrast examination and evaluation.
- Identify the elements of patient history.
- Compare the two types of pain scales used frequently in physical therapy practice.
- List the forms of data collected during the examination.
- Describe specialized examinations and interventions for the pediatric, geriatric, and women's health specialty practice areas.
- Describe the purpose and use of a plan of care.
- Discuss the therapeutic exercises used in physical therapy, including a home exercise program.
- Describe basic physical agents used in physical therapy.
- Discuss patient education.

## KEY TERMS

| | | |
|---|---|---|
| APGAR screening | evaluation | therapeutic exercises |
| cryotherapy | examination | thermotherapy |
| dementia | frequency | Visual Analog Scale (VAS) |
| duration | hydrotherapy | |

## Overview

Based on the patient/client management model outlined in Chapter 3, an episode of care within physical therapy follows a structured plan of care (POC). For example, physical therapy care always begins with the physical therapist (PT) making a physical therapy diagnosis. "A diagnosis is a label encompassing a cluster of signs and symptoms commonly associated with a disorder or syndrome or category of impairments in body structures and function, activity limitations, or participation restrictions."[1] The PT uses

---

1 https://www.apta.org/apta-and-you/leadership-and-governance/policies/diagnosis-by-physical-therapist

the examination and evaluation process to develop a physical therapy diagnosis and create an individualized patient care plan that includes intervention, prognosis, and expected outcomes.

# Examination and Evaluation

The PT performs the examination and evaluation. Specific data collection can be performed by the physical therapist assistant (PTA) at the request of the PT.

## What Is an Examination?

The **examination** involves obtaining a history, performing relevant systems reviews, and selecting and administering specific tests and measures. The specific examinations for the various body systems are described in Chapter 12.

## What Is an Evaluation?

An **evaluation** is a dynamic process in which the PT makes clinical judgments based on data gathered during the examination.

Creating a physical therapy diagnosis hinges on thoughtful consideration of all aspects of the patient's health and consideration toward possible medical concerns that warrant referral to another healthcare professional.

## Examination

The examination is a comprehensive process that must be carried out properly and systematically. The purpose of the examination is for the PT to fully understand the patient's problems from the patient's and clinician's perspectives. Initial information from a patient is often collected before the PT meets the patient for the first time. Initial information gathering includes reading the medical chart in the acute care setting or reviewing intake sheets given to the patient in an outpatient setting.

The patient history is a complete medical history of the patient's chief complaints, current complaints, allergies, current medications, lifestyle and habits, social history, vocational and economic history, and family history. During the history, the PT develops a rapport with the patient while gathering clues about their condition. Depending on the clinician's experience, the patient interview can provide enough information to list

possible differential diagnoses—an estimated 80% of the information needed to explain the presenting problem can be provided by a thorough history [1]. The information gathered during this section is noted in the "S" portion of the SOAP note (see Chapter 10).

PTs often customize the data they collect based on the patient's referral diagnosis or area of concern while considering the patient as a whole and complex being. For example, a patient with a cervical sprain may need a musculoskeletal and neurologic examination, and a patient with a nerve entrapment of the upper extremity patient should be examined for biomechanical and orthopedic concerns. The data obtained will include the following:

- Medical diagnosis and any precautions related to physical therapy
- Patient's chief complaint, including the patient's description of their condition and the reason for seeking assistance; identification of the patient's primary problem
- Patient's present problem, including the symptoms associated with the patient's primary problem, such as the location of the problem (drawing the location on a body chart), severity, nature (such as aching, burning, or tingling), persistence (constant versus intermittent), and aggravated by activity versus relieved by rest
- The onset of the patient's primary problem, including mechanism of injury (if traumatic), sequence and progression of symptoms, date of the initial onset and status up to the current visit, prior treatments and results, and associated disability
- Patient's history, including prior episodes of the same problem; prior treatments and responses; other affected areas (or body parts); familial, developmental, and congenital disorders; general health status; medications; and X-rays or other pertinent tests
- Personal information, including the patient's age, gender, and occupation
- Patient's lifestyle, including profession or occupation, assistance from family or friends, occupational and family demands (spouse, children, job expectations), activities of daily living (ADLs), any hobbies or sports, and patient's concept of the impact of functional (including cosmetic) and socioeconomic factors

### Symptom Description

Symptom description is part of the patient's history and includes the location, extension or radiation, intensity, duration, onset, frequency, progression of the symptoms, aggravating or relieving factors, and previous test results. Any symptom description measurements should be taken before and after treatment to assess the patient's response to physical therapy interventions on the symptoms. These treatments may include physical modalities and agents, relaxation training, and patient education for behavioral modification (such as reinforcing proper body mechanics during ADLs). Pain is the most common symptom for which patients seek help. Two major pain measurements are used in physical therapy:

- The **Visual Analog Scale (VAS)** consists of a 10-cm unmarked line, either vertical or horizontal, with verbal or pictorial anchors indicating a continuum from no pain at one end to severe pain at the other. The patient is asked to mark on the line the pain they are experiencing (e.g., How bad is your pain?). This mark is then measured with a ruler and expressed in centimeters, with 10 cm representing severe pain.
- The Numerical Rating System (NRS) is easier to use than the VAS. The NRS uses a range of numbers (e.g., 0–5, 0–10) to reflect increasing degrees of pain. The patient is asked, "If zero is no pain and 10 is the worst pain imaginable, how would you rate your pain?"

Several social, biological, and psychological factors can influence how pain is experienced, interpreted, and expressed. Thus, it is common to find emotional overtones in the presence of pain, which likely result from an inhibition of the pain-control mechanisms of the central nervous system (CNS) from such causes as the side effects of medications, grief, or fear of re-injury. Nociplastic pain (called central sensitization) is the semantic term used to describe augmented CNS pain, maladaptive sensory processing, and altered pain modulation. In patients with nociplastic pain, increased activity is present in the brain areas involved in acute pain sensations and emotional representations, which can result in heightened pain levels in chronic conditions [2–5]. With these patients, it becomes more important to draw their attention away from a structural bias and help them become more aware of the biopsychosocial components involved in the pain experience [6]. A patient-reported questionnaire, the OSPRO-YF 10-Item Assessment Tool (Optimal Screening for Prediction of Referral and Outcome), is designed to estimate the multiple dimensions of psychological distress that adversely influence how people respond to musculoskeletal pain [7, 8]. OSPRO efficiently identifies yellow flags (e.g., negative mood, negative pain-coping).

## Systems Review

The systems review is a limited examination that provides additional information about the patient's general health and the continuum of patient/client care throughout their life span. The purpose of the systems review is to:

- Help determine the anatomic and physiologic status of all systems (musculoskeletal, neurologic, cardiovascular, pulmonary, integumentary, gastrointestinal, genitourinary, and genitoreproductive)
- Provide information about communication skills, affect, cognition, language abilities, education needs, and learning style of the patient
- Narrow the focus of subsequent tests and measures
- Define areas that may cause complications or indicate a need for precautions during the examination and intervention processes
- Screen for physical, sexual, and psychological abuse
- Determine the need for further physical therapy services based on an evaluation of the information obtained
- Identify problems that require consultation with, or referral to, another healthcare provider

## Tests and Measures

The tests and measures portion of the examination involves a physical examination of the patient and provides the PT with objective data to accurately determine the accuracy of the hypothesis and the degree of specific function and dysfunction [9]. Objective data collection is an important examination function to create a clear picture of the patient's problems. The type and number of the tests and measures used are modified based on the history and the systems review (see Chapter 12).

### KNOWLEDGE CHECK

Where does the physical therapist obtain information for the examination?
What is the difference between an examination and an evaluation?

### *Environmental Examination*

The environmental examination is done at the patient's home or the institution where the patient lives. For example, the institutional environmental examination checks the patient's room for clutter or unsafe furniture, whether the lighting is bright enough for reading, and dangerous areas such as bathtubs that need skid-proof surfaces [10]. The environmental examination also checks the outside environment for steps that must be clearly marked, walkways in good repair, or adequate lighting in all public areas [10]. The home examination checks the exterior and interior of the home, including the kitchen, the bathroom, and the bedroom [10].

# Plan of Care

After the PT completes the examination and evaluation, the POC can be developed. The PT develops a problem list from the evaluation (impairments, activity limitations, and participation restrictions) and identifies the diagnosis, prognosis, and interventions to help improve the problem (see **Table 5-1**). In addition, short- and/or long-term functional goals oriented to function and time-sensitivity are written using the SMART (specific, measurable, achievable, relevant, and time-bound) format to identify the

proposed outcome for the patient's episode of physical therapy care.

## PTA Role in the POC

The PTA uses the evaluation, POC, and clinical judgment to determine what to do with the patient for each physical therapy session. Communication with the patient about changes in their functional status, pain levels, visits to the physician, and perception of the previous interventions will assist the PTA in making appropriate decisions about the current visit. The PTA's decisions must ensure that safety is maintained throughout the intervention and that the correct interventions are utilized within the framework of the POC. Many plans of care are not precisely detailed about modality parameters, requiring the PTA to utilize their knowledge of each modality's indication, contraindications, precautions, and appropriate parameter settings to determine the correct intervention for the patient. The PTA will monitor the patient's response, modify as necessary based on the patient's response, and document the treatment outcomes and progress toward patient goals and outcomes. Communication with the supervising PT about choices made, responses to interventions, and the need for consultation is critical to patient care.

---

**Box 5-1 Medicare Requirements**

As a requirement of Medicare, the federal insurance plan for Americans older than 65 years of age, the plan of care must also include the physical therapy diagnosis; the type of therapy to be provided; the potential of the patient to reach the functional goals; and the intensity, frequency, and duration of the plan of care.

---

**KNOWLEDGE CHECK**

What will a plan of care include?
How will a PTA use a plan of care?

---

**Table 5-1** Plan of Care

| **Patient:** John Smith | **Date:** July 5, 2019 |
|---|---|

**Dx:** R Total Knee Arthroplasty June 20, 2019

| **Current Functional Limitation:** | **Goal:** | **Interventions** |
|---|---|---|
| The patient cannot ascend or descend stairs independently without safety concerns due to weakness, decreased ROM, and ineffective motor control. | The patient will be able to ascend and descend seven steps independently with a railing to allow them to enter and exit their home safely in 3 weeks. | Therapeutic exercises emphasizing strength and flexibility. Neuromuscular control activities to improve motor control. Therapeutic activities to improve functional mobility and safety. |

| **Duration and Frequency:** | **Discharge Plan:** | |
|---|---|---|
| Two times per week for 3 weeks | The patient will be discharged from physical therapy when they have met their goals, it has been determined that they have plateaued, or they desire to discontinue physical therapy services. | |

ROM, range of motion

# Interventions

Interventions in physical therapy may include therapeutic exercises; patient/client education; biophysical agents; thermotherapy and cryotherapy; gait training; manual therapy; the use of orthotics and prosthetics, balance and coordination activities; functional training; neurologic techniques and specialized techniques in aquatics, cardiovascular and pulmonary rehabilitation, and integumentary care (see Chapter 12).

## Therapeutic Exercise

Therapeutic exercise is the most commonly used treatment used by PTs/PTAs, especially in musculoskeletal physical therapy practice [11].

### What Are Therapeutic Exercises?

**Therapeutic exercises** use muscular contractions, movement, posture, and physical activities to improve an individual's overall function and help meet the demands of daily living.

Depending on the patient's needs, therapeutic exercises or activities can achieve different goals, such as increasing muscular strength and endurance, maintaining flexibility, improving cardiopulmonary function, or promoting functionality. Therapeutic exercises incorporate a variety of activities, actions, and techniques. Therapeutic exercise programs are designed by PTs and are individualized to each patient/client's specific needs (see **Figure 5-1**).

### *Exercise Parameters*

The PT and PTA establish exercise parameters appropriate for each patient. The parameters include frequency, duration, repetitions, sets, intensity (or difficulty of the exercise), and the mode or type of activity or exercise. The **frequency** of exercise refers to how often the exercise is performed. The HEP

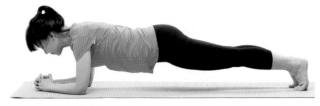

**Figure 5-1** Patient exercising to improve trunk strength and flexibility.

© rukxstockphoto/Shutterstock

An example of a home exercise program (HEP) for a patient who had a right total hip replacement 1 week ago could be:

### Exercise 1: Ankle Pumps

Slowly push your foot up and down. Do this exercise several times a day for 5 or 10 minutes.

### Exercise 2: Heel Slides

Slide your right heel toward your buttocks, bending your right knee and keeping your heel on the bed. Do not let your knee roll inward. Repeat this exercise 10 times three times a day.

### Exercise 3: Quadriceps Sets

Lying on the bed with your right leg straight and your left leg bent, press the back of your right knee into the bed (or into a rolled towel as we do in the clinic) by tightening the muscles on the top of your thigh. Count out loud to 10 while holding this position. Relax for 1 minute. Repeat this exercise five times twice a day.

Your HEP is an important part of getting better and stronger. Please do these exercises every day. Perform the exercises slowly. Stop the exercises immediately and call our office if you have any pain. Do not *increase the number* of repetitions or sets without checking with the PT or the PTA.

example instructed the patient to perform ankle pumps several times daily. **Duration** of exercise represents the length of time to perform the exercise. In the HEP example, the patient was instructed to perform the exercises daily, which means the patient was instructed to do the exercises simultaneously with physical therapy treatments as a supplement to physical therapy sessions. Repetitions and sets of exercises refer to how many exercises need to be performed and how many sets.

Classification of therapeutic exercises:
- ROM exercises to preserve flexibility and mobility of joints
- Exercises to increase strength
- Exercises to increase endurance
- Cardiopulmonary fitness exercises
- Exercises to increase coordination and control
- Exercises to increase speed
- Exercises to promote relaxation

## Patient Education

Patient education is an important intervention in physical therapy practice (see Chapter 8). The PTA should utilize a positive approach toward the patient while communicating clearly and simply.

Patient education aims to create independence, not dependence, and to foster an atmosphere of learning in the clinic. A detailed explanation should be given to the patient in a language they can understand. This explanation should include the following:

- *The name of the structure(s) involved and the cause of the problem:* Whenever possible, an illustration or model of the involved structure should be shown to the patient. The patient should be advised about the type of pain or symptoms to expect and how to manage those. Pain is, unfortunately, a necessary component of the healing process; however, the patient needs to be educated about what constitutes healing pain compared to harmful pain (an increase in pain lasting more than 2–4 hours).
- *Information about the planned interventions and the PT's prognosis for the problem:* An estimation of the healing time is useful for the patient so they do not become frustrated at a perceived lack of progress.
- *What the patient can and cannot do:* This includes the allowed use of the joint or area, a brief description of the relevant stage of healing, and the vulnerability of the various structures during the pertinent healing phase. This information makes the patient aware and more cautious when performing ADLs, recreational activities, and the HEP. Emphasis should be placed on dispelling the myth of "no pain, no gain." Instead, patients should be encouraged to respect pain. Also, patients often have misconceptions about when to use heat and ice, and it is the clinician's role to clarify such issues. Finally, education must begin about how to avoid any recurrences of the condition where applicable.
- *HEP (see later)*

## Physical Agents and Modalities

Another type of physical therapy intervention is the application of physical agents and modalities (biophysical agents) (**Table 5-2**). Physical agents and modalities use physical energy for their therapeutic effect. However, many physical agents and mechanical modalities used in physical therapy remain unproven to result in beneficial alterations in tissue physiology, except for cryotherapy and thermotherapy. However, the absence of evidence does not always mean that there is evidence of absence (of effect), and there is always the risk of rejecting valid therapeutic approaches [12].

### *Hydrotherapy*

As its name suggests, **hydrotherapy** uses warm or cold water by submerging all or part of the body and can include several types of equipment and various temperatures depending on the desired goal (**Table 5-3**).

The use of physical agents and mechanical modalities is determined by the goals of the intervention (**Tables 5-4** and **5-5**). If modalities have a role in the clinic, it is during the acute phase of healing when there is little else the clinician can do. In the remodeling or functional phase, various agents and modalities may promote blood flow to the healing tissues and prepare the tissues for exercise or manual techniques. Many texts describe all aspects of the various physical agents and electrotherapeutic/mechanical modalities.

Because of the passive nature of most physical agents or modalities, they are not prescribed by the PT indiscriminately and are given for only a short period as an adjunct, not as a substitute, to active interventions, such as therapeutic exercises and patient education (see **Figure 5-2**).

---

Why are physical agents and modalities used?
- To reduce or eliminate soft-tissue inflammation
- To speed the healing time of a soft-tissue injury
- To decrease pain
- To modify muscle tone
- To remodel scar tissue
- To increase connective tissue extensibility and length

---

## Manual Therapy

Several manual techniques are often used in orthopedic physical therapy, including soft tissue techniques, dry needling, neural mobilization, and various grades of joint mobilization (see Chapter 12).

## Motor Control and Motor Learning

In neuromuscular physical therapy, there are specific treatments to improve a patient's motor control and motor learning (see Chapter 12) (see **Figure 5-3**) [13, 14]:

- Motor control: The CNS's ability to control or direct the neuromotor system in purposeful movement and postural adjustment
- Motor learning: The acquisition of skilled movement based on previous experience

## Cardiovascular and Pulmonary Interventions

Cardiac rehab starts in the hospital and extends indefinitely into the maintenance phase (see **Figure 5-4**).

**Table 5-2** Physical Therapy Modalities

| Modality | Description |
|---|---|
| Cold/ice packs (**cryotherapy**) | Typically used in the acute stage of healing and the early subacute stage of healing. However, it can also be used at the end of a treatment session to help calm down any exacerbation of symptoms that were provoked during the session. |
| Hot packs (**thermotherapy**) | Thermotherapy is used in the later stages of healing because the deep heating of structures during the acute inflammatory stage may destroy collagen fibers and accelerate the inflammatory process. However, increased blood flow to the injured area is beneficial in the later stages of healing. |
| Paraffin (thermotherapy) | Thermostatically controlled melted wax using a paraffin bath unit to provide superficial heat to stiff or painful joints and for arthritis of the hands and feet because, by its very nature, the liquid wax can conform to all of the irregularly contoured areas found in these areas. |
| Fluidotherapy (thermotherapy) | Fluidotherapy consists of a container that provides dry heat by circulating warm air and small cellulose particles at varying degrees of agitation based on patient comfort. |
| Ultrasound (**Figure 5-2**) | Ultrasound can deliver thermal or nonthermal energy to either superficial or deep musculoskeletal tissues depending on the settings. Ultrasonic waves are delivered through a transducer with a metal faceplate and a piezoelectric crystal that vibrates rapidly, converting electrical energy into acoustic energy. |
| Electrical Stimulation | There are several types of electrical stimulation, including: Transcutaneous Electrical Nerve Stimulation (TENS): TENS is a type of electrical stimulation that uses low-frequency electrical currents to reduce pain by stimulating the nerves in the affected area. It is commonly used for musculoskeletal pain, arthritis, and neuropathic pain. Neuromuscular Electrical Stimulation (NMES): NMES is a type of electrical stimulation that uses high-frequency electrical currents to stimulate muscles. It is commonly used to help patients with muscle weakness or paralysis regain muscle strength and function. Functional Electrical Stimulation (FES): FES is a type of electrical stimulation that uses electrical currents to stimulate nerves that control muscle movements. It is commonly used to help patients with spinal cord injuries or other neurological conditions regain movement and function. Electrical Muscle Stimulation (EMS): EMS is a type of electrical stimulation that uses electrical currents to stimulate muscles. It is commonly used for muscle rehabilitation, strengthening, and relaxation. |

**Table 5-3** Clinical Applications of Whirlpool Treatment According to Temperature Ranges

| Temperature | Degrees | Use |
|---|---|---|
| Very hot | 104–110°F (40–43.5°C) | Used for a short exposure of 7–10 minutes to increase superficial structure temperature |
| Hot | 99–104°F (37–40°C) | Used to increase superficial structure temperature |
| Warm | 96–99°F (35.5–37°C) | Used to increase superficial temperature where prolonged exposure is wanted, so as to decrease spasticity of a muscle in conjunction with passive exercise |
| Neutral | 92–96°F (33.5–35.5°C) | Used with patients who have an unstable core body temperature |
| Tepid | 80–92°F (27–33.5°C) | It may be used in conjunction with less vigorous exercise |
| Cool | 67–80°F (19–27°C) | It may be used in conjunction with vigorous exercise |
| Cold | 55–67°F (13–19°C) | Used for longer exposure of 10–15 minutes to decrease the superficial temperature |
| Very cold | 32–55°F (0–13°C) | Used for short exposures of 1–5 minutes to decrease the superficial temperature |

## Table 5-4 Electrotherapeutic and Thermal Modalities

| Modality | Physiologic Responses |
|---|---|
| Cryotherapy (cold packs, ice) | Decreased blood flow (vasoconstriction)<br>Analgesia<br>Reduced inflammation<br>Reduced muscle guarding/spasm |
| Thermotherapy (hot packs, whirlpool, paraffin wax) | Increased blood flow (vasodilation)<br>Analgesia<br>Reduced muscle guarding/spasm<br>Increased metabolic activity |
| Ultrasound | Increased connective tissue extensibility<br>Deep heat<br>Increased circulation<br>Reduced inflammation (pulsed)<br>Reduced muscle spasm |
| Electrical stimulating currents: high voltage | Pain modulation<br>Muscle re-education<br>Muscle pumping contractions (retard atrophy)<br>Fracture and wound healing |
| Electrical stimulating currents: low voltage | Wound healing<br>Fracture healing |
| Electrical stimulating currents: interferential | Pain modulation<br>Muscle reeducation<br>Muscle pumping contractions<br>Fracture healing |
| Electrical stimulating currents: Russian | Muscle strengthening |
| Electrical stimulating currents: Microelectrical nerve stimulation (MENS) | Fracture healing<br>Wound healing |

## Table 5-5 Clinical Decision-Making on the Use of Various Therapeutic Modalities During Various Stages of Healing

| Clinical Presentation | Possible Modalities Used | Examples and Parameters (Where Applicable) |
|---|---|---|
| Acute: Erythema (rubor), swelling (tumor), elevated tissue temperature (calor), and pain (dolor)<br>Swelling subsides, warm to touch, discoloration, pain to touch, pain on motion | Cryotherapy<br>Electrical stimulation<br>Nonthermal ultrasound | Ice packs, ice massage, cold whirlpool (15–20°C [68°F]) |
| Subacute: Pain to touch, pain on motion, swollen | Cryotherapy/thermotherapy<br>Electrical stimulation<br>Ultrasound | Contrast baths, hot packs, paraffin wax, fluidotherapy, etc. (41–45°C [106–113°F]) |
| Chronic: No more pain to touch, decreasing pain with motion | Thermotherapy (hot packs, ultrasound, paraffin)<br>Electrical stimulation<br>Ultrasound | |

### Phases of Cardiac Rehabilitation

Cardiac rehabilitation (or rehab) is a specialized intervention for patients with a history of myocardial infarction, unstable angina, or heart transplants. The clinical presentations of cardiovascular disease are diverse. The most common cardiac diagnoses referred for direct physical therapy interventions are coronary artery disease and congestive heart failure (CHF). Cardiac rehab is multidisciplinary and may include the physician, nurse, PT, PTA, occupational

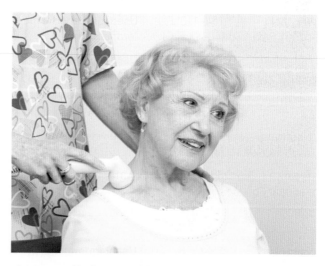

**Figure 5-2** Patient receiving an ultrasound intervention to her neck.

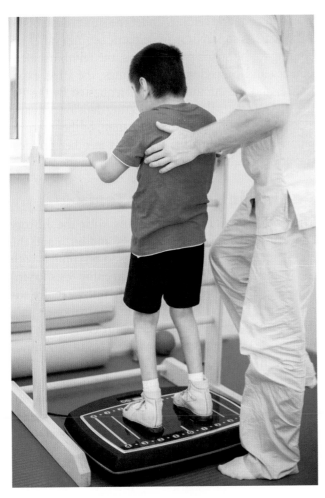

**Figure 5-3** Child working on a balance platform with a physical therapist.

© Pavel L Photo and Video/Shutterstock

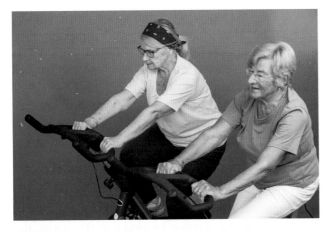

**Figure 5-4** Monitored aerobic exercise, such as stationary biking, is part of cardiac rehabilitation.

© karelnoppe/Shutterstock

therapist, certified occupational therapist assistant, social worker, nutritionist, and exercise physiologist. In cardiopulmonary rehabilitation, the PTA must be able to reassess the patient as necessary, monitor the patient's responses to treatment, monitor the patient's vital signs, and provide appropriate interventions for the patient.

The phases of cardiac rehabilitation include the following:

- Phase I takes place in the hospital. Examples of interventions in phase I of cardiac rehab are patient education about life changes; encouraging the patient's family to provide positive family support; teaching the patient bed mobility skills, the use of gentle exercises to return to basic ADLs, how to transfer with assistance, and gait training.
- Phase II takes place in outpatient settings. Examples of interventions in phase II of cardiac rehab are patient education for self-monitoring of vital signs, ADLs, upper body therapeutic exercises, treadmill activities, and stationary bicycle riding.
- Phase III occurs when the patient is discharged from outpatient programs but continues in a community-based or voluntary program of their choosing. In phase III of cardiac rehab, the patient continues a fitness program and activities of their choosing in the community or at home.

## Home Exercise Programs

The physical therapy sessions can be reinforced with home exercise programs (HEPs) by using a booklet or customized written or computer-generated instructions and drawings explaining the purpose of each activity or exercise. Before prescribing a HEP, the clinician should consider the time needed to perform the program. Also, individuals' tolerance and motivation levels vary based on their diagnosis and healing stage. For example, a short series of activities/exercises performed more frequently during the day should be prescribed when focusing on functional reeducation or for patients with poor endurance, whereas longer programs performed less frequently are aimed at building endurance or strength. Each HEP needs to be individualized to meet the patient's specific needs.

## Pediatric Examination

Pediatric physical therapy treats children with developmental dysfunctions and specific pediatric disorders. The pediatric PT is a direct care provider of pediatric physical therapy for children in hospital settings, early intervention programs, and school settings. Early intervention programs are mandated by law to provide comprehensive, multidisciplinary interventions for infants and toddlers (from birth to

3 years old) with disabilities. Individualized educational plans (IEPs) mandate comprehensive, multidisciplinary interventions for school-aged children up to age 21. The pediatric PT may also act as a school consultant by instructing teachers and teachers' assistants to facilitate the attainment of educational goals for children (from 3 to 21 years old) with disabilities. Pediatric physical therapy services depend on the child's needs and the type of physical therapy setting; for example, physical therapy will be different in an acute care hospital compared to a school environment.

The pediatric PT and the PTA are always members of a team that includes the pediatric patient's family, physicians, nurses, social workers, psychologists, occupational therapists, speech and language pathologists, certified occupational therapist assistants, special educators, and teachers.

The Academy of Pediatric Physical Therapy, a section of the APTA, has created resources for clinical practice, improving family/caregiver involvement, the use of technology, interventions, reimbursement, and specific practice setting resources. These resources are available on their website. They also publish Pediatric Physical Therapy to disseminate current research to interested readers.

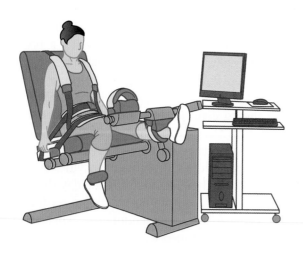

As with patients of all ages, the pediatric examination must not just consider impairments of body structures and function in isolation but also put them in context with the strengths and needs of the child and their family. In the pediatric examination, evaluation, and interventions, the PT and the PTA need specific knowledge about theories of child development, motor control, and motor learning, such as behavioral theories, principles of motor development, fetal sensorimotor development, pediatric examination, developmental sequence, preterm infant development, and pediatric pathophysiologies. As in all settings, the PTA

works in pediatric settings under the supervision of the PT. The PTA's supervision in pediatric settings varies according to the state's practice laws, the reimbursement policies and procedures, the settings, the PTA's experience, and the circumstances. If requested by the PT, the PTA supports the PT in collecting data for pediatric examinations; however, the evaluation, or the interpretation of the examination results, as in other physical therapy specialties, is performed solely by the PT.

## Pediatric Screening Tests

The pediatric examination begins with the history concerning the mother's pregnancy and birth and the child's medical history. The PT has to be familiar with the results of different pediatric screening tests for infants and children. Some screening tests, usually administered by physicians and nurse practitioners, are the **APGAR** (appearance, pulse, grimace, activity, and respiration) screening for newborns 1 and 5 minutes after birth, the Denver Developmental Screening Test, and the Bayley Scales of Infant Development. The PT also uses standardized examination tools for typically developing children with no pathology or dysfunction. These evaluation tools include the Neonatal Behavioral Assessment Scale, Movement Assessment of Infants, and Gross Motor Function Measure.

### Elements of Examination of Newborns, Infants, and Toddlers

For a newborn or an infant patient, the PT performs a neurologic examination, including stages of consciousness, skeletal system and ROM examinations, posture, and neonatal reflexes that are present at birth and that disappear later in the child's normal development. Examples of neonatal development reflexes include the flexor withdrawal reflex, crossed extension reflex, sucking reflex, plantar grasp reflex (see **Figure 5-5**), and symmetric tonic neck reflex (STNR). For example, the STNR, which is normal for an infant between 6 and 8 months of age, tests whether bending the infant's head forward causes the arms to bend and legs to straighten and if straightening of the infant's head causes the arms to straighten and legs to bend. If the STNR persists beyond 8 or 9 months, the infant will have difficulty propping on elbows while lying on the stomach and using the arms and legs in different positions.

Other examinations performed by the PT include newborn, infant, and toddler developmental milestones in gross motor development, fine motor development, social development, language development, cognitive development, and adaptive skills.

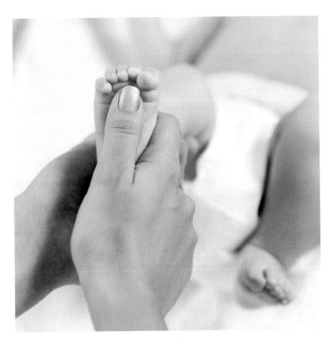

**Figure 5-5** PT checks plantar grasp reflex.
© Dmytro Vietrov/Shutterstock

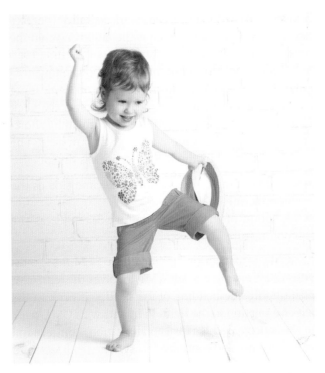

**Figure 5-6** Preschool child learning to stand on one foot.
© Evgeny Atamanenko/Shutterstock

Examples of developmental milestones for a 4- to 5-month-old infant may include the following:

- Rolls from lying on the stomach to the side and face up
- Holds the head steady while sitting supported
- Reaches for toys
- Reacts to music and their name
- Plays for 2 or 3 minutes with one toy
- Eats pureed foods
- Takes naps two to three times per day

Examples of developmental milestones for 3- and 4-year-old toddlers may include the following:

- Throws a ball overhead
- Hops 2–10 times on one foot
- Stands on tiptoe
- Draws a recognizable human figure
- Enjoys making friends and helping with adult activities
- Has a large (up to 1,000-word) vocabulary
- Learns entire songs
- Identifies colors and shapes
- Uses the toilet without help
- Brushes teeth with supervision

## Elements of Examination of Children and Adolescents

Older children with neurologic disorders may also be examined using observation and standardized tests. Older children are examined for ongoing health needs, such as monitoring of progressive diseases, for example, muscular dystrophy or scoliosis; mobility needs that need to "grow" as the child grows, for example, walkers and wheelchairs; and functional changes, as the child's growth may change the way they can accomplish school tasks and ADLs. Various standardized tests are available to compare the older child's functional abilities, such as the Peabody Developmental Motor Scales or the Bruininks–Oseretsky Test of Motor Proficiency (see **Figure 5-6**).

## Common Pediatric Conditions

Depending on the patient's age, many pediatric conditions are similar to those in the adult population, but children should not be treated as small adults. The following conditions concern the musculoskeletal, neurologic, pulmonary, and cardiovascular systems and the more common genetic conditions.

**Musculoskeletal System.** *Adolescent Idiopathic Scoliosis.* Scoliosis represents a disturbance of the intercalated series of spinal segments that produces a three-dimensional deformity (lateral curvature and vertebral rotation) of the spine. The deformity can be classified based on the location and direction of the curve. The most common location for idiopathic scoliosis is the thoracic (upper) spine, followed by the thoracolumbar (middle) and lumbar (lower) spine. The direction of the curve can be either to the left (levoscoliosis) or to the right (dextroscoliosis).

The severity of the curvature is measured in degrees using the Cobb angle, which is the angle between the most tilted vertebrae above and below the curvature.

**Congenital Muscular Torticollis.** Congenital muscular torticollis (CMT) (from the Latin *torti*, meaning twisted, and *collis*, meaning neck) refers to the neck in a twisted or bent position due to a unilateral shortening of the sternocleidomastoid (SCM) muscle. The position adopted by the head and neck is one of:

- Side bending of the neck to the same side as the contracture
- Rotation of the neck to the opposite side as the contracture

CMT is named for the side of the SCM muscle involved; for example, a left CMT involves the left SCM, resulting in side-bending of the head and neck to the left and rotation to the right. In infants with CMT, neck ROM is decreased for ipsilateral rotation, contralateral lateral flexion, and contralateral asymmetric flexion and extension. The infant cannot maintain a midline head alignment with the torso in static postures or during movement because of the neck muscle imbalance and muscle contracture. In the older child, this may result in asymmetric weight-bearing in sitting, crawling, walking, and transitional movement skills and incomplete development of automatic postural reactions.

**Arthrogryposis.** Arthrogryposis, or arthrogryposis multiplex congenita, comprises nonprogressive neurological conditions characterized by two or more joint contractures and rigid joints found throughout the body at birth. The pathogenesis of arthrogryposis has not been determined but is thought to be due to a combination of fetal abnormalities, maternal disorders (e.g., infection, drugs, trauma, and other maternal illnesses), and genetic inheritance. Although joint contractures and associated clinical manifestations vary from case to case, there are several common characteristics:

- Involved extremities are fusiform or cylindrical, with thin subcutaneous tissue and absent skin creases.
- Deformities are usually symmetric, and severity increases distally, with hands and feet typically being the most deformed.
- The patient may have a joint dislocation, especially in the hips and, occasionally, the knees.
- Distal joints are affected more frequently than proximal joints.
- ROM in the jaw is frequently limited.
- Mental intellect is not impacted.

**Talipes Equinovarus (Club Foot).** Talipes equinovarus is defined as a fixation of the foot in a handlike orientation—adduction, supination, and varus—with concomitant soft tissue abnormalities. Neurological, muscular, bony, connective tissue, and vascular mechanisms have been proposed, but the only firm evidence is that the mildest cases appear to be associated with an intrauterine posture, where the uterus restricts fetal foot movement [15].

**Congenital Hip Dysplasia.** CHD, also called developmental dysplasia of the hip (DDH), involves an abnormal growth/development of the hip, including the osseous structures, such as the acetabulum and the proximal femur, and the labrum, capsule, and other soft tissues, which prevents the femoral head from resting in the acetabulum of the pelvis so that the hip may be dislocated, dislocatable or subluxed. The condition may occur at any time, from conception to skeletal maturity. The following signs and symptoms may be found in the newborn:

- Asymmetric fat folds in the thigh
- Extra skin folds on the involved side
- Positive Ortolani test/Barlow maneuver signs: With the newborn supine, the clinician places the tips of the long and index fingers over the greater trochanter, with the thumb along the medial thigh. The infant's leg is positioned in neutral rotation with 90° of hip flexion and is gently abducted while lifting the leg anteriorly [16]. With abduction, one can feel a clunk as the femoral head slides over the posterior rim of the acetabulum and into the socket, producing the clunk originally described by Ortolani [17] and called the sign of entry as the hip relocates. From the same position, the leg is then gently adducted while gentle pressure is directed posteriorly on the knee, and a palpable clunk is noted as the femoral head slides over the posterior rim of the acetabulum and out of the socket [16]. This later clunk was originally described by Barlow [18] and is called the sign of exit, as the hip dislocates with this maneuver. Both tests detect motion between the femoral head and the acetabulum [16].

**Legg–Calvé–Perthes Disease (LCPD).** LCPD is an idiopathic osteonecrosis of the femoral head's capital femoral epiphysis with an unconfirmed etiology. Patients (most commonly, children aged 4–8 years) tend to have a limp and frequently have a positive Trendelenburg sign resulting from pain or hip abduction weakness [19]. The child complains of hip pain or pain in the medial thigh or knee (referred pain) [19]. The examination reveals a limited hip range of motion, especially in hip abduction and internal rotation.

**Slipped Capital Femoral Epiphysis (SCFE).** SCFE is a disorder of epiphyseal growth representing a unique type of proximal femoral growth plate instability due to a fracture through the proximal femoral physis. SCFE typically occurs in children between 10 and 16 and is more common in boys than girls. The exact cause of SCFE is unknown, but it is believed to be related to hormonal changes during puberty, genetics, and obesity. Stress around the hip causes a shear force to be applied at the growth plate and causes the epiphysis to move posteriorly and medially. In addition, the position of the proximal physis normally changes from horizontal to oblique during preadolescence and adolescence, redirecting hip forces from compression to shear forces. The patient usually has an antalgic limp and pain in the groin, often referred to the anteromedial thigh and knee. The leg is usually held externally rotated when supine and standing. There may be tenderness to palpation on the anterior and lateral aspects of the hip. Decreased hip motion is noted in flexion, abduction, and internal rotation.

*Juvenile Rheumatoid Arthritis (JRA).* JRA, also known as juvenile idiopathic arthritis (JIA), is a group of diseases defined as persistent arthritis, lasting at least 6 weeks, in one or more joints in a child younger than 16 years when all other causes of arthritis have been excluded. JRA can be classified as systemic (affects the whole body), pauciarticular (affects four or fewer joints), or polyarticular (affects at least five joints) disease according to onset within the first 6 months. The exact cause of JRA is unknown, but it is believed to be a combination of genetic and environmental factors. Symptoms include pain and decreased ROM, especially in the morning or after rest periods; fatigue; slow growth; postural changes; and gait deviations (limping). Periods of exacerbation and remission are common. Several standardized instruments can be used to examine a child's activities. The Childhood Health Assessment Questionnaire (CHAQ), a pediatric modification of the Stanford Health Assessment Questionnaire (HAQ), is a valid and sensitive tool in the evaluation of functional outcomes in children with chronic arthritis and is a component of the validated JRA core set criteria used to measure improvement and flare in clinical trials. Other questionnaires designed to measure physical function include the Juvenile Arthritis Functional Status Index (JASI) [20], the Juvenile Arthritis Functional Assessment Report (JAFAR) [21], the Juvenile Arthritis Quality of Life Questionnaire (JAQQ) [22], and the Pediatric Quality of Life (PedsQL):

*Osteogenesis Imperfecta (OI).* OI is an inherited condition resulting from an abnormality in type I collagen (found in bones, organ capsules, fascia, cornea, sclera, tendons, meninges, and dermis), which causes the bones to be brittle. In the most severe forms, the infant is born with multiple fractures sustained in utero or during birth.

**Neurologic System.** *Spina Bifida.* Spina bifida includes a continuum of congenital anomalies of the spine due to insufficient closure of the neural tube and failure of the vertebral arches to fuse. There are three types of spina bifida:

- Occulta: A mild form where the spinal cord and nerves are usually unaffected, and there may be a small gap in the spine without any visible signs.
- Meningocele: A moderate form where the meninges, or the protective covering around the spinal cord, protrude through the spine opening as a sac visible outside the body.
- Myelomeningocele: The most severe form, where both the meninges and the spinal cord protrude through the opening in the spine, leading to damage of the spinal cord and nerves.

The severity of the condition can vary greatly, and it may cause a range of symptoms, including weakness or paralysis in the legs, bowel and bladder problems, hydrocephalus, and learning difficulties.

*Cerebral Palsy (CP).* CP, the neurologic condition most frequently encountered by pediatric PTs, is generally considered a nonprogressive defect or lesion in single or multiple locations in the immature brain. CP is diagnosed when a child does not reach motor milestones and exhibits abnormal muscle tone or qualitative differences in movement patterns, such as asymmetry. Despite advances in neonatal care, CP remains a significant clinical problem. In most cases of CP, the exact cause is unknown but is most likely multifactorial (intracranial hemorrhage, intrauterine infection, birth asphyxia, multiple births, early prenatal, perinatal, or postnatal injury due to vascular insufficiency, or CNS malformation). There are three main types of CP:

- Spastic: The most common type, which is characterized by tight and stiff muscles, making movement difficult.
- Dyskinetic: This type of CP affects the ability to control movement, resulting in involuntary and twisting motions.
- Ataxic: This type of CP affects balance and coordination, resulting in shaky movements and difficulty with precise movements.

Additionally, CP can be classified based on the part of the body affected:

- Monoplegia: Affects one limb
- Hemiplegia: Affects the upper and lower limbs on one side of the body

- Diplegia: Affects both legs more than the arms
- Quadriplegia: CP that affects all four limbs and the torso

The severity of CP can also be classified using the Gross Motor Function Classification System (GM-FCS), which categorizes children with CP into five levels based on their ability to perform motor skills and the need for assistance:

- Level I: Children who can walk without limitations.
- Level II: Children who can walk but require assistance, such as a walker or crutches.
- Level III: Children who walk with assistance but may require a wheelchair for long distances.
- Level IV: Children who use a wheelchair for mobility and require assistance with daily activities.
- Level V: Children with the most severe impairment with limited movement requiring constant care.

Impairments in CP are problems of the neuromuscular and skeletal systems that are either an immediate result of the existing pathophysiologic process or an indirect consequence that has developed over time. Primary impairments of the muscular system include insufficient force generation, spasticity, abnormal extensibility, and exaggerated or hyperactive reflexes. Primary impairments of the neuromuscular system include poor selected control of muscle activity, poor regulation of activity in muscle groups in anticipation of postural changes and body movement (anticipatory regulation), and decreased ability to learn unique movements. The PT must be able to identify the abilities as well as participation restrictions, activity limitations, and impairment of body structure and function of the child, as children with CP have variable but significant disruptions in the accomplishment of life habits, particularly in the categories of recreation, community roles, personal care, education, mobility, housing, and nutrition, and are most associated with locomotion capabilities. Thus, the examination involves qualitative and, when possible, quantitative assessment of the single system and multisystem impairments.

*Brachial Plexus Injury*. Brachial plexus injury occurs most commonly in large babies, frequently with shoulder dystocia or breech delivery. Traumatic lesions associated with brachial plexus injury are fractured clavicle, fractured humerus, subluxation of the cervical spine, cervical cord injury, and facial palsy. The symptoms may include a lack of movement or weakness in the involved upper extremity, inability to grip or hold objects, and limited range of motion in the shoulder or arm. Early diagnosis and treatment are important for a better outcome. Physical therapy,

if prescribed, involves PROM, positioning, and tactile stimulation. The more severe cases may require surgery to repair or replace the damaged nerves.

*Developmental Coordination Disorder (DCD)*. DCD, also known as dyspraxia, is a neurological disorder that typically appears in early childhood and affects an individual's ability to plan, execute, and coordinate physical movements during everyday activities, such as dressing, grooming, writing, and participating in sports. Symptoms of DCD include difficulty with fine motor skills, such as writing, drawing, and manipulating small objects, and gross motor skills, such as running, jumping, and balancing. Individuals may also have difficulty with activities that require coordination of both sides of the body, such as riding a bike. Using task analysis and task-specific training, physical therapy treatments typically focus on helping individuals improve their motor skills, coordination, and overall physical abilities.

**Pulmonary System.** *Asthma (Hyperreactive Airway Disease)*. Asthma is a chronic inflammatory disorder of the airways characterized by (particularly at night or in the early morning) recurrent episodes of wheezing, breathlessness, chest tightness, and coughing. In susceptible individuals, the inflammation (acute, subacute, or chronic) causes airway inflammation, intermittent airflow obstruction, and an associated increase in the existing bronchial responsiveness to various stimuli. Exercise-induced asthma (EIA), or exercise-induced bronchospasm, is an asthma variant defined as a condition in which exercise or vigorous physical activity triggers acute bronchospasm in persons with heightened airway reactivity to numerous exogenous and endogenous stimuli. The diagnosis of asthma, which is not typically made until the child is 3–6 years of age, is made based on history, physical examination, auscultation and palpation, and pulmonary function tests (PFTs), especially in response to a methacholine challenge.

*Cystic Fibrosis (CF)*. CF is an autosomal recessive disorder of exocrine gland function involving multiple organ systems (lungs, liver, intestine, pancreas), chiefly resulting in chronic respiratory infections, pancreatic enzyme insufficiency, and associated complications in untreated patients. CF is caused by mutations in the *CFTR* (cystic fibrosis transmembrane conductance regulator) gene, which produces a protein that regulates the flow of salt and water in and out of cells. The failure of epithelial cells to conduct chloride and the associated water transport abnormalities result in difficulty in clearing viscous secretions in the respiratory tract (**Figure 5-7**), pancreas, gastrointestinal tract,

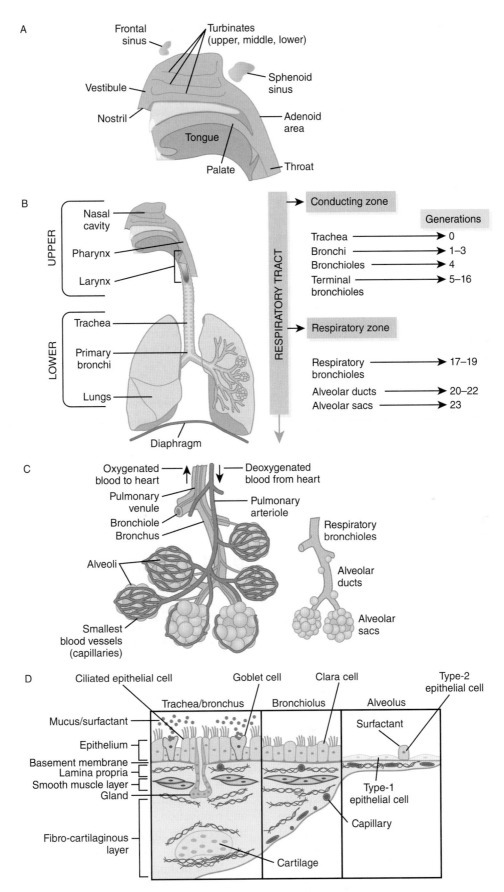

**Figure 5-7** Respiratory tract.

sweat glands, and other exocrine tissues. Symptoms of CF can include persistent coughing, wheezing, shortness of breath, frequent lung infections, poor growth and weight gain, greasy and bulky stools, and infertility in males. Sweat chloride analysis is critical to distinguish CF from other causes of severe pulmonary and pancreatic insufficiencies and to define patients requiring further analysis.

**Cardiovascular System.** *Ventricular Septal Defect (VSD)*. VSD is a congenital heart defect involving an abnormal opening of the interventricular septum between the left and right ventricles of the heart, which allows oxygen-rich blood to mix with oxygen-poor blood, putting strain on the cardiovascular system. In some cases, VSD may cause no symptoms and be detected incidentally during routine medical exams, while in other cases, it may cause fatigue; rapid breathing; poor feeding and weight gain; and cyanosis of the skin, lips, and nails. VSD is typically diagnosed using an echocardiogram.

**Genetic Conditions.** *Down Syndrome*. The extra chromosome 21 that occurs in Down syndrome affects almost every organ system, resulting in a wide spectrum of phenotypic consequences, including hypotonia, decreased force generation of muscles, congenital heart defects, visual and hearing losses, difficulties with fine and gross motor skills, and intellectual deficits, including motor, speech and language, cognitive, and social delays.

*Duchenne Muscular Dystrophy (DMD)* [23–25]. DMD, the best-known form of muscular dystrophy, is due to a mutation in a gene on the X chromosome that prevents the production of dystrophin, a normal protein in muscle. DMD affects boys and, very rarely, girls. DMD typically manifests with weakness in the pelvis and upper limbs, resulting in clumsiness, frequent falling, an inability to keep up with peers while playing, and an unusual gait (lateral trunks sway—waddling). Around the age of 8 years, most patients notice difficulty climbing stairs or rising from the ground. Because of this proximal lower back and extremity weakness, parents often note that the child pushes on his knees to stand (Gower sign). The posterior calf is usually enlarged due to fatty and connective tissue infiltration or by compensatory hypertrophy of the calves secondary to weak tibialis anterior muscles. Respiratory muscle strength begins a slow but steady decline. The forced vital capacity gradually wanes, leading to symptoms of nocturnal hypoxemia, such as lethargy and early morning headaches. As DMD progresses, a wheelchair may be needed.

*Spinal Muscular Atrophy (SMA)*. SMA is characterized by primary spinal cord and brainstem motor neuron degeneration, resulting in skeletal muscle atrophy and weakness. Classification of SMA in the pediatric population into three groups is based on clinical presentation and progression:

- Type 1 SMA (also known as Werdnig-Hoffmann disease): The most severe form presents with onset in the first few months of life. Infants with type 1 SMA typically have very weak muscle tone and difficulty with feeding, breathing, and movement. Without treatment, life expectancy is typically less than 2 years.
- Type 2 SMA: This form typically presents in early childhood, with symptoms ranging from mild to severe muscle weakness and atrophy. Children with type 2 SMA may be able to sit independently but may require a wheelchair for mobility.
- Type 3 SMA (also known as Kugelberg–Welander disease): This form typically presents in late childhood or adolescence, with symptoms ranging from mild to moderate muscle weakness and atrophy. Individuals with type 3 SMA may be able to walk independently but may experience difficulty running, jumping, and climbing stairs.
- Type 4 SMA has its onset in adulthood and is the mildest form, with symptoms of mild muscle weakness and atrophy and no significant impact on life expectancy.

## Pediatric Interventions

Pediatric treatments depend on the presenting pediatric pathology with the understanding that children are not small adults, so the focus is not on helping to restore an individual's prior level of function (rehabilitation) but on helping the child learn new skills (habilitation). To enhance task performance and increase a child's ability to perform meaningful tasks, recent research supports a goal-directed, task-oriented approach rather than interventions that address underlying impairments [26]. The interventions must be engaging, age-appropriate, fun and functional, appropriate to the circumstances, and inclusive of the family and social unit. Personal goals enhance performance and motivation, so to increase a child's motivation, the interventions should be based on their priorities and needs [26].

Most pediatric interventions use neurologic treatments of sensory stimulation to influence the motor response. For example, neurologic interventions such as the neurodevelopmental treatment or the motor control approach influence the inborn postural

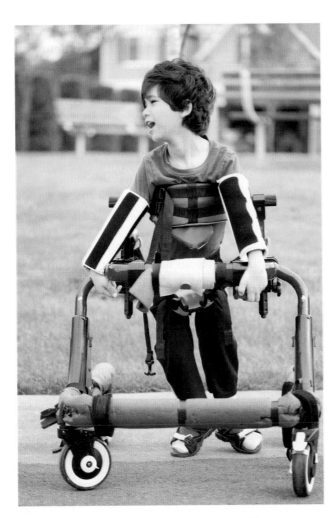

**Figure 5-8** Child walking using a rolling walker.

© Jaren Jai Wicklund/Shutterstock

reflexes and affect the child's functional motor skills. Pediatric orthopedic interventions may use strengthening exercises (as in kicking or swimming) and functional skill training, such as walking and transfers.

Functional activities can be encouraged through play using mobility and standing positioning devices. Some mobility devices in pediatric physical therapy are the rollator and posterior rolling walkers (see **Figure 5-8**). Walkers promote independence in mobility skills by strengthening the musculoskeletal system through active weight-bearing in the lower limbs. The standing positioning devices are the prone stander, standing frame, and parapodium. The prone stander and the standing frame stimulate the child to hold up the head and trunk and to stand upright. The parapodium allows the child to move while standing at the same visual height as their peers. Other mobility devices, such as the manual and power wheelchair and power scooter, can be used in multiple environments, including school and family activities.

## Rehabilitation for Specific Pediatric Conditions

***Adolescent Idiopathic Scoliosis***. Treatment for idiopathic scoliosis depends on the curve's severity, the patient's age, and the likelihood of the curve worsening over time.

- The younger the patient at diagnosis, the greater the risk of progression.
- Double-curve patterns have a greater risk of progression than single-curve patterns.
- The risk of progression in females is approximately 10 times that of males with curves of comparable magnitude.

Mild curves may require only monitoring with appropriate intermittent radiographs to check for the presence or absence of curve progression, while bracing is typically used for curves between 25° and 45° in children who are still growing to prevent the curve from worsening. Surgery (fusion) may be necessary for curves greater than 45° or if bracing is ineffective. Physical therapy intervention for scoliosis is based on the child's skeletal maturity, growth potential, and curve magnitude. With bracing, the active theory of orthotics is that curve progression is prevented by muscle contractions responding to the brace wear. Exercises to be performed while wearing a brace, such as pelvic tilts, thoracic flexion, and lateral shifts, are often taught to patients to improve the active forces

***Congenital Muscular Torticollis (CMT)***. Outcomes are best when infants are diagnosed early and start comprehensive physical therapy management before 3 months of age [27]. If untreated or treated after early infancy, CMT can lead to craniofacial deformities and painful limited cervical motion, requiring more invasive interventions, such as botulinum neurotoxin injections and surgery. The infant requires a comprehensive program of cervical stretching, cervical and trunk strengthening, activities promoting symmetrical movement, postural control exercises, environmental adaptations, and parent or caregiver education and support to provide a daily, intensive home program [27].

***Arthrogryposis***. Physical therapy typically involves a combination of soft tissue mobilization, ROM and strengthening exercises, gait training, the use of assistive technology, and environmental modifications

***Talipes Equinovarus (Club Foot)***. Most cases of clubfoot are successfully treated with nonsurgical methods consisting of reducing the talonavicular joint by moving the navicular laterally and the head of the talus medially, bracing (Ponseti brace), and serial casting, which is most effective if started immediately after birth.

*Congenital Hip Dysplasia (CHD)*. The treatment of this condition depends on the child's age. From birth to 9 months, the Pavlik harness has traditionally been used. The harness restricts hip extension and adduction and allows the hip to be maintained in flexion and abduction, the "protective position" [19]. The position of flexion and abduction enhances normal acetabular development, and the kicking motion allowed in this position stretches the contracted hip adductors and promotes the spontaneous reduction of the dislocated hip [19]. In infants older than 9 months of age who are beginning to walk independently, an abduction orthosis can be used as an alternative to the Pavlik harness [19].

*Legg–Calvé–Perthes Disease (LCPD)*. Controversy exists regarding the appropriate treatment or whether treatment is even necessary. The goal of treatment is to relieve pain, maintain the spherical shape of the femoral head, and prevent extrusion of the enlarged femoral head from the joint. Treatment methods include observation only, range of motion exercises in all planes of hip motion (especially internal rotation and abduction), bracing, Petrie casts (two long-leg casts with a bar between, holding the hips abducted and internally rotated), and surgery. Specific procedural interventions can relieve the forces incurred during weight-bearing (crutch training, aquatic therapy). Gait training may be initiated with an orthosis or with bracing. The specific gait pattern and assistive devices depend on the type of orthosis.

*Slipped Capital Femoral Epiphysis (SCFE)*. The treatment goals are to keep the displacement to a minimum, maintain motion, and delay or prevent premature degenerative arthritis [19]. Following surgical fixation, using one or two pins or screws, usually in situ, the PT completes a careful and thorough examination of the motion of the hip joint, and subsequent measurements should be taken after every operation and removal of the cast. Range of motion exercises for the hip should be done in all planes, emphasizing hip flexion, internal rotation, and abduction. Gait training post surgery is initiated once lower extremity strength and range of motion are adequate for ambulation skills. The weight-bearing status can vary but is usually non-weight-bearing or touch-down weight-bearing. Full weight-bearing is permitted when the growth plate has fused (within approximately 3–4 months).

*Juvenile Rheumatoid Arthritis (JRA)*. PTs are essential members of the pediatric rheumatology team, which includes the rheumatologist, nurse, occupational therapist, ophthalmologist, orthopedist,

and pediatrician. Other specialists, including cardiologists, dermatologists, orthotists, psychologists, and social workers, provide occasional consultation as needed. The PT develops a prioritized problem list and an intervention plan to reduce current impairments, maintain or improve function, prevent or minimize secondary problems, and provide education and support to the child and family. Specific interventions can include any or all of the following:

- Range of motion and stretching exercises
  - Acute stage: Passive and active assisted to avoid joint compression
  - Subacute/chronic stages: Active exercises
- Strengthening: Avoid substitutions, and minimize instability, atrophy, deformity, pain, and injury.
  - Acute and subacute stages: Isometric exercises progressing cautiously to resistive
  - Chronic stage: Judicious use of concentric exercises (see **Figure 5-9**)
- Endurance exercises: Encouragement to exercise—fun and recreational activities, swimming
- Joint protection strategies and body mechanics education
- Mobility assistive devices
- Rest, as needed—balance rest with activity levels using splinting (articular resting).
- Posture and positioning to maintain joint range of motion (see **Figure 5-10**)
  - Patients should spend 20 minutes/day prone to stretch the hip and knee flexors.
- Assess leg length discrepancy in standing and avoid scoliosis.
- Therapeutic modalities for pain control
- Instructions on the wearing of warm pajamas, a sleeping bag, an electric blanket
- Paraffin for hands

*Osteogenesis Imperfecta (OI)*. Typical participation restrictions for an infant with OI depend on the severity of the case. The PT should know the infant's

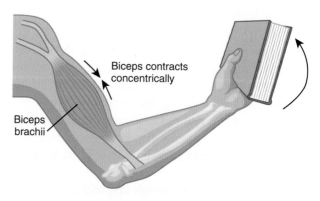

**Figure 5-9** Concentric exercise of the biceps

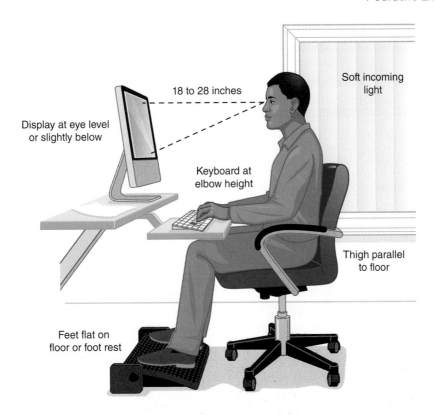

18 to 28 inches

Display at eye level
or slightly below

Soft incoming
light

Keyboard at
elbow height

Thigh parallel
to floor

Feet flat on
floor or foot rest

**Figure 5-10** Correct workstation posture

medical history of past and present fractures and know the types of immobilizations employed before beginning the examination. Pain is assessed using the FLACC (face, legs, activity, cry, and consolability), an observational scale assessing pain behaviors quantitatively with preverbal patients. Assessing active, but not passive, ROM is essential. Functional ROM may prove more useful because it will assist in visualizing the whole composite of motion needed in functional abilities. Assessing muscle strength is done by observing the infant's movements and palpating contracting muscles rather than using formal muscle tests. Caregiver education on proper and safe handling, positioning, and facilitation of movement is provided. Bathing, dressing, and carrying the infant are critical times when the infant is at risk for fractures. An aquatic exercise program is an excellent therapeutic program for a child with OI. The degree of ambulation attainable varies for preschool children with OI. Surgical interventions include intramedullary rodding, basilar impression surgery, and scoliosis correction.

*Spina Bifida*. The treatment for spina bifida varies depending on the severity of the condition. The mild forms, such as occulta, may not require any treatment, but the more severe forms, such as myelomeningocele, require prompt surgical intervention within the first few days of life to prevent further damage to the spinal cord and nerves. After surgery, ongoing management is needed to prevent complications, such as infections, hydrocephalus, and tethered spinal cord (when the spinal cord is pulled down and tethered to scar tissue). Physical therapy focuses on correct positioning, bracing, orthotics, ROM exercises, and gait as appropriate.

*Cerebral Palsy (CP)*. The intervention for the patient with CP is highly individualized and is usually part of a multidisciplinary team comprising the family, various allied health professionals, and appropriate school staff. The more one practices, the more one learns; therefore, activities should be repeated multiple times during each treatment session and throughout each day [28]. The foremost set of goals for all ages is to educate families about CP, to provide support in their acceptance of their child's problems, and to assist when parents make decisions about managing their own and their child's lives. From infancy to adulthood, physical therapy goals for clients with CP should focus on promoting participation by maximizing the gross motor activity allowed by the organic deficits and helping the child compensate for activity limitations when necessary. This necessitates a cognizance of environmental and personal factors that could enhance activity or participation or, conversely, that could increase existing activity limitations and participation restrictions. Habilitation interventions should include purposeful, relevant, developmentally appropriate, active, voluntarily regulated, goal-directed, and meaningful tasks for the child [28].

*Brachial Plexus Injury*. Physical therapy, if prescribed, involves PROM, positioning, and tactile stimulation. The more severe cases may require surgery to repair or replace the damaged nerves.

*Developmental Coordination disorder (DCD)*. Using task analysis and task-specific training, physical therapy treatments typically focus on helping individuals improve their motor skills, coordination, and overall physical abilities.

*Asthma (Hyperreactive Airway Disease)*. Physical therapy intervention for asthma may include patient education on breathing exercises (specific diaphragmatic training from recumbent to upright positions, and, eventually, to sporting conditions), postural education, relaxation techniques, endurance, and strength training, and teaching the patient how to self-monitor symptoms and patterns, and responses to medications. The medical intervention for asthma may include pharmacologic therapy.

*Cystic Fibrosis (CF)*. Patients with CF often require management by a multidisciplinary team, including physicians, nurses, nutritionists, PTs, respiratory therapists, counselors, and social workers. The goals of the intervention are to maintain adequate nutritional status, prevent pulmonary and other complications, encourage physical activity, and provide adequate psychosocial support. Physical therapy aims to improve exercise tolerance with continued attention to secretion clearance techniques (postural drainage, percussion vibration, huffing, and positive expiratory pressure [PEP]), correction and maintenance of proper postural alignment, and continued education of the caregivers. Exercise is a useful therapeutic modality for secretion clearance, peak oxygen consumption increases, maximal work capacity, and expiratory flow rates [29, 30]. Advances in pharmacology and gene-based therapies have increased life expectancy for individuals with CF, with many living well into adulthood. However, CF remains a chronic and progressive disease that requires ongoing care and management.

*Ventricular Septal Defect (VSD)*. Treatment for VSD depends on the size and location of the defect, as well as the severity. Small VSDs may close independently without treatment, while larger VSDs may require medication, surgery, or other interventions to close the opening and prevent further complications. In some cases, VSD may be treated with a catheter-based procedure that uses a small device to close the opening without surgery.

*Down Syndrome*. There is no cure for Down syndrome, but early intervention and appropriate medical care can help individuals with Down syndrome reach their full potential and live fulfilling lives. The role of physical therapy varies according to the severity of the symptoms and includes:

- Minimizing gross motor delay
- Encouraging oral motor function
- Emphasis on exercise and fitness for the management of obesity
- Balance and coordination exercises
- Maximizing respiratory function
- Motor skill acquisition
- A nutritional consult

*Duchenne Muscular Dystrophy (DMD)*. One of the primary considerations in the early management program of the young school-age child is to retard the development of contractures through ROM exercises and using night splints. Strength training may be beneficial in DMD, although the evidence remains uncertain, but if it is used, it should avoid high-impact, high-intensity, eccentric activity and focus on low-intensity shortening contractions without resistance. Braces, such as ankle–foot orthoses and knee–ankle–foot orthoses, are important adjuncts in prolonging the period of ambulation/mobility and delaying wheelchair dependency, which usually occurs during adolescence. However, using orthoses for a standing program or continuing supported walking is inappropriate for all individuals. However, a standing program may help address the issue of decreased bone mineral density and subsequent increased risk of fracture [31]. Independent walking usually ceases by age 10–12. A power scooter should be considered as an initial power wheelchair prescription for the child who is hesitant to use a power wheelchair when walking is no longer possible [31]. Once wheelchair dependency becomes inevitable, attention should shift to prevention against the harmful consequences of immobility.

*Spinal Muscular Atrophy*. The primary impairment in all forms of SMA is muscle weakness. Secondary impairments include postural compensations resulting from muscle weakness, contractures, and occasionally scoliosis. Respiratory distress is present early in acute childhood SMA. The goals of physical therapy are to improve the quality of life and to minimize disability. Therapeutic exercise, functional use of orthoses and adaptive equipment, and strategies to minimize disabilities secondary to the impairments are included to provide a comprehensive intervention.

# CASE STUDY

You are a pediatric therapist working in a school system where you provide physical therapy in the student's school environment, including the classroom, playground, and cafeteria. Your new patient is a 3-year-old boy who has spastic hemiplegic cerebral palsy. The different classifications of CP are based on two things: the distribution of the impairment, and the impairment. The distribution can be hemiplegic, diplegic, or quadriplegic. The impairment can be spastic, dyskinetic, or ataxic.

Spastic: Caused by damage to the cortex. The child will be stiff in one or more limbs and may have involuntary movements.
Dyskinetic or athetoid: Caused by damage to the basal ganglia or cerebellum. The main symptom is low muscle tone resulting in one or more floppy limbs.
Ataxic: Caused by damage to the cerebellum; results in shakiness and random movements.

Regardless of the classifications, all CP sufferers have a degree of decreased mobility and are significantly weaker than their able-bodied counterparts. In addition, they often have joint deformities, with scoliosis being the most common deformity, followed by hip deformities.

The patient's previous interventions include home physical therapy and occupational therapy services through early intervention, but he is still presenting with delays in his development relative to age-matched peers. His family has decided to transition services from the home-based, family-centered individualized family service plan (IFSP), under Individuals with Disabilities Act (IDEA), to a school-based, student-centered individualized education plan (IEP).

Your examination reveals the following:

- The patient wears glasses, and his eyes are very sensitive to bright lights.
- Increased muscle tone in the right upper and lower extremities
- Voluntary and involuntary movements in both upper and lower extremities
- Impaired protective balance reactions
- Decreased trunk, shoulder, and pelvic girdle mobility
- Able to maintain static stance with external support

The gait examination reveals that although the patient is beginning to take steps with manual assistance and ankle–foot orthoses (AFOs), his hips and knees are flexed. On occasions, the patient walks on his toes. Outside of the clinic, the patient uses a posterior walker for short distances and a manual wheelchair for longer distances.

Some of the potential barriers include:

- Environmental (e.g., appropriate facilities and equipment)
- Organizational (e.g., appropriate staff, class size, and health and safety)
- The level of disability (e.g., assistive devices and wheelchair requirements)
- Attitudinal (e.g., of the child, peers, and staff)

Based on the school environment, the goals tend to be more participation related rather than activity or body structure and function. For example, an outpatient activity goal might be "to ambulate 100 feet independently with the posterior walker with verbal cueing in 4 weeks," whereas a school environment-related goal should focus on the patient being able "to ambulate independently with the posterior walker from the classroom to the cafeteria in 12 weeks."
In a small group, discuss:

- Some of the other participation goals you might include and how you would achieve them while keeping the patient motivated
- Any specific potential barriers and how you would address them
- What principles of motor learning and types of feedback would be the most effective to encourage classroom activity
- How you could involve the classroom support staff to increase frequency of practice
- What you think would be an appropriate frequency and duration for treatment

# CASE STUDY

You are about to examine a 7-year-old boy diagnosed with Duchenne muscular dystrophy (DMD). According to his medical history, the patient was diagnosed when he was 4 years old after his mother noticed signs of clumsiness and difficulty climbing stairs. At 6 years old, the patient was prescribed glucocorticoids. At present, the patient is enjoying and is participating fully in grade 3 activities, but his mother has reported more frequent falls at home and school, which is embarrassing him, and he is taking longer to walk up and down the stairs of their house.

During the examination, which you completed over two sessions to help with the patient's fatigue levels, you noticed the following:

- A PedsQL score revealed low ratings in the physical and social functioning scales as rated by the parent and child.
- A Faces Pain Scale-Revised revealed a current pain level of 3/10, 5/10 over the past day, and 7/10 after playing during recess.
- Postural observation in standing revealed a hyper-lordotic lumbar curve, with an anterior pelvic tilt and a wide base of support. There was no evidence of the hyper-lordotic curve in sitting, but there was a noticeably increased thoracic kyphosis with winging and anterior tilting of both scapulae. Finally, the patient had bilateral pronounced calf muscles.
- Gross muscle strength testing revealed generalized muscle weakness in both lower limbs.
- Good joint range of motion for most movements except for ankle dorsiflexion and the 90-90 SLR
- Positive Gower's sign
- Functionally, the patient was able to sit without support and could cope with mild external perturbations but needed to put a hand down with moderate forces. In standing, a recovery step was required when mild external perturbations were applied in all directions.
- The gait analysis revealed a wide base of support and in-toeing during the stance phase and a diminished heel strike during initial contact, with more weight being placed on the midfoot. Also, there was a bilateral Trendelenburg with gait.
- Using the Six-Minute Walk test (6MWT), the patient walked 349 m.
- Reflex testing revealed Grade 1 for L4 and S1/S2.
- Palpation revealed decreased muscle tone of the quadriceps and hamstrings.

Based on these findings, the physical therapy diagnosis is Duchenne muscular dystrophy, showing weakness and decrease in range of motion in lower extremities, an increase in falls during activities and challenges with balance and mobility, and a risk of decreased participation in school activities.

In your groups, create:

- A problem list for this patient, and design both short-term (1-month) and long-term (6-month) goals.
- Interventions to increase range of motion, strength, balance, and respiration
- A list of potential orthotics

# Geriatric Examination

Aging is the accumulation of diverse adverse changes that increase the risk of death [32]. These aging changes are responsible for the commonly recognized sequential alterations that accompany advancing age beyond the early period of life and the progressive increases in the chance of disease and death associated with them [32].

Gerontology is the study of the aging process and the science related to the care of older adults. Geriatric physical therapy specializes in treating older individuals who present with musculoskeletal and neuromuscular conditions and dysfunction common to older adults. Generally, geriatric physical therapy focuses on health promotion and the prevention and treatment of disease and disability in later life with patients who present with musculoskeletal and neuromuscular conditions and dysfunction common to older adults. Like other specialized physical therapy areas, geriatric rehabilitation requires understanding the patient's individuality and unique developmental issues. The initial clinical examination and evaluation should focus on careful and accurate examinations (see **Figure 5-11**).

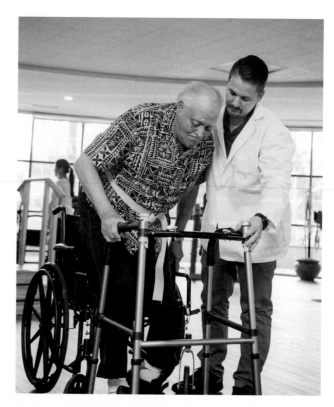

**Figure 5-11** An older adult monitored for safe mobility.

© Erik Isakson/Tetra images/Getty Images

Geriatric physical therapy settings can vary, depending on the needs of the patient and the type of care required, and include home health, outpatient clinics, skilled nursing facilities, assisted living facilities, and hospitals. The PT and the PTA help elderly patients to be in control of their own decisions whenever possible. Cultural and ethnic sensitivities are also significant aspects of geriatric rehabilitation. The whole patient should be considered, and social support must be integrated into the rehabilitation and the demands for continuity of care. Many changes are associated with aging throughout adulthood and into old age (**Table 5-6**).

In geriatric physical therapy, the PTA's role is important not only for delivering treatments but also for ongoing reexaminations to determine the following:

- The patient's capacity for safe function
- The effects of inactivity on the patient versus activity
- The effects of normal aging on the patient versus disease pathology

**Table 5-6 Summary of Multisystem Changes in the Older Adult**

| System | Changes |
|---|---|
| Musculoskeletal | Muscle mass and strength decrease by about 30% between 60 and 90 years.<br>Change in muscle fiber type, white and red. Type II fibers (fast twitch) decrease by about 50%.<br>Decrease in the recruitment of motor units<br>Decreased tensile strength of bone (more than 30% of women over 65 have osteoporosis)<br>Joint flexibility is reduced by 25–30% over 70 years. |
| Neuromuscular | Atrophy of neurons; nerve fibers decrease and change in structure.<br>Myoneural junction decreases in transmission speed.<br>Decreased nerve conduction velocity by about 0.4% a year after age 70<br>Slowing of motor neuron conduction, which contributes to alterations in the autonomic system<br>Decreasing reflexes result from decreased nerve conduction. Ankle jerk is absent in about 70%, and knee and biceps jerks are absent in about 15%.<br>Overall slow and decreased responsiveness in reaction time (simple reflexes less than complex)<br>Increased postural sway (less in women than in men, with linear increase with age) |
| Neurosensory | Decrease in sweating (implications for modalities and exercise)<br>10–20% decrease in brain weight by age 90<br>Decrease in mechanoreceptors<br>Decrease in visual acuity and ability to accommodate lighting changes resulting from increased lens density<br>Decrease in hearing capabilities (presbycusis), affecting one-third of adults aged 65–74 and one-half of people over 75 |
| Cardiovascular and pulmonary | Decrease in cardiac output by about 0.7% a year after 20 years of age<br>Increased vascular resistance<br>Decreased arterial elasticity<br>Decreased cardiac reserve and decreased physical and psychological response to stress<br>Increased irritation of the myocardium contributes to an increased risk of atrial fibrillation and arrhythmias.<br>Decrease in lung function (from age 25 to age 85, as much as 50% decrease in maximal voluntary ventilation due to an increase in air resistance; get about 40% decrease in vital capacity)<br>Respiratory gas exchange surface decreases at about 0.27 m² a year (maximum oxygen consumption for sedentary individuals of any age is 0.62–0.7 mL per minute).<br>Decreased elastin in the lungs (increased rigidity) and chest wall soft tissues, which decreases chest wall compliance.<br>A decrease in vital capacity and a decrease in pulmonary blood flow contribute to lower oxygen saturation levels.<br>Decreased cough reflex |

*(continues)*

**Table 5-6** **Summary of Multisystem Changes in the Older Adult** *(continued)*

| System | Changes |
|---|---|
| Urogenital/renal | Gradual overall structure changes in all renal components<br>Decreased glomerular filtration rate and creatinine clearance<br>Change in response to sodium intake<br>Muscle hypertrophy in the urethra and bladder |
| Gastrointestinal | Decreased peristalsis<br>Diminished secretions of pepsin and acid in the stomach<br>Decreasing hepatic and pancreatic enzymes |
| Immunologic | Decrease in overall function concerning infection<br>Decreased temperature regulation<br>Decrease in T cells |

Data from: Bottomley JM: The Geriatric Population, in Boissonnault WG (ed): Primary Care for the Physical Therapist: Examination and Triage. St Louis, Elsevier Saunders, 2005, pp 288–306
Bottomley JM: Summary of System Changes. Comparing and Contrasting age-related changes, in Bottomley JM, Lewis CB (eds): Geriatric Rehabilitation: A Clinical Approach, 2nd ed. Upper Saddleback, NJ, Prentice-Hall, 2003, pp 50–75.

## Elements of Examination of Older Adults

The geriatric physical therapy examination and evaluation focus mostly on the patient's functioning level and ability to remain independent. The POC in the initial examination is developed with the patient and/or the caregiver.

The elements of a geriatric initial examination and evaluation include the following:

- Patient and or family/caregiver interview
- Pain assessment
- Physical examinations dependent on the patient's pathology (which can be orthopedic, neurologic, and/or cardiopulmonary)
- Psychosocial assessment, including depression and **dementia** examinations
- Balance and falls risk assessment
- Functional examination, including gait and transfers
- Environmental examination for the patient's home or for the institution where the patient resides

A psychosocial assessment may include a mini-mental state examination, a mental questionnaire, a depression assessment, and a stress assessment scale. The mini-mental state examination checks the patient's cognitive changes in orientation, attention, mathematical calculation, recall, and language [10]. The Mental Status Questionnaire, composed of 10 questions, has been used in rehabilitation for a long time and is quick and easy to administer. In addition, several depression-screening instruments are used in physical therapy to assess depression in the older population. Some, such as the Geriatric Depression Scale, have better sensitivity than others.

The geriatric patient's function is examined in terms of the whole individual and not specific impairments. For example, the patient's function may be evaluated for the following [33]:

- Physical function, including sensory and motor
- Mental function, including intelligence, cognitive ability, and memory
- Social function, including the patient's interaction with family members and the community, as well as economic considerations
- Emotional function, including the patient's ability to cope with stress and anxiety and the patient's satisfaction with life

Some of the more common conditions that occur in older adults include the following:

*Osteoarthritis (OA).* OA, a *degenerative joint disease*, is a clinical condition of synovial joints. OA is characterized by cracks and general thinning of articular cartilage and synovial inflammation, especially in the weight-bearing areas of the large joints. Two types of OA are commonly recognized: primary, the most common form, which appears to be related to aging and heredity, and secondary, which may occur in any joint due to articular injury. The characteristics of OA include pain, muscle atrophy, deformity, impaired function, crepitus, swelling, inflammation, and joint effusion. OA is typically diagnosed through the history and radiographs.

*Osteoporosis*. This is a systemic skeletal disorder characterized by decreased bone mass and deterioration of bony microarchitecture resulting from a combination of genetic and environmental factors that affect both peak bone mass and the rate of bone loss. These factors include medications, diet, race, sex, lifestyle, and physical activity. Osteoporosis is typically diagnosed through medical history, physical examination, and diagnostic tests, including a bone density scan, also known as dual-energy X-ray absorptiometry (DXA or DEXA), a special type of X-ray of the spine, hips, and other parts of the body. The FRAX (Fracture Risk Assessment Tool) is a computer-based tool that uses an individual's medical history, physical examination, and other risk factors to estimate their risk of experiencing a fracture due to osteoporosis over the next 10 years. While there is no cure for osteoporosis, early diagnosis and appropriate treatment can help prevent further bone loss and reduce the risk of complications, such as fractures.

*Proximal Femur/Hip Fracture*. Hip fractures result in significant mortality, morbidity, and costs and are an increasingly common injury among older people, who usually experience significantly worse mobility, independence in function, health, quality of life, and high institutionalization rates. Studies have shown that only 40–60% of participants recover their prefracture level of mobility and ability to perform instrumental ADLs, while for those who are independent in self-care before the fracture, 20–60% still require assistance for various tasks 1 or 2 years after the fracture [34]. Apart from age, osteoporosis is the other major risk factor for a hip fracture. Other risk factors include those that increase the risk of falling, including muscle weakness and balance problems, medications that provoke dizziness, poor vision, environmental hazards, alcohol consumption, and poorly fitting or inappropriate footwear.

Symptoms of a proximal hip fracture may include pain in the hip, groin, or thigh; difficulty bearing weight on the affected leg; swelling; bruising; and limited hip range of motion.

*Diabetes Mellitus (DM)*. DM is a chronic disorder of carbohydrates, fats, and protein metabolism caused by a deficiency or absence of insulin secretion by the beta cells of the pancreas or by defects of the insulin receptors. The morbidity and mortality associated with diabetes are related to short- and long-term complications. Complications of DM include hypoglycemia, hyperglycemia, increased risk of infections and skin ulcerations, microvascular disease and complications (e.g., retinopathy, nephropathy), neuropathic complications that often lead to foot ulceration and eventual amputation, and blindness.

Resources for geriatric physical therapy are available at the Academy of Geriatric Physical Therapy. They offer information on payment, policy, and resources for continuing education. Research is published in the *Journal of Geriatric Physical Therapy*, and a magazine, *GeriNotes*, publishes articles of interest to physical therapy professionals. The group has also defined entry-level and advanced skills for PTs and PTAs working in geriatric settings, which can be found on their website.

### Geriatric Interventions

Physical therapy intervention goals are geared toward the patient as a whole person and the patient's functionality within the care environment. The geriatric patient's optimal health is contingent on health-conducive behaviors, prevention of disability, and compensation for health-related losses and impairment of aging. The PTA works closely with the PT and is involved in the ongoing reexamination of the geriatric patient.

The interventions used in geriatric physical therapy depend on the disease process. Rehabilitating the aged adult is very challenging for the PT and the PTA. Understanding the normal aging process and pathologies common to aged patients can assist the PTA in creating appropriate interventions within the POC [10]. To maintain the highest level of function for the longest time, the PT and the PTA must consider the patient's neurologic decline and physical functioning capabilities. In many situations, the geriatric patient has multiple conditions that must be treated simultaneously. Multiple diagnoses can negatively impact impairments that complicate ADLs and hinder maximal functional capabilities.

*Osteoarthritis (OA)*. The goals of a physical therapy intervention include the reduction of pain and stiffness through the use of thermal modalities, therapeutic exercises to maintain or improve range of motion and correct muscle imbalances, improve balance and ambulation, provide assistive devices (canes, walkers, orthotics, reachers, etc.) as needed, and patient education about joint protection strategies and promotion of a healthy lifestyle, for example, weight reduction. The medical intervention for OA includes nonsteroidal anti-inflammatory drugs (NSAIDs), corticosteroid injections, topical analgesics, and surgical joint replacement.

*Osteoporosis*. Physical therapy's primary role in osteoporosis is prevention through weight-bearing exercises and other interventions to help improve balance, strength, and mobility and reduce the risk of falls.

*Proximal Femur/Hip Fracture*. Physical therapy is important in preventing hip fractures by identifying individuals who are fall risks and addressing activity level, weight-bearing activities, flexibility,

strengthening, and education regarding a safe physical environment.

*Diabetes Mellitus (DM)*. Physical therapy can address many aspects of DM, including patient/family education on proper diabetic foot care, controlling risk factors (obesity, physical inactivity, prolonged stress, and smoking), injury prevention and self-management strategies, and prescriptive exercises. Exercise has been shown to delay the disease onset, improve blood glucose levels and circulation, reduce cardiovascular risk, and aid in weight control and strength gains [35, 36].

## CASE STUDY

You are examining an 80-year-old male patient whose main diagnosis is phase IV peripheral arterial disease (PAD), intermittent claudication in the right lower extremity, and septic necrosis of the right heel. The patient's past medical history is extensive and includes hypertension, type II insulin-dependent diabetes, peripheral polyneuropathy, retinopathy, a left trans-tibial amputation (2 years post), and right trans-tibial amputation (last year), two saphenous vein bypasses, and three angioplasties.

Your examination revealed the following:

- The patient lives with his wife in a bungalow with wheelchair access. The patient uses a wheelchair inside the home but is able to walk outside with a four-wheel roller walker and his prostheses for short distances.
- Patient/ family goals: He already knows the process of fitting and rehabilitation and he aims to walk, with a prosthesis, the same way as "before". The family supports him.
- Memory, attention, orientation, perception, initiative, and multitasking functions are moderately limited.
- Cardiovascular functions include PAD.
- Sensory functions are impaired (sight and sensitivity on the right side).
- Proprioceptive function and balance are low, if tested sitting in the bed without prostheses, but transfers to wheelchair with transfer board need minimal assistance, as well as donning/doffing the prostheses and wheelchair use.
- Pain is medicated, but phantom pain is noted.
- Joint mobility measures show bilateral loss of hip flexion (flexion 10° L, and 0° R) and a tendency to posture in knee flexion, on both sides.
- Strength loss is 3/5 throughout left and right lower extremities and 4/5 throughout left and right upper extremities.
- Scar and skin are very fragile.

Based on the examination findings, the physical therapy diagnosis is a double lower extremity amputation with resultant poor function and balance, placing the patient at a high fall risk.

In your groups, create:

- A problem list for this patient, and design both short-term (1-month) and long-term (6-month) goals.
- Interventions to increase range of motion, strength, balance, function, and stump care.
- A gait training program

## Oncology

PTs and PTAs may specialize in the care of patients with cancer or secondary impairments due to cancer or cancer treatments, including cardiopulmonary, integumentary, musculoskeletal, and neurologic conditions. Working with this group of people aims to maximize their function and promote wellness.

*Rehabilitation Oncology* is a journal published by the Academy of Oncologic Physical Therapy. In addition, students can find continuing education offerings and special interest groups on their website.

## Women's Health

Specialization in conditions that affect women may include incontinence, pregnancy and postpartum care, mastectomy and cancer recovery, and pelvic pain. PTs and PTAs in this practice area utilize their knowledge of muscle structure and function to assist patients in relieving pain and promote living a full and active lifestyle.

Research has demonstrated that women have distinct physiological differences and are more prone to certain conditions than men, such as myocardial infarction and ovarian and breast cancer. Pregnancy, which is gender-based; urinary incontinence; and breast cancer–related lymphatic dysfunction provide their own challenges.

### Pregnancy

Some physiologic changes occur within the various body systems during pregnancy and postpartum, requiring an assessment of the various systems (see **Figure 5-12**).

- *Endocrine*. Changes that occur in the endocrine system include, but are not limited to, the following:
  - The adrenal, thyroid, parathyroid, and pituitary glands enlarge.
  - Hormone levels increase to support the pregnancy and the placenta and to prepare the mother's body for labor. During pregnancy, a female hormone (relaxin) is released that assists in the softening of the pubic symphysis so that, during delivery, the female pelvis can expand sufficiently to allow birth. However, these hormonal changes are also thought to induce a greater laxity in all joints. This laxity can result in joint hypermobility, especially throughout the pelvic ring, which relies heavily on ligamentous support, symphysis pubis dysfunction (SPD), and sacroiliac joint (SIJ) dysfunction.

- *Musculoskeletal*. Changes that occur in the musculoskeletal system include, but are not limited to, the following:
  - Stretching and weakening of the abdominal muscles as the pregnancy develops
  - An increase in the incidence of low back pain (LBP) and pelvic pain
  - Pelvic floor weakness: The weakness can develop with advanced pregnancy and childbirth owing to the increased weight and pressure directly over these muscles—the pelvic floor drops as much as 2.5 cm (1 inch) as a result of pregnancy and can result in a condition called *stress incontinence*.

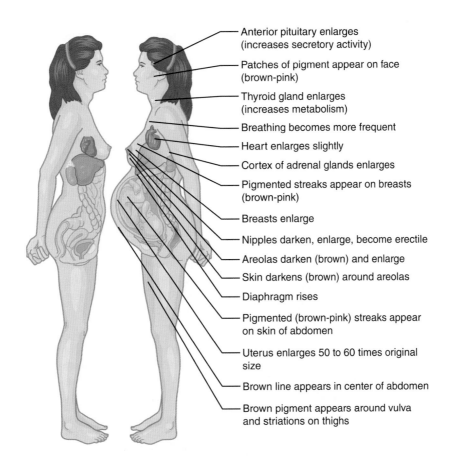

Anterior pituitary enlarges (increases secretory activity)

Patches of pigment appear on face (brown-pink)

Thyroid gland enlarges (increases metabolism)

Breathing becomes more frequent

Heart enlarges slightly

Cortex of adrenal glands enlarges

Pigmented streaks appear on breasts (brown-pink)

Breasts enlarge

Nipples darken, enlarge, become erectile

Areolas darken (brown) and enlarge

Skin darkens (brown) around areolas

Diaphragm rises

Pigmented (brown-pink) streaks appear on skin of abdomen

Uterus enlarges 50 to 60 times original size

Brown line appears in center of abdomen

Brown pigment appears around vulva and striations on thighs

**Figure 5-12** Physical changes during pregnancy

- Postural changes: These changes are related to the weight of growing breasts and the uterus and fetus, resulting in a shift in the woman's center of gravity in an anterior and superior direction, requiring postural compensations to maintain stability and balance.

- *Neurologic.* Swelling and increased fluid volume can cause peripheral nerve entrapments, such as thoracic outlet syndrome due to brachial plexus compression, carpal tunnel syndrome due to median nerve compression, or meralgia paresthetica due to compression of the lateral femoral cutaneous nerve of the thigh.

- *Gastrointestinal.* Nausea and vomiting may occur in early pregnancy and are confined to the first 16 weeks of pregnancy but occasionally remain throughout the entire 10 lunar months. Other gastrointestinal changes include a slowing of intestinal motility, constipation, abdominal bloating, hemorrhoids, esophageal reflux, heartburn (pyrosis), and an increase in the incidence and symptoms of gallbladder disease.

- *Respiratory.* Adaptive changes in the pulmonary system during pregnancy include increased ventilation as the rib cage circumference expands, producing a natural state of hyperventilation to meet oxygen demands.

- *Cardiovascular.* The pregnancy-induced changes develop primarily to meet the increased metabolic demands of the mother and fetus, including increased blood and plasma volume and an overall increase in cardiac output.

- *Metabolic.* The metabolic rate increases during both exercise and pregnancy, resulting in greater heat production. Because of the increased demand for tissue growth, insulin is elevated from plasma expansion, and blood glucose is reduced for a given insulin load. Fats and minerals are stored for maternal use.

- *Genitourinary.* During pregnancy, there is an increase in sodium and water retention [37]. Anatomic and hormonal changes during pregnancy place the pregnant woman at risk for lower and upper urinary tract infections and incontinence [37]. As the fetus grows, stress on the mother's bladder can occur, resulting in urinary incontinence.

In addition to the foregoing conditions, pregnancy can produce some or all of the following complications:

- *Hypertension.* Hypertensive disorders complicating pregnancy are the most common medical risk factor responsible for maternal morbidity and death related to pregnancy [37]. Hypertensive disorders complicating pregnancy have been divided into five types (**Table 5-7**).

- *Symphysis Pubis Dysfunction.* This disorder can occur during pregnancy or, more commonly, due to trauma during vaginal delivery. The symptoms vary from person to person, but typically, the patient reports pain with any activity that involves lifting one leg at a time or parting the legs. Lifting the leg to put on clothes, getting out of a car, bending over, turning over in bed, sitting down or getting up, walking upstairs, standing on one leg, lifting heavy objects, and walking are all painful. The amount of symphyseal separation does not always correlate with the severity of symptoms or the degree of disability; therefore, the intervention is based on the severity of the symptoms. Patient education is essential in providing advice on how to avoid stress in the

**Table 5-7** **Summary of Types of Hypertension During Pregnancy**

| Disorder | Signs/Symptoms |
|---|---|
| Gestational hypertension | Epigastric pain, thrombocytopenia, headache. |
| Preeclampsia | The more severe the hypertension or proteinuria, the more certain the severity of preeclampsia; symptoms of eclampsia, such as a headache, cerebral visual disturbance, and epigastric pain, can occur. |
| Eclampsia | The mother may develop abruptio placentae, neurological deficits, aspiration pneumonia, pulmonary edema, cardiopulmonary arrest, or acute renal failure, which may cause maternal death. |
| Superimposed preeclampsia on chronic hypertension | The risk of abruptio placentae; fetus at risk for growth restriction and death. |
| Chronic hypertension | The risk of abruptio placentae; the fetus is at risk for growth restriction and death; pulmonary edema; hypertensive encephalopathy; renal failure. |

Data from Boissonnault JS, Stephenson R: The Obstetric Patient, in Boissonnault WG (ed): Primary Care for the Physical Therapist: Examination and Triage. St Louis, Elsevier Saunders, 2005, pp 239–270.

area. Some of the suggestions to provide include the following:

- Use a pillow between the legs when sleeping.
- Move slowly and without sudden movements. Keep the legs and hips parallel and symmetrical when moving or turning in standing and in bed. Silk/satin sheets and night garments may make it easier to turn over in bed.
- When standing, stand symmetrically, with the weight evenly distributed through both legs. Avoid "straddle" movements.

Most exercises that do not stress the pubic symphysis are safe to perform. The recommended activities are swimming (avoiding the breaststroke), gentle walking (taking short strides), indoor stationary cycling, and elliptical machines. Deep-water aerobics or deep-water running using floatation devices may also be helpful.

- *Peripartum Posterior Pelvic Pain (PPPP)*. Over 50% of women experience peripartum PPPP during pregnancy, with one-third experiencing severe pain [38]. The etiology of PPPP has been linked to the physiological adaptation of the pelvis in preparation for childbirth, which is accomplished through connective tissue softening around the pelvis, pubic symphysis, and sacroiliac joint. Patient education should be provided about posture/body mechanics and equal weight bearing through both lower extremities (avoiding one-legged standing).
- *Diastasis Recti Abdominis (DRA)*. DRA is defined as a lateral separation of greater than two fingertip widths of the two bellies of the rectus abdominis at the linea alba (or linea nigra, in pregnancy) that can occur during pregnancy or delivery, resulting in a decreased ability of the abdominal musculature to stabilize the pelvis and lumbar spine with subsequent functional limitations. If DRA is confirmed, corrective exercises must be performed to prevent further muscle trauma.
- *Supine Hypotension*. This condition (inferior vena cava syndrome) may develop in the supine position, especially after the first trimester. The decrease in blood pressure is thought to be caused by the occlusion of the aorta and inferior vena cava by the increased weight and size of the uterus. Spontaneous recovery usually occurs on a change of maternal position.

## Urinary Incontinence

Urinary incontinence may be defined as an involuntary loss of urine sufficient to be a problem and occurs most often when bladder pressure exceeds sphincter resistance. The following four categories can be used to classify urinary incontinence [39]:

- *Functional incontinence:* Includes people who have normal urine control but are unwilling to use a toilet (impaired cognition) or who have difficulty reaching a toilet in time because of muscle or joint dysfunction or environmental barriers.
- *Stress incontinence:* The loss of urine during activities that increase intra-abdominal pressure, such as coughing, lifting, or laughing.
- *Overflow incontinence:* The constant leaking of urine from a bladder that is full but unable to empty due to anatomic obstruction (e.g., pregnancy) or neurogenic bladder (e.g., spinal cord injury).
- *Urge incontinence:* The sudden unexpected urge to urinate and the uncontrolled loss of urine, often related to reduced bladder capacity, detrusor instability, or hypersensitive bladder.

Physical therapy is important in assessing and treating urge and stress urinary incontinence, particularly in pelvic floor muscle rehabilitation. The pelvic floor muscles work in a coordinated manner to increase intra-abdominal pressure, provide rectal support during defecation, inhibit bladder activity, help support the pelvic organs, and assist in lumbopelvic stability [40]. Medical management of urinary incontinence is aimed at prevention and may include the following:

- Nutritional counseling to help prevent constipation and to encourage adequate hydration
- Medications to relieve urge incontinence, such as estrogen replacement therapy (ERT), anticholinergics, alpha-adrenergic blockers to increase bladder outlet/sphincteric tone, antispasmodics, and combination therapy with tricyclic antidepressant agents and antidiuretic hormone [41–44]
- Surgical intervention can include catheterization and surgically implanted artificial sphincters and bladder generators (sends impulses to the nerves that control the bladder function).

## Breast Cancer-Related Lymphedema

With early diagnosis, effective treatment of lymphedema can prevent numerous problems, including infection, loss of mobility, and long-standing physical and psychosocial problems [45]. The lymphatic system is a network of strategically placed lymph nodes connected by a substantial network of lymphatic vessels, which act as the circulatory system for the immune system. Lymphedema is an incurable, chronic, progressive, and often debilitating disease caused by intrinsic or acquired defects accumulating protein-rich fluid in the lymphatic system [46]. Breast cancer–related dysfunction of the lymphatic system and subsequent lymphedema of the upper extremity can occur as a complication of the treatment for breast cancer. Clinicians use a variety of strategies to diagnose upper extremity (UE) lymphedema. Lymphoscintigraphy is considered the gold standard for identifying lymphatic insufficiency in patients in whom the cause of swelling is unclear [46]. The most widely used strategy is circumferential UE measurements using specific anatomical landmarks. Arm circumference measurements estimate volume differences between the affected and unaffected UEs. A more accurate measure of volume difference is the water displacement technique.

Resources in women's health physical therapy include the APTA Section of Women's Health, the Section on Women's Health Student Interest Group, the *Journal of Women's Health Physical Therapy*, and the APTA's Physical Therapy Health Center for Women webpage.

Physical therapy interventions depend on the pathophysiology of the skin disorder or dysfunction. For other skin disorders, the treatment may consist of the following (see Chapter 12):

- Patient education about the disorder
- Therapeutic exercises
- Functional training for ADLs and skin and joint protection
- Modalities such as light therapy, ultrasound, aquatic therapy, whirlpool, pulsed lavage, heat, paraffin baths, fluidotherapy, tilt table, and compression therapy

## Women's Health Interventions

Interventions for women's health vary depending on the presenting condition.

## Exercise During Pregnancy

Both exercise and pregnancy are associated with a high demand for energy as the caloric demands with exercise during pregnancy are very high. The competing energy demands of the exercising mother and the growing fetus traditionally raised concern that excessive exercise might adversely affect fetal development, but several studies suggest the opposite [47, 48]. Although it is strongly recommended that all women participate in mild to moderate exercise,

based on prepregnancy fitness level, for both strength and cardiopulmonary benefits, exercise activity should occur at a moderate rate during a low-risk pregnancy. Contraindications to exercise during pregnancy include [49]:

- An incompetent cervix (early dilation of the cervix before pregnancy is full-term)
- Vaginal bleeding (especially in the second or third trimester)
- Placenta previa (the placenta is located in the uterus in a position where it may detach before the baby is delivered)
- History of multiple gestations with a risk of premature labor
- Pregnancy-induced hypertension
- Premature labor (labor beginning before the 37th week of pregnancy)
- Maternal heart disease
- Maternal type I diabetes
- Intrauterine growth retardation

Increases in joint laxity due to changes in hormonal levels may lead to a higher risk of strains or sprains, so weight-bearing exercises should be prescribed judiciously. Adequate hydration and appropriate ventilation are important in preventing the possible teratogenic effects of overheating. The goals of therapeutic exercise during pregnancy are to improve muscle balance and posture, help provide support for the growing uterus, stabilize the trunk and pelvis, and maintain function for more rapid recovery after delivery [50].

### Urinary Incontinence

A typical physical therapy intervention for pelvic floor dysfunction includes:

- Patient education, which should include:
  - Visual aids, with emphasis placed on both the sling/hammock (anterior–posterior) orientation of the fibers and the figure of eight (circumferential) orientation
  - Advising the patient to avoid the Valsalva maneuver
  - Advising the patient to avoid activities that strain the pelvic floor and abdominal muscles
  - Education to preserve acceptable skin condition [51]:
    - Education about adequate protection—adult diapers, underpads
    - Maintenance of a toileting schedule
  - The importance of psychological and emotional support

- Exercise to improve control of the pelvic floor and to maintain abdominal function, including pelvic floor muscle exercises, emphasizing both fast-twitch and slow-twitch muscle fibers, so there is a significant increase in the force of the urethral closure without an appreciable Valsalva effort. These exercises include two types of Kegel exercises [52–54]:
  - *Type 1:* Works on holding contractions, progressing to 10-second holds and resting 10 seconds between contractions.
  - *Type 2:* Works on quick contractions to shut off urine flow. The patient should perform 10–80 repetitions daily while avoiding buttock squeezing or contracting the abdominals. The patient should be encouraged to incorporate Kegel exercises into everyday life, especially when lifting, coughing, laughing, changing positions, and so on. Exercises should also include progressive strengthening of the pelvic floor musculature with weighted vaginal cones and pelvic floor exerciser.
- Biofeedback to reinforce active contraction and relaxation of the bladder [55]
- Functional electrical stimulation for muscle reeducation of the bladder and pelvic floor muscles [55]
- Noninvasive pulsed magnetic fields (extracorporeal magnetic innervation) for pelvic floor muscle strengthening [51]

### Breast Cancer–Related Lymphedema

Current treatment for breast cancer usually involves removing a portion or all of the breast accompanied by excision or radiation of the adjacent axillary lymph nodes, the principal site of regional metastasis [56]. Axillary dissection places a patient at risk for upper extremity lymphedema and loss of shoulder mobility and limited arm and hand function [57].

Complete decongestive therapy (CDT) is the company-recognized standard of care for lymphedema. The essential components of CDT include the following [56]:

- Compression and exercise: Exercise encourages skeletal muscle contractions to provide the primary pumping mechanism for lymphatic and venous drainage and, therefore, should stimulate the contraction of lymph vessels because the sympathetic nervous system innervates these vessels. Progressive resistance training (using light weights initially and progressing as tolerated) while wearing fitted compression sleeves should include the following exercises: seated row, bench press, latissimus dorsi muscle pull-down, one-arm bent-over rowing, triceps muscle extension, and biceps curl [58]. After 2 weeks, an additional progressive upper-body aerobic exercise at moderate intensities can be implemented on an arm ergometer.
- ROM exercises to address any muscle imbalances listed in the POC
- Manual lymphatic drainage (MLD): The sessions, which typically use the Vodder techniques (see Chapter 9), last 30–90 minutes, and subsequent bandaging helps to maintain and improve the decongestion. The techniques use specific circular and spiral-shaped movements with gentle skin-to-skin contact. These methods increase and decrease pressure, creating a pumping effect, and the direction of the increase in pressure lies in the direction of the lymph flow.

**KNOWLEDGE CHECK**

What pediatric screening tool is common in elementary school–aged children?
Why are environmental examinations important?

## Discussion Questions

1. The patient is returning home after a cerebrovascular accident (stroke). They can walk independently with a walker but have difficulty with stairs. Their home has the same layout and conditions as your current home. What changes must be made to create a safe home for this patient?
2. Make a list of examination categories and discuss how these will be assessed. Identify any examination skills that people in your group already know how to perform.
3. Discuss the components of the POC and how the PTA will utilize this information with a patient.
4. The PTA is teaching the patient about avoiding a recurrence of LBP. Discuss strategies that will help ensure that the patient understands the information.

5. Discuss with your classmates the different types of therapeutic exercise and how each is used: isometric, isotonic, and isokinetic resistance exercises; flexibility exercises; and ROM exercises (PROM, AAROM, and AROM).

6. Share with your classmates the opportunities and experiences you have had in each practice area of physical therapy: orthopedic, neurologic, geriatric, pediatric, cardiopulmonary, and integumentary.

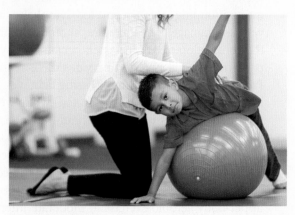

© FatCamera/E+/Getty Images

## Learning Opportunities

1. The PTA is creating an intake form for new patients. Create a list of questions to obtain a patient history.
2. Observe a PTA performing examination activities. Interview the PTA about the rationale for collecting the information, and describe how the information will be used.
3. Perform an internet search to identify websites or videos that can assist the PTA in learning examination skills, such as obtaining blood pressure, assessing skin sensation, and performing standardized balance examinations.

4. Using the APTA website and the APTA Section websites (www.apta.org), develop a list of resources to develop skills in the physical therapy practice areas.
5. The PTA works with a 3-year-old patient who needs an assistive device to stand and ambulate. Utilizing the internet, explore the options for standing positioning and mobility devices.
6. Utilize commercial websites to find examples of different types of assistive devices used for gait: walkers, canes, and so on. Consider what would be appropriate for different age groups (pediatric versus geriatric).

## References

1. Goodman CC, Snyder TK: Introduction to Screening for Referral in Physical Therapy, in Goodman CC, Snyder TK (eds): Differential Diagnosis in Physical Therapy. Philadelphia, Saunders, 2012, pp 1–30
2. Seifert F, Maihofner C: Central mechanisms of experimental and chronic neuropathic pain: findings from functional imaging studies. Cell Mol Life Sci 66(3):375–390, 2009
3. Palsson TS, Graven-Nielsen T: Experimental pelvic pain facilitates pain provocation tests and causes regional hyperalgesia. Pain 153(11):2233–2240, 2012
4. Kmiecik MJ, Tu FF, Silton RL, et al: Cortical mechanisms of visual hypersensitivity in women at risk for chronic pelvic pain. Pain 163(6):1035–1048, 2022
5. Li W, Gong Y, Liu J, et al: Peripheral and central pathological mechanisms of chronic low back pain: a narrative review. J Pain Res 14:1483–1494, 2021
6. Grzesiak AJ, Bailey T: Coming to our senses with chronic pain. Ortho Phys Ther Pract 31(2):74–77, 2019
7. Lentz TA, Beneciuk JM, Bialosky JE, et al: Development of a Yellow Flag Assessment Tool for orthopaedic physical therapists: results from the Optimal Screening for Prediction of

Referral and Outcome (OSPRO) cohort. J Orthop Sports Phys Ther 46(5):327–343, 2016
8. Salathe CR, Trippolini MA, Terribilini LC, et al: Assessing psycho-social barriers to rehabilitation in injured workers with chronic musculoskeletal pain: development and item properties of the Yellow Flag Questionnaire (YFQ). J Occup Rehabil 28(2):365–376, 2018
9. O'Sullivan SB: Clinical Decision-Making, in O'Sullivan SB, Schmitz TJ (eds): Physical Rehabilitation. Philadelphia, FA Davis, 2007, pp 3–24
10. O'Sullivan SB: Stroke, in O'Sullivan SB, Schmitz TJ (eds): Physical Rehabilitation. FA Philadelphia, Davis, 2007, pp 705–776
11. American Physical Therapy Association: Guide to Physical Therapist Practice 3.0. Alexandria, VA, American Physical Therapy Association, 2014
12. Watson T: The role of electrotherapy in contemporary physiotherapy practice. Man Ther 5:132–141, 2000
13. Shumway-Cook A, Woollacott MH: A Conceptual Framework for Clinical Practice, in Shumway-Cook A, Woollacott MH (eds): Motor Control – Translating Research into Clinical

Practice. Philadelphia, Lippincott Williams and Wilkins, 2007, pp 137–153

14. Shumway-Cook A, Woollacott MH: Motor Learning and Recovery of Function, in Shumway-Cook A, Woollacott MH (eds): Motor Control – Translating Research into Clinical Practice. Philadelphia, Lippincott Williams and Wilkins, 2007, pp 21–45

15. Miedzybrodzka Z: Congenital talipes equinovarus (clubfoot): a disorder of the foot but not the hand. J Anat 202(1):37–42, 2003

16. Aronsson DD, Goldberg MJ, Kling TF Jr, et al: Developmental dysplasia of the hip. Pediatrics 94(2 Pt 1):201–208, 1994

17. Ortolani M: Un segno poco noto e sue importanza per la diagnosi precoce di prelussazione congenita dell'anca. Pediatria 45:129–136, 1937

18. Barlow TG: Early diagnosis and treatment of congenital dislocation of the hip. J Bone Joint Surg [Br] 44:292–301, 1962

19. Leach J: Orthopedic Conditions, in Campbell SK, Vander Linden DW, Palisano RJ (eds): Physical Therapy for Children. St. Louis, Saunders, 2006, pp 481–515

20. Wright FV, Law M, Crombie V, et al: Development of a self-report functional status index for juvenile rheumatoid arthritis. J Rheumatol 21(3):536–544, 1994

21. Howe S, Levinson J, Shear E, et al: Development of a disability measurement tool for juvenile rheumatoid arthritis. The Juvenile Arthritis Functional Assessment Report for Children and their Parents. Arthritis Rheum 34(7):873–880, 1991

22. Duffy CM, Arsenault L, Duffy KN, et al: The Juvenile Arthritis Quality of Life Questionnaire—development of a new responsive index for juvenile rheumatoid arthritis and juvenile spondyloarthritides. J Rheumatol 24:738–746, 1997

23. Deconinck N, Dan B: Pathophysiology of Duchenne muscular dystrophy: current hypotheses. Pediatr Neurol 36(1):1–7, 2007

24. Eagle M, Bourke J, Bullock R, et al: Managing Duchenne muscular dystrophy—the additive effect of spinal surgery and home nocturnal ventilation in improving survival. Neuromuscul Disord 17(6):470–475, 2007

25. Sussman M: Duchenne muscular dystrophy. J Am Acad Orthop Surg 10(2):138–151, 2002

26. Vroland-Nordstrand K, Eliasson AC, Jacobsson H, et al: Can children identify and achieve goals for intervention? A randomized trial comparing two goal-setting approaches. Dev Med Child Neurol 6(58):589–596, 2016

27. Kaplan SL, Coulter C, Sargent B: Physical Therapy Management of Congenital Muscular Torticollis: a 2018 evidence-based clinical practice guideline from the APTA Academy of Pediatric Physical Therapy. Pediatr Phys Ther 30(4):240–290, 2018

28. Clayton-Krasinski D, Klepper S: Impaired Neuromotor Development, in Cameron MH, Monroe LG (eds): Physical Rehabilitation: Evidence-Based Examination, Evaluation, and Intervention. St Louis, MO, Saunders/Elsevier, 2007, pp 333–366

29. Zach MS, Purrer B, Oberwaldner B: Effect of swimming on forced expiration and sputum clearance in cystic fibrosis. Lancet 2(8257):1201–1203, 1981

30. Orenstein DM, Franklin BA, Doershuk CF, et al: Exercise conditioning and cardiopulmonary fitness in cystic fibrosis. The effects of a three-month supervised running program. Chest 80(4):392–398, 1981

31. Stuberg WA: Muscular Dystrophy and Spinal Muscular Atrophy, in Campbell SK, Vander Linden DW, Palisano RJ (eds): Physical Therapy for Children. St. Louis, Saunders, 2006, pp 21–451

32. Harman D: Aging: phenomena and theories. Ann N Y Acad Sci 854:1–7, 1998

33. Lewis CB, Bottomley JM: Geriatric Physical Therapy: A Clinical Approach. Norwalk, CT, Appleton & Lange, 1994

34. Solou K, Tyllianakis M, Kouzelis A, et al: Morbidity and mortality after second hip fracture with and without nursing care program. Cureus 14(3):e23373, 2022

35. Mota GAF, Gatto M, Pagan LU, et al: Diabetes mellitus, physical exercise and heart rate variability. Arq Bras Cardiol 120(1):e20220902, 2023

36. Hall LG, Thyfault JP, Johnson JD: Exercise and inactivity as modifiers of beta cell function and type 2 diabetes risk. J Appl Physiol (1985) 134(4):823–839, 2023

37. Boissonnault JS, Stephenson R: The Obstetric Patient, in Boissonnault WG (ed): Primary Care for the Physical Therapist: Examination and Triage. St Louis, Elsevier Saunders, 2005, pp 239–270

38. Hall J, Cleland JA, Palmer JA: The effects of manual physical therapy and therapeutic exercise on peripartum posterior pelvic pain: two case reports. J Man Manip Ther 13(2):94–102, 2005

39. Boissonnault WG, Goodman CC: The Renal and Urologic Systems, in Goodman CC, Boissonnault WG, Fuller KS (eds): Pathology: Implications for the Physical Therapist. Philadelphia, Saunders, 2003, pp 704–728

40. Markwell SJ: Physical therapy management of pelvi/perineal and perianal pain syndromes. World J Urol 19:194–199, 2001

41. Blackwell RE: Estrogen, progestin, and urinary incontinence. JAMA 294(21):2696–2697, 2005; author reply 2697–2698

42. Bren L: Controlling urinary incontinence. FDA Consum 39(5):10–15, 2005

43. Castro-Diaz D, Amoros MA: Pharmacotherapy for stress urinary incontinence. Curr Opin Urol 15(4):227–230, 2005

44. Kelleher C, Cardozo L, Kobashi K, et al: Solifenacin: as effective in mixed urinary incontinence as in urge urinary incontinence. Int Urogynecol J Pelvic Floor Dysfunct 17(4):382–388, 2006

45. Rockson SG: Causes and consequences of lymphatic disease. Ann N Y Acad Sci 1207 Suppl 1:E2–E6, 2010

46. Warren AG, Brorson H, Borud LJ, et al: Lymphedema: a comprehensive review. Ann Plast Surg 59(4):464–472, 2007

47. Wang C, Wei Y, Zhang X, et al: A randomized clinical trial of exercise during pregnancy to prevent gestational diabetes mellitus and improve pregnancy outcome in overweight and obese pregnant women. Am J Obstet Gynecol 216(4): 340–351, 2017

48. Barakat R, Perales M, Cordero Y, et al: Influence of land or water exercise in pregnancy on outcomes: a cross-sectional study. Med Sci Sports Exerc 49(7):1397–1403, 2017

49. Settles-Huge B: Women's Health: Obstetrics and Pelvic Floor, in Kisner C, Colby LA (eds): Therapeutic Exercise. Foundations and Techniques. Philadelphia, FA Davis, 2002, pp 797–824

50. Strauhal MJ: Therapeutic Exercise in Obstetrics, in Hall C, Thein-Brody L (eds): Therapeutic Exercise: Moving Toward Function. Baltimore, MD, Lippincott Williams & Wilkins, 2005, pp 259–281

51. Wilson MM: Urinary incontinence: selected current concepts. Med Clin North Am 90(5):825–836, 2006

52. Borello-France DF, Zyczynski HM, Downey PA, et al: Effect of pelvic-floor muscle exercise position on continence and quality-of-life outcomes in women with stress urinary incontinence. Phys Ther 86(7):974–986, 2006

53. Neumann PB, Grimmer KA, Deenadayalan Y: Pelvic floor muscle training and adjunctive therapies for the treatment

of stress urinary incontinence in women: a systematic review. BMC Womens Health 6:11, 2006

54. Hay-Smith EJ, Dumoulin C: Pelvic floor muscle training versus no treatment, or inactive control treatments, for urinary incontinence in women. Cochrane Database Syst Rev (1):CD005654, 2006

55. Anders K: Treatments for stress urinary incontinence. Nurs Times 102(2):55–57, 2006

56. Kisner C, Colby LA: Management of Vascular Disorders of the Extremities, in Kisner C, Colby LA (eds): Therapeutic Exercise. Foundations and Techniques, 5th ed. Philadelphia, FA Davis, 2002, pp 825–849

57. Bicego D, Brown K, Ruddick M, et al: Exercise for women with or at risk for breast cancer-related lymphedema. Phys Ther 86(10):1398–1405, 2006

58. Johansson K, Tibe K, Weibull A, et al: Low intensity resistance exercise for breast cancer patients with arm lymphedema with or without compression sleeve. Lymphology 38(4):167–180, 2005

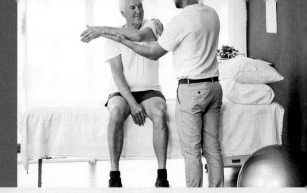

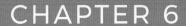
CHAPTER 6

# Ethics and Professionalism

## OBJECTIVES

- Define morals and ethics.
- Delineate the difference between medical law and medical ethics.
- List six biomedical ethical principles and their roles in health care.
- Discuss patient confidentiality.
- Describe the Health Insurance Portability and Accountability Act (HIPAA) of 1996.
- Discuss the patient's bill of rights and its importance to physical therapy practice.
- Explain cultural competence in health care and physical therapy.
- List the elements of full informed consent.
- Explain the guidelines for professional conduct physical therapists are morally bound to follow.
- Explain the guidelines for the conduct of the affiliate member that physical therapist assistants are morally bound to follow.
- Identify at least five directive ethical provisions expected of the physical therapist assistant.
- Discuss the eight value-based behaviors for the physical therapist assistant.

## KEY TERMS

autonomy
cultural competence
ethics

ethnocentrism
Health Insurance Portability and
    Accountability Act (HIPAA)

informed consent
morals
protected health information (PHI)

## Medical Ethics versus Medical Law

Medical ethics and medical law are disciplines with frequent areas of overlap, yet each discipline has unique standards. Medical law and medical ethics aim to create and maintain social good. They are both dynamic and in a constant state of change. For example, new legislation and court decisions occur, and medical ethics respond to challenges created by new laws by providing new ethical standards.

## Medical Ethics

**Ethics** is a system of moral principles or standards governing a person's conduct. **Morals** are the basis for ethical conduct. They are an individual's beliefs, principles, and values about right and wrong. Morals are personal to each individual. If individuals want to do the "right thing," they try to act with moral virtue or character. Morals are culture based, culture driven, and time dependent.

    Medical ethics is a system of principles governing medical conduct. It deals with a physician's relationship with the patient, the patient's family, fellow physicians, and society. Also, medical ethics refers to how other healthcare providers conduct themselves professionally. For example, in physical therapy, we can say that physical therapy ethics is a system of principles governing a physical therapist (PT) or a physical therapist assistant (PTA). For the PTA, ethics deals with the relationship of a PTA to the patient, the patient's family, PTs, fellow PTAs, associates, and society at large.

The professional organization, the American Physical Therapy Association (APTA) (see Appendix E and H), derives physical therapy ethics for PTs and PTAs through its policies. These ethical policies, or guidelines, set standards of conduct the members of the APTA must adhere to. Generally, the ethics statements are significant professional and moral guides, but are unenforceable by law.

## Medical Law

Medical law is the establishment of social rules for conduct. A violation of medical law may create criminal and civil liability. Lawmakers frequently turn to policy statements, including medical ethics statements of professional organizations, when creating laws affecting that profession. In this way, healthcare providers may influence legal standards when creating professional ethics standards.

On many occasions, ethics and law can blend into common standards of professional conduct. Often, a breach of ethics may also constitute a violation of the law, and a violation of the law may also infringe on specific ethical principles. For example, in physical therapy, the 5A standard of the Standards of Ethical Conduct for PTAs states, "Physical therapist assistants shall comply with applicable local, state, and federal laws and regulations." Therefore, a PTA representing themselves as a PT violates the fifth standard of the Standards of Ethical Conduct and the professional licensing laws enacted by all states.

> ### KNOWLEDGE CHECK
>
> What is the difference between medical ethics and medical law?

# Biomedical Ethical Principles

Healthcare providers are guided by six fundamental biomedical ethical principles: beneficence, nonmaleficence, justice, integrity, confidentiality, and autonomy.

Healthcare providers use these ethical principles when working with patients, conducting clinical research, or educating students to care for patients. Various clinical situations can cause ethical dilemmas. Adherence to certain biomedical ethical principles can be controversial for some healthcare providers, depending on their moral values and social conditioning. Also, ethical principles may be debatable for people from other cultures or with different religious or civic beliefs. For example, being confronted with the truth about a grave medical condition can be extremely painful and even unacceptable to a patient or a patient's family from another culture. Nevertheless, traditional biomedical ethicists believe that ethical dilemmas should only be resolved by applying the most rational and objective rules and principles to each situation.

## Beneficence

Beneficence is the ethical principle that emphasizes doing the best for the patient. It means that healthcare providers must promote the health and welfare of the patient above other considerations. For PTs and PTAs, it means that they are bound to act in the patient's best interests in physical therapy clinical practices. An example of the ethical principle of beneficence for PTs and PTAs would be a genuine display of concern for the physical and psychological welfare of their patients and clients.

## Nonmaleficence

Nonmaleficence is the ethical principle that urges practitioners not to do anything that causes harm to any patient. Hippocrates, who lived around 400 BCE, the father of medicine, was the first physician to express ethical principles of beneficence and nonmaleficence in his Hippocratic Oath. Hippocrates felt nonmaleficence was one of the most important principles of medical practice. For PTs and PTAs, nonmaleficence means they cannot intentionally cause harm to patients/clients under their care. For example, a breach of the ethical principle of nonmaleficence would be to exploit the patient financially by selling the patient an unnecessary assistive device or one at an inflated price.

## Justice and Veracity

Justice is an ethical principle that mandates that a healthcare provider distribute fair and equal treatment to every patient. In the context of receiving health care justice requires that everyone receives equitable access to the basic health care necessary for living a fully human life. An example of the ethical principle of justice in physical therapy would be to advocate for legislatures, regulatory agencies, and insurance companies to provide and improve access to necessary healthcare services for all individuals (with and without health insurance).

Veracity is an ethical principle that binds the healthcare provider and the patient in a relationship to tell the truth. The patient must tell the truth concerning their history and symptoms for the healthcare provider to apply appropriate care, while the healthcare provider must tell the truth for the patient to exercise personal autonomy. PTs and PTAs must provide the patient with ethical and truthful information. For example, a breach of the ethical principle of integrity would be a PTA identifying themselves as a PT.

<hr>

**KNOWLEDGE CHECK**

How are beneficence and nonmaleficence alike, and
  how are they different?
What do the terms justice and veracity mean?

## Confidentiality

Confidentiality is an ethical principle that requires a healthcare provider to maintain privacy by not sharing or divulging to a third party privileged or entrusted patient information. The healthcare provider holds matters discussed by the patient in confidence, except in rare instances when the information poses a clear threat to the well-being of the patient or another person, or when public health may be compromised. Confidentiality is a fundamental ethical principle in health care, and a breach of confidentiality can be a reason for disciplinary action.

Maintaining patient confidentiality encourages patients to fully divulge relevant information so that the healthcare professional can properly assess the patient/client's condition. Occasionally, there may be circumstances where the public interest outweighs the interest in maintaining confidentiality. For example, disclosing confidential information without a patient/client's consent to prevent a crime might be justified.

In physical therapy, as with any health profession, a patient's information is confidential and should not be communicated to a third party not involved in that patient's care without the patient's prior consent. A PTA should refer all requests to release confidential information to the supervising PT. A PT may disclose information to appropriate authorities when it is

Examples of federal statutes that require disclosure of confidential information (that would otherwise be breaches of confidentiality):

- The Police and Criminal Evidence Act of 1984 indicates that the police can access medical records for a criminal investigation by applying to a circuit judge.
- The Public Health (Control of Disease) Act of 1984 and Public Health (Infectious Diseases) Regulations of 1988 indicate that a doctor must notify the relevant local authority if they suspect a patient of having a notifiable disease. AIDS and HIV are not notifiable diseases. Examples of notifiable diseases (in 2010) include anthrax, botulism, cholera, diphtheria, or gonorrhea.
- The Abortion Regulations of 1991 indicate that a doctor carrying out a termination of pregnancy must notify the relevant chief medical officer, including giving the name and address of the involved patient.
- The Births and Deaths Registration Act of 1953 indicates that a healthcare professional or a midwife normally must inform the district medical officer of a birth within 6 hours; stillbirths must also be registered. Healthcare professionals attending patients during their last illness must sign a death certificate and give a cause of death.
- The Children Act of 1989 regulates many aspects of childcare, including a healthcare professional's duties to report suspicion of child abuse.

necessary to protect an individual's or the community's welfare or when required by law.

Even without ethical principles and standards, healthcare providers are bound by state and federal laws to maintain patient/client confidentiality. A breach of confidentiality can include disclosure to a third party without patient consent by various media, such as orally, written, telephone, fax, electronically, or via email. State and federal laws protecting patients' confidentiality include:

- Federal and state constitutional privacy rights
- Federal legislation and regulation governing medical records and licensing of healthcare providers
- Specific federal legislation designed to protect sensitive information, such as HIV test results, genetic screening information, drug and alcohol abuse rehabilitation, and mental health records

On rare occasions, when a patient accepts treatment or hospitalization or is transferred from one practitioner or facility to another, a patient's consent to the disclosure of confidential information can be

A patient's written authorization for the release of information is required for:

- Patient's attorney or insurance company
- Patient's employer (unless a workers' compensation claim is involved)
- Member of the patient's family (except where a member of the family received durable power of attorney for healthcare agencies)

implied from the circumstances. In such situations, disclosing confidential patient information is necessary to *ensure the patient's emergency* treatment or continuation of patient care. State and federal laws allow or require disclosing medical records to healthcare providers involved in the patient's treatment or on patient transfer from one facility to another.

## Health Insurance Portability and Accountability Act of 1996 (HIPAA)

In 1996, the **Health Insurance Portability and Accountability Act (HIPAA)** created additional patient confidentiality considerations. HIPAA mandates the adoption of federal privacy protections for individually identifiable health information. In response to this mandate, the US Department of Health and Human Services (DHHS) published the privacy rule in the Federal Register in December 2000. Subsequently, in August 2002, the DHHS issued final rulemaking modifications to the privacy rule. In addition, the Health Information Technology for Economic and Clinical Health (HITECH) Act was passed in 2009. This law describes how electronic data must be safeguarded under HIPAA regulations.[1]

**Privacy Rule.** As per the DHHS, the HIPAA privacy rule created rules to protect individuals' medical records and other personal health information. The privacy rule applies to health plans, healthcare clearinghouses, and healthcare providers conducting transactions electronically. The rule requires appropriate safeguards to protect the privacy of personal health information and sets limits/conditions on the uses and disclosures that may be made of such information without patient authorization. The rule also gives patients rights over their health information, including the right to examine and obtain a copy of their health records and to request corrections. However, the rule does not replace federal, state, or other laws that provide individuals with even greater privacy protections.

The privacy rule requires covered entities to implement appropriate administrative, technical, and physical precautions to reasonably safeguard protected health information (PHI) from any intentional or unintentional use or disclosure that violates the privacy rule. Covered entities are healthcare providers (such as PTs), health plans (such as Medicare or Blue Cross/Blue Shield), and healthcare clearinghouses (which process nonstandard health information from another entity into a standard format).

In certain situations, a patient or client may ask the covered entity for more protection than the privacy rule affords. The covered entity can agree or disagree with the patient/client's request. If the covered entity agrees with the request to add further restrictions to the privacy rule, the covered entity is bound by HIPAA to add those restrictions to the privacy rule. For example, if the patient/client asks the PT or PTA not to call their place of employment about the confirmation of an appointment for physical therapy services, the PT/PTA must agree with the patient/client's request. If the PT or the PTA inadvertently calls the patient at work, they violate HIPAA.

## Protected Health Information (PHI)

### What is PHI?

**Protected health information (PHI)** includes individually identifiable health information in any form, including information transmitted orally or in written or electronic form. PHI represents information in any form or medium that is created or received by a healthcare provider, health plan, public health authority, employer, life insurer, school or university, or healthcare clearinghouse and relates to the past, present, or future physical or mental health of an individual; the provision of health care to that individual; or future payment for the provision of health care to an individual.

PHI is part of standard transactions, including the use of electronic media to do the following:

- File claims for reimbursement
- File requests for payments or remittance advice
- Check on a claim's status
- Coordinate benefits
- Check enrollment and disenrollment in a health plan

1  https://www.hhs.gov/hipaa/for-professionals/privacy/index.html

- Determine health plan eligibility
- Make or receive referral certifications and authorizations
- Make or receive health plan premium payments
- Submit health claims attachments
- File a first report of injury
- Transmit other information (prescribed by the secretary of the DHHS)

## Notice of Privacy Practices for PHI

### What is notice of privacy practices?

The privacy rule gives an individual (a patient/client) the right to adequate notice of how a covered entity (a healthcare provider) may use and disclose the individual's PHI. The covered entity must give the notice of privacy practices to the individual on the first service delivery date, involving face-to-face exchange with the patient/client.

Thus, the PT must give the notice of privacy to the patient/client on the first date of service (usually, on the initial examination and evaluation). However, another covered entity, such as a radiologist who did not see the patient/client but only read the X-ray and therefore did not have face-to-face contact with the patient/client, does not need to give notice of privacy to the patient/client. The healthcare provider (such as the PT) must also make a "good faith" effort to get the individual's (patient/client's) written acknowledgment that they received the privacy notice.

The privacy rule does not require an individual's signature on the notice. Consequently, the individual (patient/client) can sign a separate sheet or initial a cover sheet of the notice, depending on their choice.

## Incidental Uses and Disclosures of PHI.

Many healthcare providers express concern about their inability to engage in confidential conversations with other providers or patients if there is a chance of being overheard. However, DHHS stated that the privacy rule does not intend to prevent customary and necessary healthcare communications or practices from occurring. Thus, it does not require the risk of incidental use or disclosure to be eliminated to meet the standards. An incidental use or disclosure is permissible if the covered entity (healthcare provider) has applied reasonable safeguards and implemented the minimum necessary standards, meaning that the covered entity must have in place appropriate administrative, technical, and physical safeguards that limit incidental uses and disclosures.

Examples of reasonable safeguards that a covered entity (such as a physical therapy provider) needs to implement may include:

- Avoiding the use of the patient's name in public hallways
- Speaking quietly in the waiting room when discussing a patient's condition with the patient/patient's family
- When making private phone calls, verifying the identity of the person you are speaking to
- Leaving limited voice mail information
- Locking file cabinets or records rooms
- Requiring additional passwords on computers used by all employees working in the facility; this can better protect the patient's identity (see **Figure 6-1**)

For example, if a PTA wants to discuss a patient's treatment with a PT (or another assistant) in a public area, they should move to a more private place and speak softly. When talking to a patient in a semiprivate room, the PTA should pull the curtain, lower their voice, and be discreet.

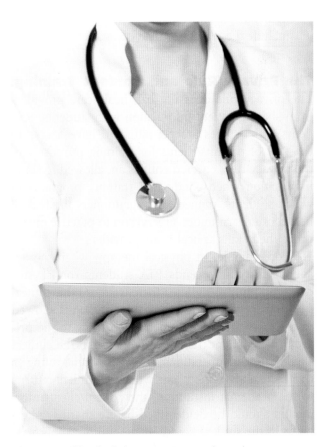

**Figure 6-1** Physical therapy personnel need to safeguard electronic documentation.

Regarding safeguarding PHI, the DHHS specifies:

- Providers (such as PTs) do not need to retrofit their offices, have private rooms, or install soundproof walls to avoid the possibility of a conversation being overheard. In physical therapy, cubicles, dividers, shields, or curtains may constitute reasonable safeguards. Gyms, where several patients receive exercise therapy simultaneously, may not constitute reasonable safeguards.
- Providers can leave messages for patients on their answering machines, but they have to limit the amount of information disclosed on the answering machine (such as confirming the patient's appointment by mentioning only the patient's name and no other information related to the type of provider, etc.). The same applies when leaving a message with someone who answers the phone.
- Providers must take safeguards limiting access to areas where the patient's chart is located by ensuring the area is supervised, keeping the chart face down or facing a wall if stored vertically, or escorting nonemployees in the area.
- Having patients sign in or calling out patient names in a waiting room is acceptable as long as the information disclosed is appropriately limited. For example, the sign-in sheet should not include the reason for the visit.

### The Privacy Rule and Student Training.

The privacy rule does not ban healthcare providers from sharing patient information with students. Students and trainees are permitted to have access to the PHI of patients/clients for training purposes. In the privacy rule, covered entities are allowed to share information when conducting training programs in which students, trainees, or practitioners in areas of health care learn under supervision to practice or improve their skills as healthcare providers.

For example, in physical therapy, when the academic institution sends PTA students (or PT students) to clinical sites for their training, the clinical site, and specifically the clinical instructor, is allowed to disclose PHI to the student. According to the privacy rule, student training is included in the clinical site's healthcare operations, having the same ruling as treatment and payment, and when the student returns to the academic institution, the patient/client information should be deidentified before sharing. Alternatively, the student could obtain authorization from the patient/client to utilize (for training purposes) the patient/client's PHI at the academic institution. Covered entities should take reasonable safeguards by encouraging their students to protect the identity of patients/clients during discussions and be mindful of the minimum necessary standard.

### The Privacy Rule and Family Members.

Under the privacy rule, it is permissible for a provider to disclose PHI to a family member or other person involved in the patient's care. Where the patient is present during a disclosure, the provider may disclose PHI if it is reasonable to infer that the patient does not object. The provider may do the following:

- Obtain the patient's agreement
- Allow the patient to object (and they do not object)
- Decide from the circumstances and based on professional judgment that the patient does not object

When the patient is not present (or is incapacitated), the provider may disclose relevant information if (based on professional judgment) the disclosure is in the patient's best interest.

### Patient/Client Authorization for Uses and Disclosures of PHI

Patient/client authorization is not needed for the following:

- Patient/client seeking their own PHI
- Disclosure to the DHHS
- Uses and disclosures required by laws other than HIPAA (vital statistics, infectious diseases, product recalls, and certain employer reporting of Occupational Safety and Health Administration–related workplace surveillance)
- Victims of domestic violence or elder abuse, as required by law
- Judicial and administrative proceedings (such as court of law orders and subpoenas for relevant information)
- Use and disclosure of health oversight activities (such as state licensure or government benefits programs in Medicare audits)
- Law enforcement activities
- Specialized government functions (such as when the Secret Service needs information about a patient to protect the President of the United States)
- Emergency situations with serious threats to health or safety
- Workers' compensation (exempted only to the extent required by state law)

Patient/client authorization is needed for research activities. Certain institutional review boards (IRBs) waive the requirement of written authorization depending on the minimal privacy risks and if the research is impractical if authorization is required. HIPAA's privacy rule for clinical research conducted by universities and government agencies is complex. The privacy rule states that a researcher may use or disclose PHI from existing databases or repositories for research purposes either with the patient/client's authorization or with a waiver of authorization from an IRB.

## Minimum Necessary Standards for Disclosure of PHI.
The privacy rule requires covered entities to make reasonable efforts to limit the disclosure of PHI to the minimum necessary to accomplish the intended purpose.[2]

Exceptions to the minimum necessary rule include:
- Uses or disclosures required by law
- Disclosures to the individual who is the subject of the information
- Uses or disclosures for which the covered entity has received authorization that meets the appropriate requirements; the authorization must identify the minimum requirements
- Uses or disclosures to requests by a healthcare provider for treatment purposes; for example, a PT is not required to apply the minimum necessary standards when discussing a patient's plan of care with a PTA.
- Uses or disclosures required for compliance with the regulations implementing the other administrative simplification provisions of HIPAA or disclosures to DHHS for purposes of enforcing the privacy rule

## Personal Representatives of Patients/Clients.
When the patient/client cannot exercise their privacy rights, that patient/client may designate another individual to act on their behalf concerning these rights. According to the privacy rule, a person authorized to act on behalf of a patient/client in making health care-related decisions is the patient/client's representative. Concerning uses and disclosures, the personal representative must be treated by the covered entities as the patient/client themselves by exercising the patient/client's rights. For example, the PT or the PTA must provide the patient/client's representative with any requests for disclosure or any authorization for disclosure of the patient/client's PHI.

## Parent Access to a Minor's PHI.
The privacy rule defers to the state or other applicable law regarding a parent's access to health information about a minor. The state or other applicable law explicitly requires, permits, or prohibits access to PHI about a minor to a parent. Most states have the parent as the personal representative of a minor patient/client.

A parent is not the personal representative of a minor patient/client under the following conditions:
- When a court of law determines someone other than the parent will make decisions for the minor
- When a state or other law does not require the consent of a parent or other person before a minor can obtain a particular health service, and the minor consents to the health service (for example, there are state laws where a minor can obtain mental health treatment without parental consent)
- When a parent agrees to a confidential relationship between the minor and the physician (or healthcare provider)
- When the minor has been legally emancipated from their parents

## Patient/Client Access to PHI.
An individual (such as a patient/client) has the right to access their PHI and any information that reflects a provider's decision regarding the patient/client. The patient/client can examine their chart and other records, even records the provider thinks the patient will never see. For example, if the provider sends a letter to a collection agency to collect the copayment for a patient/client's visit, the patient/client has the right, upon request, to get a copy of the letter in 30 days (if the records are on-site) or 60 days (if the records are off-site). The provider can charge a reasonable copying cost. Some state laws require the provider to charge a certain amount per copy per page. A patient/client also has the right to receive an accounting of disclosures of PHI made by the covered entity if the patient/client requests such an accounting.

The patient/client can receive the following information from a covered entity:
- PHI that was generated during the 6 years before the date of the request
- An accounting of disclosures that includes the date of each disclosure, the name of the entity or person who received the PHI, a brief description of the PHI disclosed, and a brief statement of the purpose of the disclosure

The covered entity (healthcare provider) may charge the patient/client a reasonable accounting cost for the disclosure of PHI if the patient/client requests more than one accounting in 12 months. The covered entity cannot terminate the patient for requesting many accountings of disclosure of PHI because it is a federal right of the patient/client, and the provider cannot take retaliatory action.

**Marketing of PHI.** A covered entity cannot use PHI in marketing without prior written and specific authorization from the patient/client. The privacy rule defines marketing as communication about a product or service that encourages recipients of the communication to purchase or use the product or service. Marketing is also an arrangement where a covered entity discloses PHI to another entity in exchange for direct or indirect remuneration. Marketing is not considered a communication describing a health-related product or service the covered entity provides. For PTs, a health-related product could be a cervical pillow or a home traction device. Describing a health-related product to the patient/client in a pamphlet does not constitute marketing. Also, communication made during a face-to-face patient/client encounter, even if it is marketing, does not require authorization. In addition, giving patients/clients promotional gifts of nominal value (such as pens or magnets) does not require authorization. For example, if the PT gives the patient a sample of therapeutic gel to use at home, it does not require authorization because the communication was face-to-face and the gel was of nominal value. However, prior patient authorization is required if the PT wants to sell that patient's name to the company that sells the therapeutic gel (so the company can contact the patient to encourage them to buy it).

**Security of Electronic PHI.** All entities that gather PHI must have policies and procedures to safeguard the confidentiality, integrity, and availability of information. The policies should address how the electronic PHI will be created, received, maintained, and transmitted to other parties. In addition, all entities must analyze their risks of security breaches and create appropriate solutions. Some examples of safeguards include staff training and monitoring, electronic firewalls, appropriate electronic equipment to monitor for breaches, and the use of password protection and encryption software. While the administrative burden of electronic protection is best left to computer engineers, each PT and PTA will be expected to perform their vigilance by frequently changing passwords, logging off computers when not in use,

positioning monitors to prevent accidental viewing of the screen, being aware of malware and malicious infections from websites and email and refraining from utilizing personal devices that may not have the appropriate safeguards in place.

In addition to outlining the need for security, the HITECH Act outlines the Breach Notification Rule. Any entity with a system breach, including incidents of lost, stolen, improperly disposed of PHI, hacking, or inappropriate viewing, must notify individuals, DHHS, and sometimes the media of the breach. Enforcement and penalties relate to the level of negligence and can include civil penalties. In addition, criminal penalties may also be possible.

**Penalties for Violation of HIPAA.** The DHHS Office for Civil Rights oversees and enforces HIPAA's privacy rules. Breaking HIPAA's privacy rule means either a civil or a criminal sanction. Civil penalties are imposed for inadvertent violations not resulting in personal gain; they are usually fines. Criminal sanctions involve monetary penalties and jail time.

The enforcement of the transactions and standard code sets is primarily complaint-driven. For example, when the Centers for Medicare and Medicaid Services (CMS) receives a complaint about a covered entity, it notifies the entity in writing that a complaint has been filed. The entity has the opportunity to demonstrate compliance or to submit a corrective action plan. Organizations that exercise reasonable diligence and make efforts to correct problems, and implement changes required to comply with HIPAA, are unlikely to be subject to civil or criminal penalties. If the covered entity does not respond to CMS, fines could be imposed as a last resort.

---

**KNOWLEDGE CHECK**

What does confidentiality mean?
What protections are contained in HIPAA?
What information is considered personal health information?
What are good practices to prevent breaking confidentiality and HIPAA?

---

## Autonomy and Patients' Rights

**Autonomy** is an ethical principle in health care that means a form of personal liberty or self-governance. The principle of respect for patient autonomy acknowledges a patient's right to control their life (including deciding who should access their personal information). The patient is free to decide to act on their decisions, and their decisions must be respected. An example of the ethical principle of autonomy in physical therapy would be the PT's obligation not to restrict a patient's freedom to select their provider of physical therapy services.

In our society, a patient's autonomy and ultimate control over treatment are reflected in the patient's bill of rights. The Patient's Bill of Rights was adopted by the American Hospital Association in 1973 and revised in 1992. Patient rights evolved with the expectation that hospitals and healthcare institutions would support these rights to deliver effective patient care. A designated surrogate or proxy decision-maker can exercise a patient's rights on their behalf if the patient lacks decision-making capacity, is legally incompetent, or is a minor.

Regarding patients' rights in physical therapy practice, the APTA's position states that the individual referred or admitted to the physical therapy service has rights, including but not limited to the following[3]:

- Selection of a PT of one's choosing to the extent that it is reasonable and possible
- Access to information regarding practice policies and charges for services
- Knowledge of the identity of the PT and other personnel providing or participating in the program of care
- The expectation that the referral source has no financial involvement in the service; if that is not the case, knowledge of the extent of any financial involvement in the service by the referring source
- Involvement in the development of anticipated goals and expected outcomes and the selection of interventions
- Knowledge of any substantial risks of the recommended examination and intervention
- Participation in decisions involving the physical therapy plan of care to the extent reasonable and possible
- Access to information concerning their condition
- The expectation that any discussion or consultation involving the case will be conducted discreetly and that all communications and other records about the care, including the sources of payment for treatment, will be treated as confidential
- The expectation of safety in the provision of services and safety concerning the equipment and physical environment

- Timely information about impending discharge and continuing care requirements
- Refusal of physical therapy services
- Information regarding the practice's mechanism for the initiation, review, and resolution of patient/client complaints

# Understanding Cultural Competence

The first guideline in the patient's bill of rights is the patient's right to considerate and respectful care. From the cultural competence perspective, it means that patients who are racially, ethnically, culturally, and linguistically diverse have the right, the same as other patients, to receive effective, understandable, and respectful care that is provided in a manner compatible with their cultural health beliefs and practices and preferred language (see **Figure 6-2**). Patients also have the right to accessible and appropriate healthcare services and to evaluate whether healthcare providers can offer these services. Healthcare organizations and providers can offer accessible and appropriate healthcare services if they become culturally and linguistically competent.

Cultural and linguistic competence is a set of congruent behaviors, attitudes, and policies in a system, an agency, or among professionals that enable effective work in cross-cultural situations. Culture means the integrated patterns of human behavior, including the language, thoughts, communications, actions, customs, beliefs, values, and institutions of racial, ethnic, religious, and social groups.[4] Culture,

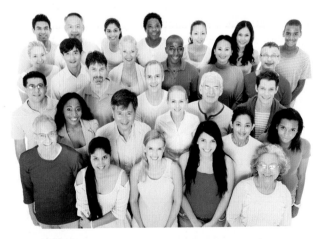

**Figure 6-2** Cultural diversity requires respect for everyone.

© Rawpixel/Shutterstock

---

3 https://www.apta.org/apta-and-you/leadership-and-governance/policies/access-admission-patient-client-rights
4 https://minorityhealth.hhs.gov/omh/browse.aspx?lvl=2&lvlid=53

learned from the earliest age, enables humans to connect and interact meaningfully with others and the surrounding environment. Connecting with others allows people to recognize and share knowledge, attitudes, and values, resulting in a shared perception of the world and how to act within it. Culture can also profoundly influence an individual's values, beliefs, and behaviors.

**Cultural competence** is also an awareness of, sensitivity to, and knowledge of the meaning of culture. Cultural competence implies having the capacity to function effectively as an individual and an organization within the context of the cultural beliefs, behaviors, and needs presented by consumers and their communities. Cultural competence includes openness and willingness to learn about cultural issues and the ability to understand a person's own biases, values, attitudes, beliefs, and behaviors.

### What is cultural competence?

- An evolving process
- An acceptance of and respect for differences
- A continuing self-assessment regarding culture
- Vigilance toward the dynamics of differences
- The ongoing expansion of cultural knowledge and resources
- Adaptations to services

The development of cultural competence depends more on attitude than on specific knowledge of the culture, and the outcome is respect and sensitivity for other cultures.

## Ethical and Legal Perspectives of Cultural Competence

From an ethical perspective, cultural competence is vital to all levels of healthcare practice. Ethnocentric approaches to healthcare practice can be ineffective in meeting the healthcare needs of diverse cultural groups of patients and clients. Healthcare providers' cultural and linguistic competence can strengthen and broaden healthcare delivery systems. The DHHS Office of Minority Health has issued 14 national standards for culturally and linguistically appropriate services in health care. The national standards, intended to be inclusive of all cultures, are proposed to correct inequities currently existing in health services and to make these services more responsive to the individual needs of all patients and clients. Although the national standards are directed primarily at healthcare organizations, individual healthcare providers are encouraged to use them to make their practices more culturally and linguistically accessible.

As both an enforcer of civil rights law and a major purchaser of health services, the federal government has a pivotal role in ensuring culturally competent

The 14 governmental standards for culturally/linguistically accessible healthcare service are:

- Patients and clients receive effective, understandable, and respectful care from all staff members compatible with their cultural health beliefs and practices and preferred language.
- Healthcare organizations implement strategies to recruit, retain, and promote at all levels of the organization a diverse staff and leadership that represent the demographic characteristics of the service area.
- Healthcare organizations ensure that staff at all levels and disciplines receive ongoing education and training in culturally and linguistically appropriate service delivery.
- Healthcare organizations offer and provide language assistance services, including bilingual staff and interpreter services, at no cost to each patient/consumer with limited English proficiency at all points of contact, promptly during all hours of operation.
- Healthcare organizations provide to patients/consumers in their preferred language both verbal offers and written notices informing them of their right to receive language assistance services.
- Healthcare organizations assure the competence of language assistance provided to limited English-proficient patients/consumers by interpreters and bilingual staff. Family and friends should not be used to provide interpretation services (except on request by the patient/consumer).
- Healthcare organizations make available easily understood patient-related materials and post signage in the languages of the commonly encountered groups and groups represented in the service area.
- Healthcare organizations develop, implement, and promote a written strategic plan that outlines clear goals, policies, operational plans, and management accountability and oversight mechanisms to provide culturally and linguistically appropriate services.
- Healthcare organizations conduct initial and ongoing organizational self-assessments of culturally and linguistically appropriate services and are encouraged to integrate cultural and linguistic competence into their internal audits, performance improvement programs, patient satisfaction assessments, and outcome-based evaluations.

- Healthcare organizations ensure that data on the individual patient/consumer's race, ethnicity, and spoken and written language are collected in health records, integrated into the organization's management information systems, and periodically updated.
- Healthcare organizations maintain a current demographic, cultural, and epidemiologic profile of the community and a needs assessment to accurately plan for and implement services that respond to the cultural and linguistic characteristics of the service area.
- Healthcare organizations develop collaborative partnerships with communities and utilize a variety of formal and informal mechanisms to facilitate community and patient/consumer involvement in designing and implementing culturally and linguistically appropriate services.
- Healthcare organizations ensure that conflict and grievance resolution processes are culturally and linguistically sensitive and capable of identifying, preventing, and resolving cross-cultural conflicts or complaints by patients/consumers.
- Healthcare organizations are encouraged to regularly inform the public about their progress and successful innovations in implementing culturally and linguistically appropriate services standards and to provide public notice in their communities about the availability of this information.

healthcare services. For example, Title VI of the Civil Rights Act of 1964 mandates that no person in the United States shall, on the ground of race, color, or national origin, be excluded from participation in, be denied the benefits of, or be subjected to discrimination under any program or activity receiving federal financial assistance. The standards for culturally and linguistically appropriate services are current federal requirements for all recipients of federal funds. State and federal agencies increasingly rely on private accreditation entities to set standards and monitor compliance with these standards. Both the Joint Commission, which accredits hospitals and other healthcare institutions, and the National Committee for Quality Assurance, which accredits managed care organizations and behavioral health managed care organizations, support the standards for culturally and linguistically appropriate services. In physical therapy, the Commission on Accreditation in Physical Therapy Education also supports the standards, promoting incorporating cultural and linguistic competence into physical therapy education curricula. In addition, the Maternal and Child Health Bureau has cultural and linguistic competence training programs emphasizing cultural competency as an integral component of health service delivery.[5]

## Developing Cultural Competence in Health Care

The makeup of the American population is changing due to immigration patterns and significant increases among racially, ethnically, culturally, and linguistically diverse populations already residing there. Despite similarities, fundamental differences among people arise regarding nationality, ethnicity, culture, family background, and individual experience. These differences affect the health beliefs and behaviors that both patients and providers have and expect of each other.

The delivery of accessible, effective, and cost-efficient high-quality primary health care requires healthcare practitioners to deeply understand the sociocultural background of patients, their families, and the environments in which they live. Culturally competent primary health services facilitate clinical encounters with more favorable outcomes, enhance the potential for a more rewarding interpersonal experience, and increase the satisfaction of the individual receiving healthcare services.

Healthcare providers should realize that addressing cultural diversity means more than knowing the values, beliefs, practices, and customs of Asians,

Cultural diversity can be addressed through awareness/acceptance of the following patient/client characteristics:

- Racial characteristics and national origin
- Religious affiliations
- Physical size
- Spoken language
- Sexual orientation
- Physical and mental disability
- Age
- Gender
- Socioeconomic status
- Political orientation
- Geographic location
- Occupational status

5 https://mchb.hrsa.gov/programs-impact/focus-areas/building-mch-leaders-mch-workforce/leadership-competencies

African Americans, Hispanics, Latinos, Alaskan Natives, Native Americans, and Pacific Islanders.

Healthcare providers must strive to achieve the ability and availability to work effectively within the cultural context of a patient/client, the patient/client's family, and the community. Cultural desire involves caring for patients/clients, being open and flexible with them, accepting their differences, and being willing to learn from others about their culture. Healthcare providers must possess a cultural desire involving commitment to care for all patients and clients, regardless of their cultural values, beliefs, customs, or practices.

A culturally competent healthcare provider values diversity with awareness, acceptance, and observance of differences in life views, health systems, communication styles, and other life-sustaining elements. Cultural knowledge must be incorporated into the delivery of services to minimize misperception, misinterpretation, and misjudgment. Although it is impossible to learn all there is to know about all cultural subgroups, culturally competent healthcare providers must be aware of the relevant beliefs and behaviors of their patients/clients and their patients'/clients' families and must be able to adapt to diversity to create a better fit between the needs of the people requiring services and the people meeting those needs.

Strategies to improve patient–provider interaction include the following:

- Providing training to increase cultural awareness, knowledge, and skills
- Recruiting and retaining minority staff
- Providing interpreter services
- Providing linguistic competency that extends beyond the clinical encounter to the appointment desk, advice lines, medical billing, and other written material
- Coordinating evaluations and treatments with traditional healers
- Using community health workers
- Incorporating culture-specific attitudes and values into health promotion tools
- Including family and community members in healthcare decision-making
- Locating clinics in geographic areas that are easily accessible to certain populations
- Expanding hours of operation

Healthcare providers must focus on enhancing attitudes in the following areas:

- Become aware of the influences that sociocultural factors have on patients, clinicians, and the clinical relationship

- Be willing to make clinical settings more accessible to patients
- Be able to accept responsibility and understand the cultural aspects of health and illness
- Be able to recognize personal biases against people of different cultures
- Be able to respect and have tolerance for cultural differences
- Be willing to accept responsibility to combat racism, classism, ageism, homophobia, sexism, and other kinds of biases and discrimination that occur in healthcare settings

Healthcare providers are continuously striving to increase their cultural competence, responding to the needs of racial and ethnic minorities. The reasons may be the state and federal guidelines that encourage or mandate greater responsiveness of health systems to the growing population diversity and meeting the federal government's Healthy People 2020 goal of eliminating racial and ethnic health disparities. In addition, many healthcare systems find that developing and implementing cultural competence strategies are good business practices for increasing providers' and patients' interest and participation in their health plans among racial and ethnic minority populations. For example, when increasing cultural competence, the most successful efforts of healthcare providers have been directed at eliminating language and literacy barriers. Bilingual and bicultural services have been developed to serve Asian American and Latino communities. Within the Latino community, peer educators (called *promotores*) were so successful that more and more ordinary people from other diverse and hard-to-reach populations began to act as bridges between their community and the world of health care. These peer educators learn about healthcare principles from physicians, nonprofit organizations, or other healthcare providers and share their knowledge with their communities. The peer education model is becoming extremely effective in reaching populations that find the healthcare information more credible from someone with a familiar background than a healthcare provider.

## Developing Cultural Competence in Physical Therapy

PTs and PTAs must develop culturally competent communication skills and understanding to interact with patients/clients from diverse cultures effectively. In physical therapy, the primary healthcare teams working with primary care physicians on an outpatient encounter the most cultural diversity. However, all physical therapy clinicians encounter some degree of cultural diversity because culture is so complex, involving cultural diversity experiences and other patients'/clients' cultural and socially unique characteristics.

> PTs and PTAs can increase their cultural competence by utilizing the following steps [1]:
> 1. Identify personal cultural biases.
> 2. Understand general cultural differences.
> 3. Accept and respect cultural differences.
> 4. Apply cultural understanding.

## Identifying Personal Cultural Biases

Identifying personal cultural biases is the first step in becoming culturally competent. Many people do not comprehend their attitudes and values in connection to others, especially people from diverse populations. Every person has ethnocentrism and personal values and beliefs contributing to cultural misalignments. **Ethnocentrism** is judging another culture based on one's cultural customs and standards. For example, in physical therapy, a PT or a PTA can label a patient "noncompliant" with a physical therapy home exercise program when, in reality, the patient did not understand the instructions relating to the exercises. A blind ethnocentric approach to this "noncompliant patient" will not lead to an effective solution. In this example, the misalignment is the attempt of the therapist to simplify a complex world. People tend to identify similarities and commonalities to manage diversity and ignore the differences. Oversimplification leads to generalization, which may lead to stereotyping, an oversimplified conception, opinion, or belief about people. Knowingly or unknowingly, the therapist, as with most healthcare providers, imposes their expectations on the patient to accomplish the desired task. Rather than labeling the patient as noncompliant, the PT or PTA should identify the language barrier, whether linguistic, jargon, or comprehension issues.

## Understanding General Cultural Differences

An understanding of general cultural differences is the second step in becoming culturally competent. It involves actively seeking knowledge regarding different cultures to deal with diverse patient/client populations. When identifying a patient/client from another culture, the PT and the PTA can refer to appropriate resources to address the situation positively and effectively. For example, consider a patient of Hispanic descent who continuously arrives late for physical therapy treatments. The therapist, whose dominant US culture values timeliness, expects the patient to arrive on time for their scheduled appointment. The therapist misinterprets the patient's lateness as disinterest in physical therapy treatment and possibly noncompliance. In this example, the therapist must refer to the appropriate resources about the Hispanic culture to discover that punctuality is not necessarily a high priority. The therapist may either ignore the patient's lateness or modify the patient's schedule, allowing the patient enough time to arrive late.

## Accepting and Respecting Cultural Differences

Accepting and respecting cultural differences is the third step in becoming culturally competent. It involves acknowledging, accepting, appreciating, and valuing diversity. The natural human tendency is to respond to differences with discomfort, apprehension, and fear. People tend to avoid or minimize situations of cultural diversity, perhaps tolerate them but do not acknowledge and respond to them. PTs and PTAs should be able to accept, value, and adjust physical therapy care to culturally suitable standards. For example, an older Asian American patient is not performing the recommended home exercise program and is labeled noncompliant. In reality, the older patient, as the "family leader" in Asian American culture, often could not perform any activity or task without the family helping them. In this example, the therapist should discuss the situation with the older patient's family, adjusting the home exercise program and incorporating it into the family's activities and tasks.

## Applying Cultural Understanding

Applying cultural understanding is the fourth step toward increasing cultural competence and involves implementing culturally competent healthcare practices. The PT and the PTA have identified personal culture and biases, recognized diversity as worthy, acquired an understanding of various cultural differences, and are now prepared to apply cultural competence in physical therapy clinical practice.

The development of cultural competence is an ongoing learning process. During this learning process, in clinical settings, the PT and the PTA may make mistakes; however, the therapist should be able to learn from these mistakes. Research [1] has shown that the acquisition of cultural competency has proven elusive

When applying cultural competence, we must accept, value, and understand:

- The beliefs, values, traditions, and practices of a culture
- The culturally defined health-related needs of individuals, families, and communities
- The culturally based belief systems regarding the etiology of illness and disease and those related to health and healing
- The culture's attitudes toward seeking help from healthcare providers

to healthcare professionals; therefore, clinicians, educators, and students must develop, implement, and promote a strategic plan outlining clear goals, policies, operational plans, and management accountability to provide culturally and linguistically appropriate services. Cultural and linguistic competence is typically incorporated into the PT or PTA's curricula in school and training.

Physical therapy educators can promote:

- Increase student awareness about the impact of culture and language on healthcare delivery
- Provide education about the importance of recruitment and retention of diverse students to faculty, administrators, and staff
- Offer continuing education and training about cultural and linguistic competence to faculty, administrators, and staff

## KNOWLEDGE CHECK

What is the first step to identifying cultural competence?

What patient/client characteristics make up cultural diversity?

What are the strategies for developing cultural competence?

What is ethnocentrism?

## Informed Consent

The third principle of the patient's bill of rights states that the patient has the right to receive information from their certified healthcare provider to make informed consent before any procedure and/or treatment starts. The informed consent includes information such as the medically significant risks involved with any procedure, probable duration of incapacitation, and, where medically appropriate, alternatives for

care or treatment. **Informed consent** is the process by which a fully informed patient can participate in choices about their health care.

Elements of informed consent to be discussed with the patient/client include:

- The nature of the decision or the procedure (such as a clear description of the proposed intervention)
- Reasonable alternatives to the proposed intervention
- The relevant risks, benefits, and uncertainties related to each alternative
- Assessment of patient understanding
- The patient's acceptance of the intervention

For the informed consent to be valid, the patient must be considered competent to decide, and the consent must be voluntary. Healthcare providers (such as PTs) should not coerce patients into making uninformed decisions about their health, especially considering that patients feel powerless and vulnerable when facing illness or affliction. PTs should involve the patient in decision-making by explaining that they are active participants in their healthcare resolutions. All the necessary information has to be explained to the patient in layperson's terms, and the patient's understanding has to be continuously assessed. In addition, the information must be delivered in terms the patient can understand (including translating the material into another language) and be free of professional jargon [2]. As in any communication with the patient, the PT and the PTA must consider the following basic communication elements [3]:

- Talking clearly and simply (using everyday words)
- Repeating the information as necessary
- Breaking down the information into a series of steps
- Taking into consideration the patient's difficulties in understanding (such as speaking another language, having visual or hearing impairments, and/or having difficulty reading or understanding the material)

In emergencies, when the patient is unconscious (especially when the patient's life is in danger) or incompetent, and no surrogate decision-maker is available, the healthcare provider must use the principle of beneficence and act on the patient's behalf. The type of consent used in emergencies is called presumed or implied consent.

In physical therapy, the PT is solely responsible for providing information to the patient and obtaining informed consent during the first visit before starting the initial examination/evaluation. This process is per jurisdictional law. When the patient is a minor or an adult who is not competent, a legal guardian (or a designated surrogate) or a parent (in the case of a minor) receiving the information has to understand the information and be able to give or refuse informed consent. The PTA also has to provide information to the patient and obtain informed consent when applying reassessments (as directed by the PT) and intervention(s).

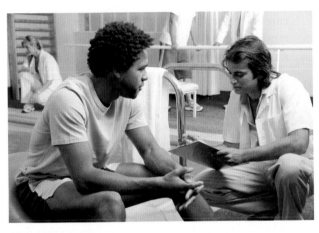

© Fuse/Corbis/Getty Images

# Ethics Documents for PTs

The APTA has developed ethical principles to assist PT and PTA members in understanding how to act morally and professionally. In addition, the APTA's ethical principles can help PTs and PTAs with the following:

- Identifying and clarifying moral issues [2]
- Evaluating moral reasons and forming moral viewpoints
- Acquiring awareness of alternative viewpoints [2]
- Strengthening attitudes of care and respect for patients/clients and oneself
- Maintaining integrity and acting in morally responsible ways [2]

For PTs who are members of the APTA, the Association has created a code of ethics and a guide for professional conduct. The code of ethics for PTs provides ethical principles for maintaining and promoting ethical practice. The purpose of the guide for professional conduct is to interpret the ethical principles of the code of ethics. The guide contains mostly directive ethical provisions and only eight nondirective ethical provisions regulating the official conduct of member PTs. Currently, the general framework of the guide for professional conduct contains 11 principles having the following topics:[6]

- Principle 1: Attitudes of a physical therapist
- Principle 2: Patient–physical therapist relationship: truthfulness, confidential information, patient autonomy, and consent
- Principle 3: Professional practice, just laws and regulations, and unjust laws and regulations
- Principle 4: Professional responsibility, direction and supervision, practice arrangements, and gifts and other considerations
- Principle 5: Scope of competence, self-assessment, and professional development
- Principle 6: Professional standards, practice, professional education, continuing education, and research
- Principle 7: Business and employment practices, endorsement of products or services, and disclosure
- Principle 8: Accurate and relevant information to the patient and accurate and relevant information to the public
- Principle 9: Consumer protection
- Principle 10: Pro bono service and individual and community health
- Principle 11: Consultation, patient–provider relationships, and disparagement

These ethical documents govern members within the APTA. While the APTA cannot sanction nonmembers for ethical violations, these documents guide best-practice guidelines and can be utilized in legal and regulatory proceedings when ethical and legal issues arise in practice.

# Ethics Documents for Physical Therapist Assistants

The APTA also has created Standards of Ethical Conduct of PTAs and a Guide to the Conduct of the PTA. The purpose of the standards of ethical conduct is to maintain and promote high standards of conduct for PTAs who are affiliate members of the APTA. The guide for conduct helps PTAs interpret the standards of ethical conduct. The Standards of Ethical Conduct of the PTA include the following tenets:

- Standard 1: Physical therapist assistants shall respect the inherent dignity and rights of all individuals.

- Standard 2: Physical therapist assistants shall be trustworthy and compassionate in addressing the rights and needs of patients/clients.
- Standard 3: Physical therapist assistants shall make sound decisions in collaboration with the physical therapist and within the boundaries established by laws and regulations.
- Standard 4: Physical therapist assistants shall demonstrate integrity in their relationships with patients/clients, families, colleagues, students, other healthcare providers, employers, payers, and the public.
- Standard 5: Physical therapist assistants shall fulfill their legal and ethical obligations.
- Standard 6: Physical therapist assistants shall enhance their competence through the lifelong acquisition and refinement of knowledge, skills, and abilities.
- Standard 7: Physical therapist assistants shall support organizational behaviors and business practices that benefit patients/clients and society.
- Standard 8: Physical therapist assistants shall participate in efforts to meet the health needs of people locally, nationally, or globally.

Generally, the standards and the guide also promote the following seven ethical principles for PTAs:

- Provide respectful and compassionate care for the patient, including sensitivity to individual and cultural differences
- Act on behalf of the patient/client while being sensitive to the patient/client's vulnerability
- Work under the direction and supervision of the PT
- Comply with laws and regulations governing physical therapy
- Maintain competence in the provision of selected physical therapy interventions
- Make judgments commensurate with one's educational and legal qualifications
- Protect the public and the profession from unethical, incompetent, and illegal acts

All the guidelines for PTs and PTAs are issued by the ethics and judicial committee of the APTA and are amended to remain current with changes in the physical therapy profession and new patterns of healthcare delivery.

Other professions, such as occupational therapy, orthotics and prosthetics, psychology, respiratory care, and nursing, also have ethical guidelines for professional conduct. Most commonly, the codes of ethics within many health professions specialties contain vague language regarding expected performance levels. This may be because it is difficult to include technical aspects of a profession's medical or clinical practice in the code of ethics.

# Confronting Ethical Dilemmas

At some point in a healthcare worker's career, they will likely face an ethical dilemma. Some examples of ethical scenarios in health care include:

- Confidentiality: A patient confides in their healthcare provider about a sensitive issue but explicitly requests that the information not be shared with anyone else. However, the provider believes sharing the information with other healthcare professionals involved in the patient's care would be of benefit. Should the provider break the patient's confidentiality to improve their care?
- Informed consent: A patient is considering a treatment option but hesitates due to potential risks and side effects. The healthcare provider wants to proceed with the treatment and pressures the patient to give informed consent. Should the provider prioritize the patient's autonomy and allow them to decide or push for the treatment they believe is best?
- Resource allocation: A hospital has limited resources, and multiple patients require the same life-saving treatment. The provider must decide which patient to treat, knowing that not all patients will survive without it. Should the provider prioritize the patient with the highest chance of survival or provide the treatment on a first-come, first-served basis?
- Conflict of interest: A healthcare provider has a financial interest in a medical device company and recommends that patients use the company's products, even when other options may be more appropriate. Should the provider prioritize the patient's well-being or their own financial gain?

It is important to recognize that ethical dilemmas occur and to be prepared to plan to work through the process to make the best decision based on legal and ethical principles. Realm-Individual-Process-Situation (RIPS) is a problem-solving framework commonly used in health care that provides a structured approach to clinical decision-making by considering the complex interplay among the person, their environment, and their occupation. The four components of RIPS are as follows:

1. Realm refers to the overarching context or environment in which the person's occupation

occurs. It includes the physical, social, cultural, and institutional factors that shape the person's experiences.

2. Individual: refers to the person engaging in the occupation. It includes their unique characteristics, such as their personality, values, interests, and abilities.
3. Process: refers to the dynamic interaction between the person and their environment. It includes the sequence of events that occur as the person engages in their occupation and the strategies they use to overcome challenges and achieve their goals.
4. Situation: refers to the specific circumstances of the person's occupation. It includes the physical and social context in which the occupation occurs and any constraints or barriers that may affect the person's ability to participate.

The RIPS is a flexible and adaptable framework that emphasizes the importance of client-centered care, which is tailored to a person's individual needs and preferences and can be applied across a wide range of clinical settings and patient populations. An article published in the HPA Review in 2005 explains the RIPS model about not just what to do but why (see **Table 6-1**).[7]

### KNOWLEDGE CHECK

When asking a patient for informed consent, what should be included?
To act ethically and professionally, what standards should a PT/PTA adhere to?

## Table 6-1 RIPS Model of Ethical Decision-Making

| Step 1: | Investigate the Situation |
| --- | --- |
| Realm: | The individual realm is concerned with the people involved in the situation. For example, the patient, the patient's caregiver, and the PT/PTA may all be affected in an ethical situation.<br>The organizational realm is concerned with the effect decisions will have on the institution.<br>An example of the organizational realm is the PT department or the hospital.<br>The societal realm concerns how a situation may affect the population, including the local, national, or global society. |
| Individual Process: | This process requires the PT/PTA to consider what is occurring and their role in the situation. There are four questions to be asked.<br>■ Should I be morally sensitive to the situation? This is a level of situational awareness.<br>■ Should I be making a moral judgment? This requires deciding what is "right" versus "wrong."<br>■ Do I have the moral motivation to do something about the situation? This requires that one place the moral value affecting the situation above other values.<br>■ Do I have the moral courage to do something about the situation? This requires considering whether they are willing to do something about the situation. |
| Situation: | This step in the process requires that the PT/PTA classify the situation. There are five classes:<br>■ Issue/Problem: Ethical values are part of the situation.<br>■ Dilemma: At least two choices could be made, both of which may be "right" decisions.<br>■ Distress: While a "right" choice exists, the power to implement the solution is not yours.<br>■ Temptation: In this situation, there is a "right" versus "wrong" choice; however, you may benefit from choosing the "wrong" choice.<br>■ Silence: No one is speaking out about the situation. This may lead to distress later. |
| Step 2: | Reflect |
| | It is important to consider and weigh each aspect of the RIPS in Step 1. Some may carry more weight in the situation, thus impacting the decision more. One should also consider if the situation is unethical or illegal, "feels" like it is wrong, or could withstand the scrutiny of the public or family. |

*(continues)*

7 https://www.s3-live.kent.edu/s3fs-root/s3fs-public/file/RIPS_DecisionMaking_0.pdf?VersionId=Lcmfbo1Y_vJGpw20Wi_cYHs48emzFTpJ

**Table 6-1** RIPS Model of Ethical Decision-Making *(continued)*

| Step 3: | Make a Decision |
|---|---|
| | If the situation is "right" versus "wrong," one can go directly to Step 4: Implementation. If the situation has multiple "right" choices, the PT/PTA must consider the best choice by weighing other factors. <ul><li>Are there rules that help to make this decision? Examples would be laws, regulatory decisions, and policies and procedures.</li><li>For each choice, make a list of the pros and cons of the decision. This will help you weigh the choices of each for all people affected.</li><li>How will this affect the relationships that have been established?</li></ul> |
| **Step 4:** | **Implement, Evaluate, and Reassess** |
| | The implementation steps will have little value if the person does not follow up with an assessment of its effectiveness. So the PT/PTA should ensure that the implementation has successfully solved the situation and, if not, consider whether or not there was a fault in the RIPS process or implementation or if the situation changed and needs reassessment. |

Data from Swisher, L, Arslanian, L, Davis, C. The realm-individual processsituation (RIPS) model of ethical decision making. HPA Resource. October 2005; 1–8. Accessed July 2015, at: www.apta.org

# Professionalism

Professionalism is difficult to define because it involves many variables. In addition to the previously mentioned ethical principles and reasoning, elements of professionalism may include the following values/attributes:

- Responsibility. The state or quality of being accountable or answerable for something, including the obligation to take action, make decisions, and accept the consequences of one's actions. The concept of responsibility is closely linked to ethics, as it involves making choices and taking actions that align with one's moral values and principles.
- Critical thinking. The process of actively and objectively analyzing information, arguments, and evidence by examining and evaluating arguments to determine the validity and soundness of a conclusion.
- Problem-solving. The process of finding a solution to a problem or a set of problems by defining the problem, generating and evaluating potential solutions, and implementing a chosen solution. Effective problem-solving requires analyzing information, identifying patterns and relationships, and thinking creatively to generate potential solutions.

- Decision-making. The process of selecting a course of action from a set of alternatives to achieve a desired outcome by identifying a problem or opportunity, generating and evaluating options, and choosing the best course of action based on available information.
- Behavior. Professional behavior refers to the actions, attitudes, and conduct expected of individuals in the workplace and encompasses a range of behaviors, including ethical behavior, effective communication, teamwork, punctuality, responsibility, and respect for others.
- Communication. Communication is the exchanging of information, ideas, thoughts, or feelings between individuals or groups. It involves transmitting and receiving messages through various channels, including verbal (spoken or written), nonverbal (gestures, facial expressions, body language), and visual (images, symbols, graphs). The various types of communication are described in detail in Chapter 8.
- Interpersonal skills. The ability to effectively communicate, interact, and collaborate with others, including a range of abilities such as active listening, empathy, conflict resolution, negotiation, and the ability to adapt to different personalities and communication styles.

# Core Values

The APTA describes professionalism as a systematic and integrated set of core values. These values are identified as the following (in alphabetical order)[8]:

- Accountability
- Altruism
- Compassion/caring
- Excellence
- Integrity
- Professional duty
- Social responsibility

Although the seven core values represent PT professionalism, as physical therapy team members, PTAs must also be receptive to these values. As active participants in the professional physical therapy environment, PTAs must employ values for self-assessment, critical reflection, and professional behaviors and attitudes concerning their colleagues, patients/clients, other professionals, the public, and the profession.

In 2009, the APTA's board of directors created a task force to identify behaviors appropriate for PTs/PTAs to display. The task force's work created the eight Value-Based Behaviors:

1. Altruism
2. Caring and compassion
3. Continuing competence
4. Duty
5. Integrity
6. PT/PTA collaboration
7. Responsibility
8. Social responsibility

## Altruism

Altruism is "the primary regard for or devotion to the interest of patients/clients, thus assuming the fiduciary responsibility of placing the needs of the patient/client ahead of the clinician's self-interest." Examples of altruism may include:

- Placing the patient/client's needs above those of the PTA
- Providing pro bono services (under the direction of the PT)
- Providing physical therapy services to underserved and underrepresented populations (under the direction of the PT)
- Completing patient/client care before attending to personal needs (under the direction of the PT)

## Caring and Compassion

Compassion (a precursor of caring) is "the desire to identify with or sense something of another's experience." Caring is "concern, empathy, and consideration for the needs and values of others." Examples of compassion and caring may include:

- Respectfully listening to the patient's concerns without judgment and interacting with the patient's needs and desires in mind
- Understanding the sociocultural, economic, and psychological influences on the individual's life in their environment
- Understanding an individual's perspective
- Communicating effectively (verbally and nonverbally) with others, taking into consideration individual differences in learning styles, language, and cognitive abilities
- Recognizing and refraining from acting on one's social, cultural, gender, and sexual biases
- Attending to the patient/client's personal needs and comfort
- Demonstrating respect for others and considering others to be unique and of value

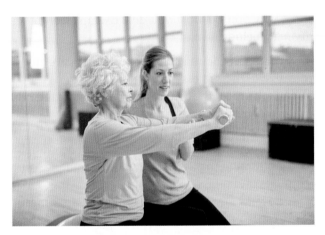

© Ammentorp Photography/Shutterstock

## Continuing Competence

Continuing competence requires conscious reflections on the clinician's current abilities and developing a plan for lifelong learning of knowledge, skills, and attitudes that will benefit patient interactions. Examples of continuing competence may include:

- Personal self-assessment practices and assessment by a PT to help create a plan for improvement
- Creating a personal goal of lifelong learning through continuing education courses, journal reading, and learning from colleagues
- Creating a plan for career advancement through education and opportunities for growth and advancement
- Engaging in the acquisition of new knowledge throughout one's career
- Sharing one's knowledge with others

## Duty

Duty is "the commitment to meeting one's obligations to provide effective physical therapy services to patients/clients to serve the profession, and to positively influence the health of society." Examples of professional duty may include:

- Demonstrating beneficence by providing optimal care
- Facilitating each individual's achievement of goals for function, health, and wellness
- Preserving the safety, security, and confidentiality of individuals in all contexts related to physical therapy
- Promoting the profession of physical therapy
- Taking pride in being a PTA

## Integrity

Integrity is "steadfast adherence to high ethical principles or professional standards; truthfulness, fairness, doing what you say you will do, and 'speaking forth' about why you do what you do." Examples of integrity may include:

- Abiding by the rules, regulations, and laws applicable to the profession
- Adhering to the profession's highest standards (ethics, reimbursement, honor code, etc.)
- Being trustworthy
- Knowing one's limitations and acting accordingly
- Confronting harassment and bias among ourselves and others
- Choosing employment situations that are congruent with ethical standards

## PT/PTA Collaboration

"The PT/PTA team works together, within each partner's respective role, to achieve optimal patient/client care and to enhance the overall delivery of physical therapy services." Examples of PT/PTA collaboration may include:

- Promoting understanding of the role of the PTA and education level, state laws, rules and regulations, and APTA guidelines for PTAs
- Creating a respectful working relationship with the PT that utilizes both team members' skills and strengths for the betterment of the patient
- Promoting physical therapy to consumers and community members

## Responsibility

Responsibility is the "active acceptance of the roles, obligations, and actions of the PT/PTA, including behaviors that positively influence patient/client outcomes, the profession, and the health needs of society." Examples of responsibility include:

- Understanding personal strengths and weaknesses and practicing ethically within the PTA's abilities
- Working conscientiously to provide accurate and timely care
- Taking responsibility for actions and consequences
- Communicating clearly with all team members (patient, PT, other healthcare providers)

## Social Responsibility

Social responsibility "promotes a mutual trust between the profession and the larger public that necessitates responding to societal needs for health and wellness" [3]. Examples of social responsibility values may include:

- Advocating for the health and wellness needs of society, including access to health care and physical therapy services
- Promoting cultural competence within the profession and the larger public
- Promoting social policy that affects the function, health, and wellness needs of patients/clients
- Ensuring that existing social policy is in the best interest of the patient/client
- Advocating for changes in laws, regulations, standards, and guidelines that affect PT service provision
- Promoting community volunteerism
- Participating in collaborative relationships with other health practitioners and the public at large
- Ensuring the blending of social justice and economic efficiency of services

### KNOWLEDGE CHECK

What are the eight value-based behaviors of the PT/PTA?

Which of the core values of a PT/PTA is described as the devotion to the interest of a patient/client?

## Integrity in Practice

The APTA has created the Center for Integrity in Practice as part of its Integrity in Practice initiative. The initiative grew out of recognizing fraud, abuse, and waste in health care and the desire to educate PTs and PTAs about the issues occurring in practice. Obtaining something one is not entitled to through deception or misrepresentation is fraud. Fraud is an intentional act. Providers unintentionally commit abuse when they receive payment for services they are not entitled to. Waste is any unnecessary cost or treatment. PTAs should know that under the False Claims Act, they can incur monetary fines, damages, and repayment of the claim monies received.

To assist PTs and PTAs in preventing these inappropriate billing issues, the Center provides scenarios to help identify the issues and suggestions for problem resolution. A primer on fraud, abuse, and waste learning module is available through the Center and helps PTs and PTAs learn to navigate the rules and regulations related to payment. Additionally, the Center has joined the American Board of Internal Medicine Foundation's Choosing Wisely campaign to create a list of five things PTs, PTAs, and consumers should question about physical therapy care.

## Professional Advocacy

Advocacy for the profession and the promotion of legislation for the betterment of society are important professional duties of all PTs and PTAs. Advocacy could include opportunities at the local, state, or national level. Civic organizations that advocate for specific groups may allow for volunteer involvement in awareness, sponsorship, or activism. Opportunities for civic service in city, state/district, or national leadership may allow PTs and PTAs to serve their communities. For those who choose not to serve this way, the APTA has opportunities for national advocacy, and most state chapters are organized similarly.

## Discussion Questions

1. Describe behaviors that you would find in a professional.
2. Using the behaviors described in question 1, connect each to a core value that professionals hold.
3. The PTA works for a skilled nursing facility and is frequently encouraged to bill patients for enough time so that they qualify for the highest Medicare payment allowed. The PT and PTA discuss that one of the patients cannot effectively work the amount of time the manager requests. What ethical dilemmas are presented in this scenario, and what options do the PT and PTA have regarding this situation?

## Learning Opportunities

1. Using the following chart, list things you can do to develop professional behavior.

| Professional Behavior | Practice or Skill | Core Value |
|---|---|---|
| Example: Good judgment | Continuing education | Excellence |

2. Utilizing the internet, find information regarding a cultural group in your area, and share your findings with your group. Investigate the culture's beliefs about health and accessing healthcare providers, the use of alternative health practices, social interactions that may differ from your culture, and so on. Describe how you might respectfully interact with them in a healthcare setting.
3. Utilize the following websites to perform cultural competence self-awareness.
   - https://nccc.georgetown.edu/documents/ChecklistEIEC.pdf
   - https://www.lacrosseconsortium.org/uploads/content_files/files/Awareness_self_assessment.pdf
4. Utilize the RIPS steps to analyze the following ethical situations.
   - The PT clinic employs two PTs and three PTAs. One of the PTs has gone on maternity leave for 12 weeks, and there is no one to cover her caseload and supervise one of the PTAs. The clinic manager states that it should not be a problem for the other PT to supervise all three PTAs because it is only for a few weeks. State law restricts the PT to supervising no more than two PTAs at any time.
   - The PTA works within a small clinic with their supervising PT. The PT has been having personal problems, and the PTA recently noticed that the PT smells of alcohol at work.
   - The PT manager tells the PTA that she should falsify patient improvement data to keep the person on her caseload longer.

- While at lunch in the cafeteria, the PTA discusses a patient by name. After she leaves the table, a coworker sitting behind you tells you that the person she was talking about is her neighbor.

- The PTA is working with a patient who has repeatedly asked you to give him the phone number of one of your single coworkers so he can ask her on a date.

## References

1. Black JD, Purnell LD: Cultural competence for the physical therapy professional. J Phys Ther Educ 16(1):3–10, 2002
2. Gabard DL, Martin MW: Physical Therapy Ethics. Philadelphia, PA, F.A. Davis Company, 2003
3. Dreeben O: Physical Therapy Clinical Handbook for PTAs. Sudbury, MA, Jones & Bartlett Learning, 2008

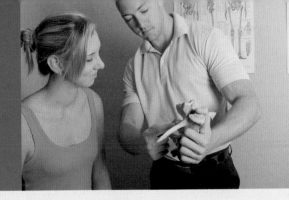

# CHAPTER 7

# Laws and Regulations

## OBJECTIVES

- Identify the four primary sources of law in the United States.
- Describe the Americans with Disabilities Act of 1990.
- List the main points of the Americans with Disabilities Act and its effect on businesses and employers.
- Discuss the Individuals with Disabilities Education Act of 1997.
- Describe the role of licensure laws.
- Identify the organization responsible for creating and managing the National Physical Therapy Examination for physical therapists and physical therapist assistants.
- Explain four minimum standards for licensure/certification to enter the profession for physical therapists and physical therapist assistants.
- Describe the Occupational Safety and Health Administration (OSHA) and its role in health care.
- Discuss the importance of the bloodborne pathogens OSHA standard in health care, including physical therapy practice.
- Identify the Violence Against Women Act of 2013 and domestic violence issues in the United States.
- Describe domestic violence responses in health care and physical therapy.
- Identify two types of malpractice laws that can affect physical therapist assistants.
- Compare and contrast the principles of negligence and malpractice.

## KEY TERMS

Americans with Disabilities Act (ADA)
bloodborne pathogens standards (BPS)
disability

domestic violence
economic abuse
emotional abuse
Occupational Safety and Health Administration (OSHA)

physical abuse
psychological abuse
sexual abuse

## Overview

Numerous laws and regulations impact physical therapy services. There are four primary sources of such obligations in society: constitutional law authority, statutory law authority, common law authority, and administrative or regulatory law authority. A legislature comprises legislators elected by the country's population. Laws enacted by legislatures are usually known as primary legislation. Most laws are designed to protect the public from harm. Constitutional laws have superiority because they were created from the federal Constitution, which is the supreme law of the land. Members of society have to fulfill most of the federal constitutional obligations, which are found in the amendments to the Constitution. For example, the first 10 amendments, or the Bill of Rights, delineate individual protections from overreaching by federal, state, and local governmental. A statute, also known as an act, is a law passed by a legislature. Federal statutes are divided by general subjects into titles. Examples of important federal statutes that affect physical therapy practices are Medicare and Medicaid laws, workers' compensation acts, the Americans with Disabilities Act (ADA) of 1990, the 1973 Rehabilitation Act, the Individuals with Disabilities Education Act (IDEA) of 1997, and licensure laws.

Statutory laws have the second priority after constitutional laws. Congress and state legislatures enact statutes within their spheres of legal authority. State constitutional laws offer citizens greater rights than federal constitutional laws; however, state constitutional laws are subordinate to federal constitutional laws. State statutes typically regulate education, insurance, and professional licensure. For example, each state has a physical therapy practice act that covers the scope and protection of physical therapist (PT) practice, the definition of providers who may legally provide physical therapy services, and the state's definition of PT practice (see Licensure Laws later).

Common laws, decrees handed down by judges, have a third priority as legal tenets. In the United States, some common laws remain based on early English common laws. Most U.S. civil laws concerning ethical and legal issues in health care are derived from common laws. An example of common law affecting physical therapy practice is malpractice law.

Administrative or regulatory agencies enact administrative or regulatory laws at the local, state, and federal levels. Unlike statutes, regulations are developed by government agencies, not the legislature, and serve to promulgate administrative rules that supplement statutes and executive orders. Administrative or regulatory laws influence business conduct. For example, state regulations require continuing education for PTs and physical therapist assistants (PTAs) in regulations, or the practice act itself. Thus, through regulatory agencies, administrative or regulatory laws affect healthcare professions in practice, research, and educational settings. Federal administrative agencies with broad authority over physical therapy business affairs include the Occupational Safety and Health Administration (OSHA) and the Centers for Medicare and Medicaid Services (CMS).

Executive orders, typically issued by a governor or president, or a combination of both, direct a federal official or administrative agency to engage in or refrain from a course of action.

# Laws Affecting Physical Therapy Practice

Several federal statutes affect physical therapy practice: the Americans with Disabilities Act (incorporating mostly Titles I to V), the Individuals with Disabilities Education Act of 1997, the Health Insurance Portability and Accountability Act (HIPAA) (see Chapter 6), the Social Security Amendments of 1965 (see Chapter 11), and the Affordable Care Act (ACA) (see Chapter 11).

## The Americans with Disabilities Act

The **Americans with Disabilities Act (ADA)** of 1989 [1] is a nondiscriminatory law that marked the first explicit national goal of achieving equal opportunity, independent living, and economic self-sufficiency for individuals with disabilities [2]. The ADA prevents discrimination against persons with disabilities in employment, public accommodations (see **Figure 7-1**), state and local government services, and telecommunications.

### What is a disability (as per the ADA)?

- Physical or mental impairment substantially limits one or more major life activities.
- A person with a **disability** must have a record of such physical or mental impairment.
- A person with a disability has such an impairment.
- The major life activities include, among others, all the important activities of daily living (ADLs), including the ability to see, hear, speak, walk, care for oneself, maintain cardiorespiratory function, perform manual tasks, and engage in formal and informal learning activities.

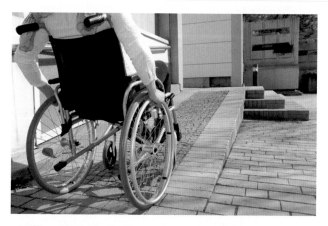

**Figure 7-1** Accessibility should not be an issue.
© RioPatuca/Shutterstock

The ADA's purpose is to ensure that people with disabilities can integrate into U.S. society by ensuring equal access to public accommodations and services and equal opportunities in employment. The ADA was modeled after the Rehabilitation Act of 1973, which prohibits employment discrimination based on disability in federal executive agencies and all institutions receiving Medicare, Medicaid, and other federal support. The ADA has five sections or titles.

### Title I of the ADA

Title I of the ADA protects people with disabilities against employment discrimination. Title I became effective in July 1992 for businesses employing 25 or more people and in July 1994 for businesses employing 15 or more people. Title I prohibits employment discrimination by private and public employers, employment agencies, or union organizations against employees and job applicants qualified to perform their jobs' essential functions. Discrimination applies to an employee's recruitment, selection, training, benefits, promotion, discipline, and retention. The qualified individual with a disability is a job applicant or employee who can perform essential functions with or without reasonable accommodations.

A reasonable accommodation means any adjustment to a job, the work environment, or the way things are usually done that would allow a person with a disability to apply for a job, perform job functions, or enjoy equal access to benefits available to other individuals in the workplace. Many accommodations may help people with disabilities work successfully. Some of the most common accommodations include:

- Making physical changes, such as installing a ramp or modifying a workspace or restroom
- Providing sign language interpreters for people who are deaf or readers for people who are blind
- Providing a quieter workspace or making other changes to reduce noisy distractions for someone with a mental disability
- Providing training and creating written materials in an accessible format, such as in Braille on audio devices
- Providing teletypewriters (TTYs) for use with telephones by people who are deaf and hardware and software that make computers accessible to people with vision impairments or who have difficulty using their hands
- Giving time off to an individual who needs treatment for a disability

The reasonable accommodations must be carried out on the request of an applicant or employee (or by the employee having a disability) unless the employer can prove that to do so would amount to an undue hardship.

Undue hardship means that the accommodation would be excessively disruptive, very costly, difficult to implement, or would fundamentally alter the nature of the employer's business operation. For example, suppose a physical therapy clinic hired a visually impaired massage therapist who needs improved lighting to complete paperwork. In that case, it may be more appropriate to install dimmable lighting in the room where the massage therapist will work. Such an accommodation would allow for appropriate lighting when he is doing paperwork but be adjustable for lower lighting when working with clients. If the employee expected excessively bright lighting all the time, that may constitute "undue hardship" for the business because it would not be conducive to the massage's relaxing effects.

### Titles II, III, IV, and V of the ADA

Title II of the ADA protects against discrimination regarding equal access to public services, including public transportation services. Title III of the ADA protects against discrimination related to equal public accommodations, including all private businesses and services. All religious organizations and some private clubs are exempt from the group requiring private accommodations. Title IV of the ADA protects against discrimination related to equal access to telecommunications services. Title V of the ADA is a miscellaneous section that discusses the ADA's relationship to other federal statutes, key definitions, and an affirmation that the states cannot claim immunity from the ADA requirements. This section includes protection from retribution for any individual who advocates for a person with a disability.

Both public and private hospitals and healthcare facilities, such as physical therapy facilities, must provide their services to people with disabilities in a nondiscriminatory manner. To do so, they may have to modify their policies and procedures, provide auxiliary aids and services for effective communication, remove barriers from existing facilities, and follow the ADA accessibility standards for new construction and alteration projects. However, when healthcare providers need to modify their policies and procedures, the ADA does not require providers to make changes that would fundamentally alter the nature of their services.

Healthcare providers must also find appropriate ways to communicate effectively with persons who have disabilities that affect their ability to communicate. Various auxiliary aids and services, such as interpreters, written notes, readers, large print, or Braille text, can be used depending on the circumstance and the individual. However, if any auxiliary aid or services would result in an undue burden or fundamentally alter the nature of services, the ADA does not require the healthcare provider to acquire these auxiliary aids and services. For example, telecommunication devices for people who are deaf or hard of hearing (TDD), such as TTYs, must be accessible where a voice telephone is made available for outgoing calls on more than an incidental convenience basis. This includes inpatient rooms and emergency department or recovery room waiting areas. Outpatient medical and healthcare facilities (such as physical therapy outpatient facilities) are not required to have TTYs for patients/clients, but they should have relay systems for making and receiving calls from patients or clients with hearing or speech impairments.

## Individuals with Disabilities Education Act (IDEA) of 1997

The Individuals with Disabilities Education Act (IDEA) was introduced in 1975. In 1997, the act was amended by then-President Clinton. IDEA is a law ensuring services to children with disabilities throughout the nation. It governs how states and public agencies provide early intervention, special education, and related services to eligible infants, toddlers, children, and youth with disabilities. Infants and toddlers (birth to 2 years of age) with disabilities and their families receive early intervention services under IDEA Part C. Children and youth (ages 3–21 years) receive special education and related services under IDEA Part B.

### Physical Therapy Services for Children with Disabilities

The American Physical Therapy Association (APTA) supports the provision of physical therapy services to children with special needs. PTs plan and implement programs to help children with various sensory and motor disabilities attain their optimal educational potential and cost-effectively benefit from special education within federally approved state plans [3]. Physical therapy's primary goal is identifying and serving the best interests of children with disabling conditions within the school setting and their overall quality of life [3]. PTs/PTAs provide:

- Early physical therapy services for infants and toddlers with disabilities
- Physical therapy services for children with disabilities in educational programs

Also, PTs assume a significant role in developing a child's individualized education program or individualized family service plans.

The purposes of the IDEA of 1997 include the following:

- To ensure that all children with disabilities have available to them a free appropriate public education that emphasizes special education and related services designed to meet their unique needs and prepare them for employment and independent living
- To protect the rights of children with disabilities and parents of such children
- To assist states, localities, educational service agencies, and federal agencies in providing for the education of all children with disabilities
- To assist states in implementing a statewide, comprehensive, coordinated, multidisciplinary, interagency system of early intervention services for infants and toddlers with disabilities and their families
- To *ensure that* educators and parents have the necessary tools to improve educational results for children with disabilities by supporting systemic change; coordinated research and personnel preparation; coordinated technical assistance, dissemination, and support; and technology development and media services
- To assess and ensure the effectiveness of efforts to educate children with disabilities

The PT's roles in early intervention for infants and toddlers with disabilities include:

- Consulting with parents, other service providers, and representatives of appropriate community agencies to ensure the effective provision of services in that area
- Training parents and others regarding the provision of those services
- Participating in the multidisciplinary team's assessment of a child and the child's family and developing integrated goals and outcomes for the individualized family service plan

## Licensure Laws

All states enact licensure laws, giving licensees the exclusive right to practice their professions. Licensure laws protect the consumer against professional

Physical therapy may include the following services:

- Screening, evaluation, and assessment of infants and toddlers to identify movement dysfunction
- Obtaining, interpreting, and integrating information appropriate to program planning to prevent, alleviate, or compensate for movement dysfunction and related functional problems
- Providing individual and group services or treatment to prevent, alleviate, or compensate for movement dysfunction and related functional problems

- Requirements for periodic relicensure
- Requirements for mandatory reporting of perceived unethical conduct within the scope of permissible practice
- Restrictions, if any, on an independent or autonomous practice called practice without referral
- Provisions establishing licensure boards to administer professional licensure
- Provisions defining grounds and procedures for disciplinary action

## KNOWLEDGE CHECK

What types of laws are utilized by the Centers for Medicare and Medicaid to apply rules and regulations?

What is included in Title I of the Americans with Disabilities Act?

What does the Individual with Disabilities Education Act of 1997 require for compliance?

incompetence. Healthcare professionals, such as physicians, surgeons, dentists, occupational therapists, PTs, and registered nurses, and technically educated healthcare providers, such as PTAs and certified occupational therapist assistants are subject to mandatory licensure requirements for practice. State licensure laws also implement regulatory practice acts that define the requirements of licensed health professional practices, such as PTs, occupational therapists, physicians, surgeons, dentists, and registered nurses.

Requirements of regulatory practice acts include:

- Requirements for licensure of professionals educated in the United States
- Requirements for licensure of foreign-educated or foreign-trained professionals
- Requirements for continuing professional education
- Requirements for practice within the state according to temporary licensure

Violations of mandatory licensure laws are punishable as criminal offenses and form the basis for administrative claims and civil healthcare malpractice lawsuits. The fact that practice acts can vary from state to state is particularly important. For example, the levels of supervision required for a PTA by the supervising PT can vary significantly. Thus, a PT or PTA license/certification cannot automatically be transferred from one state to another but requires a separate application.

### Box 7-1 Laws

- Common law. A body of law based on court decisions rather than statutes or codes (e.g., code of ethics). An example in health care includes healthcare professionals–patient confidentiality.
- Civil law. Civil law is concerned with the peaceable resolution of disputes among individuals. An example in health care includes negligence resulting in injury or death.
- Criminal law. There are two main types of criminal law offenses: felonies (serious offenses like murder, robbery, and arson) and misdemeanors (minor offenses like traffic violations or petty thefts). An example in health care includes overbilling or improper billing (fraud).

## Licensure for PTs and PTAs

The APTA established the following policies regarding the licensure of PTs and PTAs in the United States[1]:

- PTs are licensed.
- PTAs should be licensed or otherwise regulated in all U.S. jurisdictions.

---

1 American Physical Therapy Association: Consumer Protection Through Licensure of Physical Therapists and Physical Therapist Assistants. HOD 06-14-08-07 [Internet]. [cited 2023 Feb]. Available from: https://www.apta.org/apta-and-you/leadership-and -governance/policies/consumer-protection-licensure

- State regulation of PTs and PTAs should, at a minimum:
    1. Require graduation from a physical therapy education program that is accredited by the Commission on Accreditation in Physical Therapy Education (CAPTE), or
        a. In the case of an internationally educated PT seeking licensure as a PT, a substantially equivalent education, or
        b. In the case of a graduate of an international PTA program seeking licensure, certification, or registration as a PTA, a substantially equivalent education.
    2. Require passing an entry-level competency exam
    3. Provide title protection
    4. Allow for disciplinary action
- Additionally, PTs' licensure should include a defined scope of practice.
- All PTAs must work under the direction and supervision of the PT. State statute defines the supervision relationship between PTs and supervised personnel. Many states limit the number of PTAs an individual PT may supervise, while others define supervision by the number of personnel supervised, including PTAs or PT aides and technicians. The supervision rules also usually include the time between PT/PTA consultation and PT/patient visits. Some states may require a co-treatment by the PT and PTA with the patient.

Physical therapy licensure laws for PTs are enacted in 53 jurisdictions, including the 50 states, the District of Columbia, Puerto Rico, and the U.S. Virgin Islands. PTAs are licensed or certified in 50 jurisdictions. The Federation of State Boards of Physical Therapy (FSBPT) works toward desirable and reasonable uniformity in regulation and standards through strategic planning and ongoing communications among the jurisdictions. The licensure examination and related activities are the responsibility of the FSBPT. The National Physical Therapy Examination (NPTE) licensure examination has two versions: one for PTs and the other for PTAs. The jurisdictions agreed to support one passing score on the national licensure examination for PTs and PTAs. This agreement facilitates the mobility of PTs and PTAs across states and holds all PTs beginning practice in the United States to the same entry-level standard of competence. Each state determines the criteria to practice and issues a license to a PT or a PTA. Additionally, some states require that students take a jurisprudence exam to ensure they are informed about the laws and regulations governing PTs and PTAs in that state. For more information, please check the FSBPT website at www.fsbpt.org.

---

**KNOWLEDGE CHECK**

What are the requirements for practice included in regulatory practice acts?
What are the APTA policies regarding licensure?

---

# Occupational Safety and Health Administration's Federal Standards

The **Occupational Safety and Health Administration (OSHA)** is a federal government regulatory agency concerned with the health and safety of workers.

---

OSHA's role is to assure safe and healthful working conditions for working men and women by:

- Authorizing enforcement of the standards developed under the OSHA Act
- Assisting and encouraging the states in their efforts to assure safe and healthful working conditions
- Providing for research, information, education, and training in occupational safety and health

---

OSHA's services include establishing protective standards, enforcing those standards, and reaching out to employers and employees through technical assistance and consultation programs.

## The Bloodborne Pathogens Standard

This OSHA standard requires that employers protect workers who could be exposed to blood or infectious agents by:

- Creating a plan, including policies and procedures, to minimize the risks of exposure to bloodborne pathogens
- Requiring the use of universal precautions and provide personal protective equipment to employees
- Providing work areas that ensure minimized risk practices can be employed, such as the availability of sharps disposal containers, warning labels,

laundry handling containment, and appropriate cleaning products

- Providing hepatitis B vaccinations and postexposure examinations to employees
- Providing training to employees to minimize risk and enforce policies and procedures that decrease the risk

OSHA has developed factsheets on the **bloodborne pathogens standards (BPS)**. The OSHA website (www.osha.gov) has files that are downloadable and contact information for regional OSHA offices where questions about compliance and the standard can be answered. Individual employers should have a training program to inform their employees about risks and safety standards in their healthcare setting.

## Methods of Infection Control

Limiting healthcare worker exposure to bloodborne diseases is achieved by implementing the following categories of infection controls:

- Engineering controls
- Immunization programs
- Work practices, such as careful handwashing after each patient contact and procedures for handling sharps (see **Figure 7-2**)
- Disposal and handling of contaminated waste
- Use of personal protective equipment, especially gloves, gowns, and goggles
- Use of mouthpieces, resuscitation bags, or other ventilation devices
- Use of disinfectants
- Labeling and signs
- Training and education programs
- Postexposure follow-up

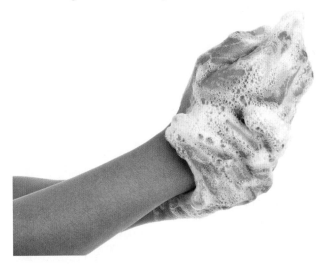

**Figure 7-2** Safety starts with washing hands.
© Samuel Borges Photography/Shutterstock

## Universal Precautions

Universal precautions represent OSHA's recommendations to control and protect employees from exposure to all human blood and other potentially infectious materials. The BPS requires all blood and other potentially infectious materials to be considered as infectious regardless of the perceived risk of an individual patient or patient population. For example, a PT/PTA who treats mostly older adults in a rural area may feel that the prevalence of human immunodeficiency virus (HIV) and hepatitis B virus (HBV) among these patients is negligible. However, the PT/PTA is required by the standards to use the same universal precautions when treating infected patients. The precautions can protect the PT/PTA and the patients from contamination.

Regarding universal precautions and respecting OSHA's rules and regulations, healthcare employees are responsible for:

- Using protective barriers and procedures consistently in all situations and for all patients.
- Understanding that the purpose of practicing universal precautions is to prevent infection from bloodborne pathogens on the job.
- Assuming that any patient or bodily fluid is potentially infectious for bloodborne pathogens such as HBV or HIV.
- Understanding that potentially infectious materials include semen, vaginal secretions, cerebrospinal fluid, synovial fluid, pleural fluid, pericardial fluid, peritoneal fluid, amniotic fluid, saliva in dental procedures, and any body fluid that is visibly contaminated with blood.
- Complying with the summaries of the universal precautions recommendations.

Universal precautions recommendations include:

- Use protective equipment and clothing whenever in contact with bodily fluids.
- Dispose of waste in proper containers using proper handling techniques for infectious waste.
- Dispose of sharp instruments and needles in proper containers.
- Keep the work area and the patient area clean.
- Wash hands immediately after removing gloves and at all times required by the agency policy.
- Immediately report any exposure to needle sticks, blood splashes, or any personal illness to the direct supervisor and receive instructions about follow-up action.

# Domestic Violence and Legal Issues

Domestic violence is a significant problem in the United States. Domestic violence statistics are frightening. Although many domestic violence assaults are never reported, the U.S. Department of Justice estimated that more than 12 million women and men are physically abused, raped, or stalked by their intimate partners each year.[2]

### What is domestic violence?

**Domestic violence**, also called domestic abuse, intimate partner violence (IPV), or battering, occurs between people in intimate relationships and takes many forms, including coercion; threats; intimidation; isolation; and emotional, sexual, and **physical abuse**.

Domestic violence may often result in death. In addition to the loss of life, medical care and productivity resulting from IPV cost the United States billions of dollars each year.

Domestic violence affects people of all ages, races, ethnicities, and religions, and there are no typical victims of domestic abuse. Domestic violence exists among people of all ages, races, ethnicities, and religions. It occurs in both opposite-sex and same-sex relationships. Economic or professional status does not indicate a likelihood of domestic violence. Abusers and victims can be laborers or college professors, healthcare professionals or judges, truck drivers or schoolteachers, store clerks, or stay-at-home moms and dads. Domestic violence can occur in the fanciest mansions or the poorest ghettos.

Domestic violence, or IPV, is a health problem of enormous proportions. In the United States, 27% of women and 11.5% of men experience physical and/or **sexual abuse** by an intimate partner at some point in their adult lives. Elderly Americans are also victims of domestic abuse. For example, research published in the *American Journal of Public Health* found that 1 in 10 Americans older than 60 experienced abuse yearly [4]. In addition, children are also exposed to IPV.

## Recognizing Domestic Violence Patterns

The relationships between the abuser and the person abused differ. In all abuse cases, the abuser aims to have power and control over their intimate partner. Anger is only one way an abuser tries to gain authority and instill fear in a relationship. The batterer can also turn to physical violence, such as kicking, punching, grabbing, slapping, or biting.

Methods the abuser may use to gain power and control over the intimate partner include the following[3]:

- Physical violence, such as hitting, kicking, or hurting the victim using physical force
- Sexual violence, such as forcing the victim to have sexual intercourse or to engage in other sexual activities against the intimate partner's will
- Using children as pawns, such as accusing the intimate partner of bad parenting, threatening to take the children away, or using the children to relay messages to the partner
- Denial and blame, such as denying that the abuse occurred or shifting responsibility for the abusive behavior onto the partner
- Coercion and threats, such as threatening to hurt other family members, pets, children, or self
- **Economic abuse**, such as controlling finances, refusing to share money, sabotaging the partner's work performance, making the partner account for money spent, or not allowing the partner to work outside the home
- Intimidation, such as using certain actions, looks, or gestures to instill fear, breaking things, abusing pets, or destroying property
- **Emotional abuse**, such as insults, criticism, or name-calling
- Isolation, such as limiting the partner's contact with family and friends, requiring permission to leave the house, not allowing the partner to attend work or school, or controlling the partner's activities and social events
- Privileges, such as making all major decisions, defining the roles in the relationship, being in charge of the home and social life, or treating the partner as a servant or possession

Data from Office of Justice Programs. 2001. Toolkit To End Violence Against Women. US Department of Justice. https://www.ojp.gov/pdffiles1/206041.pdf

---

2 https://www.cdc.gov/violenceprevention/intimatepartnerviolence/index.html
3 https://www.ojp.gov/ncjrs/virtual-library/abstracts/toolkit-end-violence-against-women

# Domestic Violence and Health Care

Domestic violence is a serious crime that substantially impacts the health and welfare of adults and children. Physical and sexual assaults by partners can result in various injuries, including cuts, broken bones, bruises, internal injuries, concussions, internal bleeding, and death. Additionally, mental health consequences of physical, sexual, and/or domestic **psychological abuse** may include posttraumatic stress disorder, depression, suicide, substance abuse, and anxiety disorders.

Physicians and healthcare professionals can play a major role in helping victims to disclose violence. They also can assure the victim that advice and support are available [5]. Domestic violence can go undetected in healthcare settings, mostly because most victims are reluctant to report domestic violence abuse.

> Reasons healthcare providers may experience difficulties identifying/helping victims of domestic violence include the following [5]:
>
> - The healthcare provider's fears or experiences of exploring the issue of domestic violence
> - The healthcare provider's lack of knowledge of community resources
> - The healthcare provider's fear of offending the victim and jeopardizing the provider–patient relationship
> - The healthcare provider's lack of time or lack of training
> - The healthcare provider's unresponsiveness caused by feeling powerless and not being able to fix the situation
> - The victim's infrequent visits as a patient
> - The victim's unresponsiveness to questions asked by the healthcare provider

The first step toward ensuring appropriate care is identifying individuals experiencing domestic violence. Healthcare providers may try the following actions [5]:

- Observe the victim for physical and behavioral clues.
- Question the victim and validate domestic abuse.
- Respect the victim's privacy and use confidentiality measures.
- Assess and treat the victim.
- Keep accurate records and concise documentation about the victim's abuse.
- Support and follow up on the victim's care.

In many situations, the victim may not realize the health impact of the abuse. The victim may or may not be symptomatic. Also, they may not disclose abuse because they cannot understand how violence affects their health. Other reasons for not disclosing may be fear of the partner, embarrassment, and fear of discussing the abuse with the healthcare provider. Consequently, the healthcare provider's role is to initiate prevention strategies. For example, the healthcare provider can educate patients about healthy relationships, parenting skills, and the warning signs of an abusive relationship. The healthcare provider may also prompt female victims regarding the following [5]:

- Social norms are changing.
- Social norms do not promote hostility or violence toward women.
- Men these days are more involved as co-parents.
- The status of women in U.S. society is growing through education and jobs.

Healthcare providers must believe that preventing domestic abuse will reduce other types of interpersonal violence, such as child abuse, elder abuse, and the physical and mental health effects of childhood exposure to domestic violence. By educating patients about the broad implications of domestic abuse and the elevated risk of multiple forms of violence in the same household, healthcare providers can help end the cycle of family violence [5].

# Domestic Violence and Physical Therapy

Because control and power are the two main issues of domestic violence, the abuser uses fear and the threat of physical harm to control the victim. The abuser may use physical and economic control to limit the victim's access to medical care, including physical therapy. The victim's regular appointments at a physical therapy clinic can pose a threat to the abuser, allowing the victim to form a relationship with the PT and the PTA and possibly reveal the cause of their injuries. The abuser may not allow the victim to continue physical therapy by limiting the victim's access to transportation or finances. As a result, the victim/patient may appear noncompliant with physical therapy. Noncompliance can also be caused by the effects of depression or fatigue caused by the abuse.

For PTs and PTAs (the same as for other healthcare providers), recognizing a victim of domestic violence is not easy. Some victims attempt to conceal their injuries from healthcare providers. However, it is possible that, if asked, the victim may reveal their situation.

Recognizable signs of abuse while the victim is accessing physical therapy services may include the following from the APTA:

- The abuser accompanies the victim to all appointments and refuses to allow the victim to be interviewed alone; also, the abuser can use verbal or nonverbal communication to direct the victim's responses during appointments
- The patient may be noncompliant with physical therapy treatment regimens and/or frequently miss appointments
- The patient's statements about not being allowed to take or obtain medications (prescription or nonprescription medication)
- The abuser canceling the victim's appointments or sabotaging the victim's efforts to attend appointments (e.g., by not providing child care or transportation)
- The patient engages in therapist-hopping
- The patient lacks independent transportation, access to finances, or the ability to communicate by phone

Signs that a patient should be screened for domestic abuse may include the following from the APTA:

- Chronic pain
- Injuries during pregnancy
- Repeated and chronic injuries
- Exacerbated or poorly controlled chronic illnesses, such as asthma, seizure disorders, diabetes, hypertension, and heart disease
- Unattended gynecological problems
- Physical symptoms related to stress, anxiety disorders, or depression
- Hypervigilant signs, such as being easily startled or very guarded, experiencing nightmares or emotional numbing
- Suicide attempts
- Eating disorders
- Self-mutilation
- Car accidents where the victim is the driver or the passenger
- Overuse of prescription pain medications and other drugs

According to the APTA, an abuser's tactics to control the healthcare providers may include:

- Intimidating healthcare professionals with a variety of threats or acts
- Portraying themselves as a good provider and caregiver and/or consistently praising healthcare professionals
- Harassing healthcare professionals by repeated phone calls, threats of legal action, and/or false reports to superiors about supposed breaches of confidentiality, inappropriate treatment, or rude behavior
- Splitting healthcare teams by creating divisiveness among professionals

- Develop objective criteria for identifying, examining, and treating patients/clients who may be victims of domestic violence.
- Have available legally required notifications and release of information to the proper authorities when evaluating/examining patients/clients who may be victims of domestic violence.
- Screen, evaluate/examine, reevaluate, and care for patients/clients who may be victims of domestic violence.
- Provide in-service training and continuing education about domestic violence to all physical therapy personnel.
- Establish a domestic violence protocol for emergencies for patients/clients who may be victims of domestic violence.
- Have a list of appropriate referrals to community agencies for patients/clients who may be victims of domestic violence.

As signs, victims may have more than one injury, including short-term injuries, such as black eyes, contusions, lacerations, and fractures. Other injuries that can be observed in physical therapy are burns, vision or hearing loss, knife wounds, or joint damage.

PTs and PTAs have an ethical duty to treat domestic violence victims, address the victims' rights, dignity, confidentiality, compliance with governing laws, and accept responsibility. If a PTA suspects a patient is a victim of domestic violence, the PTA should report their suspicions to the PT of record. PTs and PTAs could work together with other healthcare providers and their community leaders to establish the following domestic violence guidelines for their organization(s):

PTs should routinely screen for domestic violence by asking direct questions about injuries, evasive behavior, and the patient's fear of their partner. Patients must be interviewed privately, away from their intimate partner or other family members. For patients who understand terms such as abuse or battered, direct questioning is the best way to elicit a response. Indirect questioning may be more appropriate for patients who do not understand these terms. The best questioning methods are to frame the questions in the context of domestic violence being a common problem in U.S. society. This approach allows the patient to be more comfortable about the subject and to open up about their problems as a victim of domestic abuse.

Examples of direct questions for victims of domestic violence include the following from the APTA:

- I am concerned about your symptoms, especially because they may be caused by someone hurting you. Has someone been hurting you?
- Your bruise looks painful. Did someone hit you?
- Did your partner hit you?

Examples of indirect questions for victims of domestic violence include:

- You seem concerned about your partner. Are you having problems with your partner?
- What types of problems do you have with your partner?
- How does your partner feel about you having physical therapy? Does your partner resent you coming here?

Questions that PTs or PTAs should never ask victims of domestic violence include:

- Why would you stay with a person like that?
- What could you have done to defuse the situation?
- Why don't you just leave?
- What did you do to aggravate your partner?
- Did you do something to cause your partner to hit you?

Some states require healthcare providers to report injuries caused by a knife, gun, or other deadly weapons, or injuries resulting from a criminal act, act of violence, or nonaccidental act. PTs and PTAs should obtain a copy of their state's statutes and consult with legal counsel regarding individual cases and changes in state and federal laws relating to domestic violence. In cases where the PT or PTA needs to report the abuse, they should be able to work with the patient so that the report's timing allows for the patient's safety. Specific state-by-state information can be found on the U.S. Department of Health and Human Services website.

When domestic abuse is confirmed, PTs and PTAs must be able to document the abuse correctly in the patient's medical records. Although sometimes a victim may not intend to pursue legal remedies, the victim may change their mind and proceed to court. The medical records must be admissible in a court of law.

## Domestic Violence and Legal Issues

On October 28, 2000, the U.S. Congress passed the Violence Against Women Act (VAWA), which reauthorized and expanded the 1995 Violence Against Women Act. VAWA 2000 improves legal tools and

The APTA's documentation guidelines on domestic violence include:

- The medical records must be written in the regular course of business during the examination or the interview.
- The medical records must be legible.
- The medical records must be properly stored and accessed by appropriate staff only.
- The medical records must include the following information:
  - Patient's date and arrival time at the clinic or the treatment site.
  - Patient's name, address, and phone number of the person(s) accompanying the victim (if possible).
  - Patient's own words about the cause of their injuries.
  - A detailed description (with explanations) of injuries, including the type, number, size, location, and resolution; a description of a chronology of the violence asks about the first, most recent, and most serious episodes.
  - Any documentation of inconsistency between the injury and the explanation about the injury.
  - Documentation that the clinician asked about domestic violence and the patient's response.
  - Color photograph(s), including the patient's informed consent for the photograph(s); photographs should be taken from different angles, including the patient's face in at least one picture. Two pictures are necessary for each major trauma area. The photographs must be marked, including the patient's name, the injury's location, and the person taking the pictures.
- If the police were called, the investigating officer's name, badge number, phone number, and any actions taken.
- Documentation about the name of the PT, PTA, physician, or nurse who treated the patient (if applicable).

Data from American Physical Therapy Association: Documenting Domestic Violence [Internet]. [cited 2005 Apr]. Available from: www.apta.org

programs addressing domestic violence, sexual assault, and stalking. VAWA 2000 also reauthorized critical grant programs created by the original Violence Against Women Act and subsequent legislation, established new programs, and strengthened federal laws. For example, VAWA 2000 referred to the definition of dating violence as violence committed by a person who has been in a social relationship of a romantic or intimate nature with the victim. The length of the relationship, the type of relationship, and the frequency of interaction between the persons involved determine the existence of such a relationship. In 2013, further reauthorization legislation expanded protections to include immigrants, gays, lesbians, and transgender individuals. It also expanded Native American tribal court powers to prosecute perpetrators of violence.

The U.S. Department of Justice, in cooperation with the National Advisory Council on Violence Against Women and the Violence Against Women Office, educates and mobilizes the public about violence against women. These organizations are asking communities to help victims of domestic violence by:

- Engaging the media, community members, and educators
- Ensuring that services are available to those who seek help
- Creating campaigns with a grassroots-organized component
- Forming community partnerships
- Targeting education and awareness campaigns at young people and men
- Creating partnerships with the media so that antiviolence campaigns continue through changes in media ownership and leadership
- Complementing community service campaigns with aggressive free media campaigns
- Seeking corporate support for media campaigns
- Targeting education and awareness campaigns to populations that might not be reached via a general outreach
- Evaluating public education efforts rigorously

Domestic violence can be handled in three types of law courts:

- Criminal court, where the state will prosecute the abuser. The possible crimes include abuse of an intimate partner, violation of a protection order, elder abuse, murder, rape, assault, kidnapping, false imprisonment, property destruction, vandalism, trespassing, stalking, unlawful possession or concealment of a weapon, intimidating a witness, and many others.

- Divorce or family court, where family violence directly affects divorce proceedings, can be a factor in limiting or prohibiting the abuser's rights to child custody or visitation rights.
- Civil court, where the victim can address a protection order violation or sue for monetary damages. Possible civil lawsuits include sexual harassment or personal injury.

## Elder Abuse

Elder abuse occurs when someone knowingly, intentionally, or by negligence causes harm to an older adult. This abuse can take the form of physical abuse, sexual abuse, negligence, exploitation, emotional abuse, abandonment, or not confronting an older adult's self-neglect. The Elder Justice Act of 2010 established governmental authorities and funding to support Adult Protection Services in all states. Grants are available for staff training and those who oversee elderly residential facilities to identify instances of elder abuse better (see **Figure 7-3**). Because PTs and PTAs work closely with patients for extended periods, it may be easier for these healthcare professionals to recognize elder abuse. Each state has resources to assist with reporting these issues by contacting Adult Protective Services of the state where the person resides.

### KNOWLEDGE CHECK

What is a sign of domestic abuse?
Explain the types of abuse.
What behaviors might an abuser use to control the healthcare provider?
How can a healthcare provider help a person who is abused?

## Harassment

Harassment within the workplace can occur by supervisors, coworkers, and those who are not employees. In the case of healthcare environments, this can also include patient harassment of personnel. Harassment is unwanted conduct and can be due to race, color, religion, sex, age, or disability. Harassment becomes illegal when it affects continued employment or is considered intimidating or hostile. Generally, the employee must mitigate the harassment by expressing their feelings to the person directly or to a supervisor. It is the responsibility of the employer to take steps to prevent harassment from occurring. Consequences

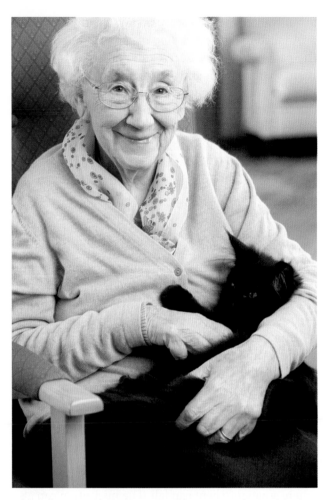

**Figure 7-3** Older adults must be cared for with respect and concern for their quality of life.
© Monkey Business Images/Shutterstock

to perpetrators of harassment can include referral for training or counseling, reprimand, demotion, reassignment, or loss of employment. In some cases, authorities may pursue a criminal case.

PTs and PTAs should consider how they might address patient harassment when it occurs so that they can have a respectful but clear response. An example of this may be a request for a date by a patient. A respectful response may include that it is not legal for practitioners and patients to date. Another example may be an inappropriate comment about the healthcare worker. A respectful response would include that those comments are not appropriate or necessary for the clinical environment.

## Malpractice Laws

Malpractice laws are civil laws derived from common laws. Malpractice occurs when a hospital or healthcare professional causes injury to a patient because of

a negligent act of carelessness. Healthcare malpractice is liability-generating conduct by a primary healthcare professional associated with the adverse outcome.

Healthcare malpractice liability may include:

- Professional negligence. Negligence deviates from the standard of care that a reasonable person would use in a particular set of circumstances
- Intentional misconduct. Misconduct is the failure to comply with the rules of conduct or professional standards in the duties of a licensed professional.
  - Patient injury from abnormally dangerous examination/treatment-related activities
  - Patient injury from any dangerously defective examination/treatment-related products

Healthcare professionals such as PTs can be sued by patients or their legal representatives for treatment-related healthcare malpractice. A PTA can also be sued, but the liability prevails with the PT of record, who was the supervisor of the PTA. A settlement or an adverse judgment against a healthcare provider for malpractice means possible practice-related sanctions, such as licensure restrictions or licensure fines. In physical therapy, PTs are personally responsible for malpractice acts involving the relationships between the PT and the PTA (or nonlicensed personnel) and between the PT and the patient. Examples of PTs' malpractice acts can include:

- Negligence
- Inadequate supervision of PTAs or nonlicensed personnel
- A violation of ethical principles
- Performances that result in harm to the patient

PTAs are also responsible for malpractice acts involving the relationships between the PTA and the patient and between the PTA and nonlicensed personnel. Examples of PTAs' malpractice acts can be negligence and performances that harm the patient.

## Negligence

PTs, PTAs, and PTA students are liable for their negligence. Negligence is failing to give reasonable care or the giving of unreasonable care. A healthcare practitioner is negligent only when harm occurs to the patient/client. For example, a PTA working in the same clinic as a PT leaves a hot pack on the patient for too long without applying the necessary toweling layers and supervising the patient. The hot pack causes burns to the patient. The PTA is liable for negligence because they did not do what another PTA would have done in the same circumstances. In this situation, the PTA disregarded the following actions:

- Applying the necessary layers of toweling
- Supervising the patient closely
- Giving the patient a bell to ring if the hot pack was too hot
- Checking the treatment area every 5 minutes

The supervisory PT is also liable for negligence because of faulty supervision of the PTA. Also, PTs and PTAs can be liable for failing to perform a duty of care, causing harm to the patient. A duty of care is an obligation of a PT or a PTA to prevent harm to the patient/client. The process known as the duty of care entitles the patient/client to safe care by making it mandatory they are treated using the common or average standards of practice expected in the community under similar circumstances.

To prove negligence for a breach of the duty of care, the patient/client must provide evidence that harm resulted from the breach of the duty of care. For example, in the case of the patient who was burned by the hot pack, a physician must examine the patient to confirm that the patient suffered skin burns from the hot pack.

To be proven by the patient, negligence requires all the following:

- The healthcare provider owed the patient a legal duty of care.
- The healthcare provider breached, violated, or failed to comply with the legal duty of care owed to the patient.
- The healthcare provider's breach of duty of care caused injury to the patient or the patient's property.
- The patient sustained or suffered legally cognizable damages, for which a court of law will award monetary judgment designed to make the patient as "whole" again as possible.

Concerning negligence, typically, the patient must show that they were harmed because the healthcare provider did something wrong or failed to do something that should normally have been done under the circumstances. For example, consider a PTA treating a patient just examined and evaluated by the PT for physical therapy (postsurgery) for a total hip replacement (THR). The PTA disregards patient education about THR precautions. After the treatment, the patient does not know about THR precautions and ends up with a dislocation of the new hip and an unwanted new THR operation. In this case, the PTA failed to perform a duty of care by not educating the patient about THR precautions. The PTA caused harm to the patient and is personally liable for a malpractice action. Depending on the circumstances and the jurisdictional practice acts, the PT may also be liable for being the PTA's direct supervisor and perhaps for not educating the patient in the initial examination and evaluation about THR precautions (and/or for not reminding the PTA to educate the patient about the precautions).

In physical therapy clinical practice, patients may contribute to their negligence by not following directions from the PT/PTA. For example, if the patient with a THR received education about the THR precautions but tried to perform activities independently and dislocated the hip, the patient contributed to their negligence. In this circumstance, the PT and the PTA must show proof that the patient received, orally and in writing, education about THR precautions and understood the precautions. The proof can be a written copy (given to the patient) of the THR precautions filed in the patient's records.

There are also situations in physical therapy clinical practice when the institution is negligent if a patient/client is harmed due to an environmental problem, such as a slippery floor or a poorly lit area where a patient/client can fall. The institution can also be liable if the PT or the PTA was incompetent (or was not licensed) or for allowing a nonlicensed person to perform the duties of a PT or a PTA.

## Malpractice Acts in Physical Therapy

Examples of malpractice acts involving PTs, PTAs, or PT/PTA students include the following [6]:

- Burns due to defective equipment (such as an ultrasound device)
- Utilization of defective equipment (such as wheelchairs or assistive devices)
- Patient falls during gait training
- Exercise injuries
- Any action or inaction inconsistent with the APTA's ethical principles and standards of practice

Patients have a statute of limitations 1–4 years after the injury to make a claim. While employers provide malpractice insurance to protect their employees and businesses, individual PTs and PTAs should consider obtaining their own personal policies. This protection is necessary for instances where the employee may have violated company policy, either intentionally or inadvertently.

Attorneys can ask PTs and PTAs to testify in a court of law as expert witnesses. To be legally competent to testify as an expert witness, a witness must meet two basic requirements: (1) the expert witness must be knowledgeable concerning the health professional product or service, and (2) the expert witness must have been directly or indirectly involved with the legal standards of care for the defendant's healthcare discipline at the time that the incident creating the legal controversy took place.

Healthcare providers, including PTs and PTAs, should participate in legal proceedings as expert witnesses to testify on behalf of patients, peers, and others to achieve justice. Being an expert witness is a civic duty, similar to voting or jury duty.

## KNOWLEDGE CHECK

What is negligence?
What are examples of malpractice?

## Discussion Questions

1. Identify accessibility barriers in your home, school, or other public places.
2. Discuss appropriate responses to a patient who appears to be in a relationship where domestic violence is occurring.
3. A PT works with a patient who has called her at home several times to ask questions and chat. The PT feels that the situation has become more than a healthcare provider/patient relationship. Discuss possible respectful responses to this situation.

## Learning Opportunities

1. Using the Federation of State Boards of Physical Therapy webpage (www.fsbpt.org), locate your state's licensing board and review the laws that govern PTs/PTAs in your state.
2. Use the internet to identify the location of the closest Adult Protective Services agency. Identify what an ombudsperson does and when you should contact one.
3. Create a brochure for the physical therapy profession about malpractice issues.

## References

1. Americans with Disabilities Act of 1989: 104 Stat 327. 1989, pp 101–336, 42 USC 12101 s2 (a) (8)
2. Waddell G, Waddell H: A Review of Social Influences on Neck and Back Pain Disability, in Nachemson AL, Jonsson E (eds): Neck and Back Pain: The Scientific Evidence of Causes, Diagnosis, and Treatment. Philadelphia, PA, Lippincott Williams and Wilkins, 2000, pp 13–55
3. American Physical Therapy Association: Physical Therapy for Individuals with Disabilities: Practice in Educational Settings [Internet]. 2012 [cited 2023 Feb 2]. Available from: https://www.apta.org/apta-and-you/leadership-and-governance/policies/pt-for-individuals-with-disabilities
4. Acierno R, Hernandez MA, Amstadter AB, et al: Prevalence and correlates of emotional, physical, sexual, and financial abuse and potential neglect in the United States: the National Elder Mistreatment Study. Am J Public Health 100(2):292–297, 2010
5. Coker AL, Smith PH, Fadden MK: Intimate partner violence and disabilities among women attending family practice clinics. J Womens Health (Larchmt) 14(9):829–838, 2005
6. Scott RW: Health Care Malpractice: A Primer on Legal Issues for Professionals. New York, McGraw-Hill, 1999

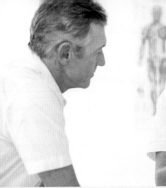
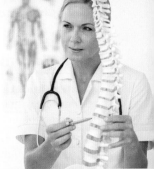

# CHAPTER 8

# Communication

## OBJECTIVES

- Discuss the role of therapeutic communication in physical therapy.
- Contrast empathy and sympathy.
- Describe the significance of verbal and nonverbal communication.
- Differentiate between verbal and nonverbal communication skills.
- Identify the elements required to establish a therapeutic relationship with the patient.
- Identify strategies for dealing with difficult patients.
- Describe components of a good physical therapist/physical therapist assistant relationship.
- Identify strategies to create trust between the physical therapist and the physical therapist assistant.
- List several listening skills and their importance to physical therapy.
- Discuss effective listening skills.
- Contrast open and closed postures.
- Describe written communication for patients and other healthcare professionals.
- Name the primary purpose of the home exercise program handout.
- Describe the main elements of the home exercise program.

## KEY TERMS

| | | |
|---|---|---|
| closed question | empathy | self-awareness |
| communication | open question | therapeutic relationship |

## Overview

Patient management involves a complex relationship among the physical therapist (PT), the physical therapist assistant (PTA), and the patient/client to develop a rapport between the physical therapy team and the patient while providing an efficient and effective exchange. This process's success involves many skills, including effective teamwork and communication skills. Becoming an effective clinician relates to communicating with the patient, the patient's family, and the other healthcare team members. Good communication involves understanding human behavior, effective listening, and detecting subtle changes in

mood, tone of voice, and body language. Nonverbal cues, such as mood and body language, are especially important because they often are performed subconsciously.

## Therapeutic Communication

Therapeutic communication occurs when a PT or a PTA interacts with a patient/client in a therapeutic or healing manner. Ideally, **therapeutic relationships** are partnerships among the PT, PTA, and patient/client. To achieve these partnerships

## What is communication?

**Communication** is the most immediate tool used to interact with others and can take many forms, including the following:

- Verbal. The exchange of information or ideas through spoken words, face-to-face conversation, or media, such as telephone, radio, or television. The effectiveness of verbal communication depends on factors such as tone, inflection, body language, and the clarity and conciseness of the message.
- Written. A form of communication in which messages are exchanged through written text, such as emails, letters, reports, medical records, memos, or text messages. Effective written communication requires understanding the audience and the purpose of the message, clear and concise language, an appropriate tone, and a well-organized structure. The use of written communication has been greatly facilitated by advances in technology, making it a widely used method of communication in the digital age.
- Nonverbal. The transfer of information or messages through means other than spoken or written. It includes a range of behaviors, such as facial expressions, eye contact, gestures, posture, tone of voice, and appearance, that can influence and complement verbal communication. Understanding and effectively using nonverbal communication is key to effective interpersonal communication.
- Electronic. The exchange of information or messages through electronic devices, such as computers, tablets, or smartphones. It includes various forms of digital communication, such as text messaging, instant messaging, email, social media, and online forums. Despite its accessibility, electronic communication has raised challenges, such as privacy concerns, difficulty interpreting tone and intent, and the potential for misunderstandings due to the lack of nonverbal cues. Effective electronic communication skills involve understanding the technology being used and the norms and conventions of the particular medium to ensure that messages received by the intended audience are clear and concise.
- Reading. A form of communication in which a reader interprets written or printed words to understand the intended message or information. Reading can take many forms, including books, newspapers, professional literature, medical documentation, magazines, websites, and digital devices. Effective reading requires active engagement and comprehension and the ability to critically identify bias and misinformation and analyze and evaluate the presented information.

and to convey positive attitudes to patients/clients, PTs and PTAs use verbal and nonverbal forms of communication.

The American Physical Therapy Association (APTA) has designed several communication-based proficiencies, including the Leadership, Administration, Management, and Professionalism (LAMP) certificate program offered by the section on Health Policy and Administration (HPA) of the APTA. For example, the first course, Leadership 101: Personal Leadership Development—The Catalyst for Leading Within, is designed for self-reflection to identify preferred leadership styles, strengths, and weaknesses.

Whatever the resource, the PT/PTA must learn to interact with others with different communication styles and personalities (**Table 8-1**).

At the initial visit, the PT, PTA, and patient/client establish a therapeutic alliance. This therapeutic alliance will be highly successful if the PT and PTA convey the attitude that they:

- Value the patient/client
- Are attentive to the patient's/client's needs
- Acknowledge the patient's/client's message
- Genuinely empathize with the patient/client
- Want to provide the patient/client with the very best care

The communication process between the healthcare provider and the patient includes other elements of interaction beyond verbal and nonverbal communication factors, including:

- The healthcare provider is self-aware, which allows communication of inner feelings, ideas, emotions, and actions between the patient and the provider.
- The healthcare provider focuses on the patient.
- The healthcare provider listens to the patient objectively without categorizing or projecting personal beliefs and values.
- The healthcare provider develops a trusting relationship with the patient without assuming a parental role but conveys expertise and confidentiality.

## Empathy

Physical therapy is a science and a healing art. PTs and PTAs should be able to interact with patients/clients using a humanistic communication style, placing the patient/client in a position of equality, with equal responsibility for positive outcomes in the rehabilitation process. A complete therapeutic relationship between the PT/PTA and the patient/client will take place if the

**Table 8-1** General Recommendations for Communication

| Verbal commands | Should focus the patient's attention on specific desired actions for intervention |
|---|---|
| Intentional pause | Using a purposeful pause can help draw out more information from the patient. |
| Instruction | Instructions should remain as simple as possible and must never incorporate confusing medical terminology.<br>Before initiating the intervention, the general sequence of events should be explained to the patient. |
| Questions | The patient should be asked questions before and during the intervention to establish a rapport and provide feedback on the current intervention's status. Open-ended questions or statements, such as "How does that feel?," encourage the patient to elaborate, help determine the patient's chief complaint, and decrease the opportunity for bias on the part of the clinician. Close-ended questions, such as "Where is your pain?," are more specific and help to focus the examination and deter irrelevant information. *Neutral* questions, such as "What activities make your symptoms worse?," are structured in such a way as to avoid leading the patient into giving a particular response. Leading questions, such as "Does it hurt more when you walk?," must be used carefully. |
| Tone of voice | The PTA should speak clearly in moderate tones and vary their tone of voice as required by the situation. |
| Nonverbal behaviors | These include expressions, mannerisms, gestures, and posture. Examples of good nonverbal behaviors include projecting a relaxed posture with arms uncrossed, good eye contact, pleasant facial expression, and nods of agreement. Examples of bad nonverbal behaviors include yawning, blank facial expressions, constantly looking at the clock, and fidgeting. |
| Empathy | Expressing empathy involves understanding the ideas being communicated and the emotion behind the ideas—seeing another person's viewpoint and what the person is experiencing. Particularly important aspects of empathy are the recognition of patients' rights, potential cultural differences, typical responses to loss, and the perceived role of spirituality in health and wellness to the patient. |
| Paraphrasing | Using words to describe something a patient says ensures a mutual understanding of what the patient has said. |
| Summarizing | Involves providing the patient with a compressed version of a verbal interaction so that the patient can get confirmation that what they have said has been understood |
| Knowledge | Knowing the importance of each question is based on the didactic background of the clinician. For example, if the patient reports that lumbar extension relieves their low back pain, but that lumbar flexion aggravates it, the clinician needs to know which structures are stressed in lumbar flexion, but unstressed in lumbar extension. |

PT/PTA can understand, develop, and use the inner abilities of self-awareness and empathy in the communication process (see **Figure 8-1**).

## What is empathy?

**Empathy** is imagining oneself in another person's place and understanding the other person's feelings, ideas, desires, and actions.

As an example of empathy, it can be said that an actor or actress empathizes with the part because he or she genuinely feels and identifies with the part being performed. Healthcare providers must genuinely

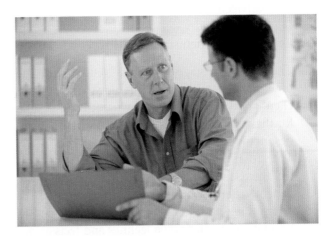

**Figure 8-1** Interacting with the patient.
© mangostock/Shutterstock

feel their patients'/clients' feelings, ideas, desires, and emotions. For PTs and PTAs, empathy also can be described as having the ability to understand the patient's/client's health problem from within the patient's/client's frame of reference.

Psychologists state that to feel empathy, one must have self-awareness; awareness of others; the ability to imagine; and accessible feelings, desires, ideas, and representations of actions. For example, when discussing the concept of self-awareness, the most important aspect of children's emotional development is a growing awareness of their emotional states and the ability to discern and interpret the emotions of others. At about 2 years of age, children become aware of their emotional states, characteristics, and abilities. This phenomenon is called **self-awareness**.

The growing awareness of, and the ability to recall, one's emotional states leads to empathy, or the ability to appreciate the feelings and perceptions of others. Empathy depends not only on an individual's ability to identify someone else's emotions but also on their capacity to imagine themselves in the other person's place and, as a result, experience an appropriate emotional response.

Empathy and social awareness are important factors in developing a person's moral sense. Moral sense or morality is an individual's belief about the appropriateness of their actions, thoughts, or feelings.

For a healthcare provider, empathy depends on one's ability to put oneself in a patient's place and experience the patient's feelings. As an example, pain can be psychologically experienced at the same time as the patient. The reason may be that the healthcare provider feels responsible for being there to treat the patient's condition. Thus, a learned reaction is activated, and the provider experiences pain. At that moment, the healthcare provider communicates this feeling to the patient and establishes an agreement of empathy between them.

Generally, empathy occurs in three stages in the relationship with patients/clients [1]:

1. The cognitive stage—Involves getting into the other person's position by listening to the patient/client and trying to imagine what it must be like for the patient/client to experience what they are describing
2. The crossing-over stage—The PT/PTA begins to feel themselves as the patient/client, living in the patient's/client's world.
3. The coming back to own feelings stage—The PT/PTA returns to their own feelings and feels a special alliance with the patient.

Empathy is important because it means the PT/PTA can do the following:

- Listen better to the patient/client
- Contribute better to the patient's/client's healing process
- Form therapeutic partnerships with the patient/client
- Become actively engaged in the patient's/client's therapeutic process
- Facilitate effective interventions by understanding the patient/client as a whole
- Involve the patient/client and their family/caregiver in the decision-making process
- Establish a therapeutic environment that encourages the patient's/client's motivation and behavioral changes

## Empathy versus Sympathy

Empathy is not the same as sympathy. When one has empathy for someone, they have similar feelings to that person. When one has sympathy, they understand and have compassion for the person but do not necessarily have the same feelings. For example, a patient tells the clinician about his wife's death, which occurred 1 month earlier. As he talks about missing his wife and his love for her, the patient's voice gradually becomes anguished, and he bursts into tears. If the clinician felt sympathy for the patient, they would think the patient remembered his wife only in pain and could say, "I feel your pain" or "I am sorry for your loss." However, if the clinician felt empathy, they would think that the patient was remembering his wife in pain and the joy of his love for her and could say to the patient, "I feel your pain and your great love for your wife." When feeling empathy, the clinician shares the grieving man's emotional pain and does not just feel sorry for him. Although sympathy is also appropriate in our relationships with patients, pity is not appropriate because it is sympathy with condescension, which conveys an inappropriate inequality between the patient and oneself.

---

**KNOWLEDGE CHECK**

What is the ability to imagine oneself in another person's place and to understand their feelings, ideas, desires, and actions?
What is the difference between empathy and sympathy?
What are the three stages of empathy?

# The Therapeutic Relationship

The first time a PT or a PTA meets a patient, they must develop a rapport and a therapeutic connection with that patient. A therapeutic alliance is a collaborative relationship between a healthcare provider and their patient. The therapeutic alliance involves several key elements, including:

- Empathy: The healthcare provider must understand the patient's experience and perspective and communicate that understanding to the patient.
- Trust: The patient must be able to trust the healthcare provider to act in their best interests and maintain confidentiality.
- Collaboration: The healthcare provider and patient must work together to set treatment goals and develop a plan of care tailored to the patient's unique needs and preferences.
- Respect: The healthcare provider must demonstrate respect for the patient's autonomy and values and avoid judgment or criticism.

## Communication Challenges

The clinician may occasionally encounter patients uninterested in forming a therapeutic relationship. The patient may sabotage the relationship by being tardy for appointments, canceling repeatedly, or making rude comments. What follows are some strategies for dealing with difficult people.

First, stay calm. When a patient or coworker becomes upset, it is easy to become upset, defensive, or reactionary. The best policy is to continue interacting respectfully. The clinician should avoid being short or abrupt with the patient or displaying irritation. The clinician may need to ignore the comment or redirect the patient back to the intervention that is occurring. Remember, people who display defensive, resistant, or noncompliant behaviors are most likely doing so unconsciously. Secondly, focus on trying to solve the problem. The clinician should start by listening carefully to what the person is saying. In the process of listening, the clinician may devise a strategy to alleviate the issue, and even if the problem cannot be fixed, the patient usually feels better that someone at least listened and tried to help. And lastly, try to let go of things you cannot control. Difficult people cannot always be helped, but it does not have to direct how the clinician acts or functions. For example, if the patient continually refuses treatment, the clinician should encourage them to participate, explain the consequences

## Box 8-1 Rapport

Rapport is a relationship of mutual trust and understanding between two or more people, which involves creating a personal connection through effective communication, empathy, and mutual respect. Rapport is essential for establishing trust, understanding and responding to the needs and perspectives of others, and collaborating effectively to achieve common goals. Several factors contribute to building rapport, including:

- Active listening. Refer to Section Effective Listening in Verbal Communication.
- Eye contact. The act of looking directly at someone when speaking to them or when they are speaking to you. Good eye contact can be an important aspect of nonverbal communication and can convey various messages, such as interest, attention, confidence, and respect. Good eye contact is a sign of respect and attentiveness in many cultures, but the importance and interpretation of eye contact can vary across cultures and in different situations. For example, in some cultures, making too much eye contact can be perceived as aggressive or threatening. Thus, finding an appropriate balance between the situation and cultural context is important.
- Mirroring body language. The act of unconsciously copying another person's posture, gestures, or movements is used as a form of nonverbal communication to help establish rapport and build trust in personal and professional interactions by sending a subconscious message that two people are on the same wavelength and in tune with each other's emotions and perspectives. However, mirroring must be used subtly and naturally, as overly obvious or deliberate mirroring can be perceived as insincere or threatening.
- Vocal tone. The clinician needs to match the volume and pacing of the patient's speech to increase rapport. The voice volume should be at a level that is sufficient for the patient to hear, and the clinician should avoid speaking loudly when possible, especially to those who are hard of hearing. For example, when talking to older adults, showing respect and patience is important, as is speaking clearly and using language they can understand. You should also ask questions, let them share their experiences and perspectives, avoid interrupting, and be mindful of their physical and emotional needs.
- Contact. The use of touch can be an important communication tool when striking the right balance between forming a connection and being too invasive.

A therapeutic alliance with the patient can be established by considering the following attributes and how a PTA may behave when displaying them:

- Punctuality. It is important to be prepared for each patient and attend to them promptly because it shows respect for them and their time.
- Friendliness. When greeting patients, clinicians should smile and introduce themselves with their names and title. When speaking to patients, speaking more formally is generally more appropriate. Examples include calling them by their surname rather than their first name. This formality may change after establishing a relationship, but the clinician should ask patients what they prefer to be called.
- Cultural competence. Cultural competence involves a combination of knowledge, attitudes, and skills that enable individuals to understand and appreciate cultural differences, communicate across cultural lines, and work effectively with people from diverse backgrounds while understanding and respecting the values, beliefs, and customs of different cultures.
- Communicative. The patient will expect that the clinician clearly explains, in a language the patient can understand, the plan of care for that physical therapy session outlining the expected outcomes of the interventions; and obtain informed consent for the interventions to be performed. Informed consent involves explaining the interventions to the patient, including benefits and risks if appropriate, and receiving confirmation from the patient that the patient will participate in these interventions.
- Communication with the patient should be at the level of understanding of the individual patient. The clinician should consider the patient's age, cognitive function, and level of sensory impairment to explain the information appropriately. Speaking in too simplistic language may appear disrespectful to a patient whose intelligence is above that level and will be just as frustrating as the clinician speaking in medical jargon that the patient does not understand.
- Patient-focused behaviors. The clinician should not appear rushed or hurried while working with the patient. By focusing on the patient, the status of the patient's impairments, and the information each member communicates, the clinician will display respect and concern for the patient. This is an important component in building a relationship with the patient. The clinician should also remember not to become distracted. While working in a busy gym area, it may be difficult to focus energy and attention entirely on the patient, but if the clinician is constantly watching others or talking to coworkers, the relationship with the patient may suffer. The patient may believe the clinician is not fully engaged with them and become distrustful or disrespected.
- Knowledgeable. The best way for the clinician to appear knowledgeable is to be prepared for the patient by reading the evaluation before interacting with the patient, asking pertinent questions, and communicating an understanding of the patient's condition. The clinician should be able to answer the patient's questions. This does not mean that the clinician has to know every answer. For example, the PTA should always look for the answer by researching or asking their supervising PT. Most importantly, the clinician must communicate their findings to the patient.
- Trustworthy. If the patient believes the clinician has the patient's best interest in mind, the relationship will flourish and build trust. The clinician must display all the above characteristics to develop this relationship.
- Helpfulness. Occasionally, the clinician may be asked to perform a job or a request that is not technically part of the job. An example would be filling an acute care patient's water glass. The patient does not forget helpfulness. The patient remembers that the clinician went out of their way to do something nice for them, which will help build rapport.
- Comfortable. The therapeutic relationship will develop rapidly if both the patient and the clinician feel comfortable with each other. Developing a comfort level requires the clinician to converse with the patient easily. While the focus of the relationship is based on the patient's impairments, the casual conversation will help to develop rapport. Talking to the patient about their family, occupation, or community events helps deepen the relationship and brings more satisfaction to the patient and the clinician. When the clinician shows interest in the patient as a person, the clinician displays caring and compassion, which are attributes expected in a therapeutic relationship.

of not completing the rehab program, and inform the physician of their efforts. If the patient still refuses, the clinician should understand that they did what they could, and the patient has the right to make choices that may not be in their best interest.

Clinicians should recognize that grieving people may display behaviors that impede therapy. Grief, much like physical pain, is a personal emotion. Sadness, tearfulness, anger, guilt, loneliness, anxiety, fatigue, and emptiness are common signs exhibited by people experiencing grief. Patients may also exhibit physical symptoms of insomnia, loss of appetite, lassitude, shortness of breath, and sensitivity to noise. Awareness of these behaviors and symptoms can help the clinician acknowledge the person's grief and support their therapeutic needs.

Another challenge clinicians may face is working with people with poorly controlled mental health illnesses. First, one must deal with their personal bias about mental health. To overcome bias, clinicians should examine their feelings about mental health illnesses. One strategy to help with this is to learn about mental health disorders. By understanding behaviors and recognizing symptoms of the illness, the clinician can put into perspective the challenges the patient faces. The clinician will recognize patient responses and behaviors as part of the illness and can interact more therapeutically by responding rather than reacting. Secondly, the clinician should employ tactics that will create consistency, honesty, friendliness, optimism, and nonjudgmental interactions with the patient. Patients will be more likely to accept physical therapy interventions by providing a nurturing relationship.

Along with mental health illnesses, patients who have cognitive impairment and dementia can be very challenging to work with. Patients with cognitive impairment may lack understanding of complex issues or be unable to problem-solve or understand cause-and-effect relationships. Patients with dementia may display disorientation, hallucinations, impulsivity, distractibility, lack of safety awareness, forgetfulness of object name and use, an unsureness of what they are supposed to do, mood swings, and general confusion. Sometimes these issues are episodic and inconsistent from one visit to the next, which adds to the difficult nature of working with patients who have dementia. Working with any of these patients requires patience and repetition. A clinician should recognize that behaviors with this group of clients will usually increase when placed under stress that they cannot cope with. Patients should be challenged with achievable interventions, but the clinician should continue to push the client with a slow progression. Simple directions focusing on functional activities will generally be more successful than therapeutic exercises that may not make sense to these individuals.

### KNOWLEDGE CHECK

What attributes assist in creating a healthy therapeutic relationship with patients/clients?
What strategies can a clinician use when working with people who do not assist in creating a healthy therapeutic relationship?

# The PT and PTA Relationship

The relationship between the PTA and the patient is critical, but another relationship requires just as much attention to provide effective physical therapy services. That is the relationship between the PT and the PTA. Depending upon the setting, a PTA may have one or more supervising PTs, and each PT may have certain expectations and preferences for patient care. The PTA and the PT must create a team based on understanding, trust, honesty, and effective communication (see **Figure 8-2**).

Each team member will come with varying degrees of understanding regarding their role. This understanding will depend upon their education and tenure in the position. A new graduate PT may not have worked with a PTA previously. In

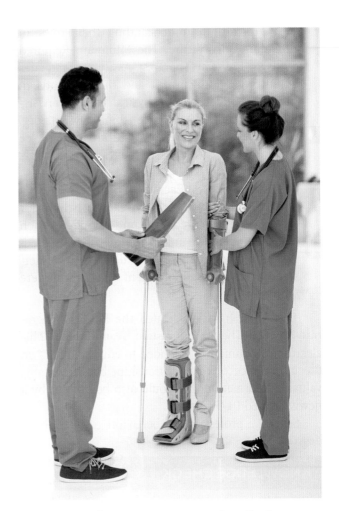

**Figure 8-2** PT/PTA relationships require effective communication.
© michaeljung/Shutterstock

this case, if the PTA has many years of experience, they must learn about each other personally and professionally.

The team members should explore the following topics to help promote unity:

- Education: The first step in creating the team would be to understand the education of each member, including the initial physical therapy degree and a discussion of specific skills that are taught. Additionally, continuing education courses should be discussed to help each other understand their skill set beyond entry-level education.

- State laws: The PT and PTA must have the same understanding of state statutes and a plan for implementing the laws and administrative rules. Because laws can vary from state to state, the team must abide by the current state in which they practice physical therapy.

- Professional and ethical aspects of care: The APTA has a variety of documents that assist the PT/PTA team in understanding their roles in providing quality care. The Minimum Required Skills of Physical Therapist Assistant Graduates at Entry-Level document and the Standards of Ethical Conduct for the Physical Therapist Assistant document are available from www.apta.org. PTA supervision guidelines and algorithms (see Appendix B) may also assist the team in creating a plan for teamwork.

- Personal attributes: Each team member will have strengths and weaknesses; it can be helpful for those to be explored and understood by each team member. An understanding of the expectations of each member can alleviate misunderstandings and disappointment that can interfere with trust.

The APTA has also created the Physical Therapist–Physical Therapist Assistant Team Toolkit. This electronic document is intended to educate others on the importance of this relationship, but it contains valuable information that could also be utilized by a newly formed PT/PTA team.[1]

Several professional behaviors have been described:

## KNOWLEDGE CHECK

What personal and professional characteristics should be explored when creating an effective PT/PTA team?

# Types of Communication Forms

The two main communication forms are verbal and nonverbal.

- Verbal or oral communication uses messages conveyed orally from a sender to a receiver.
- Nonverbal communication uses messages conveyed through methods other than orally or in writing. It is divided into two groups: communication through body language and communication through facial expressions, including gestures and eye contact.

## Verbal Communication

Verbal communication is a significant part of physical therapy clinical practice, as in other healthcare professions. Verbal communication is an important part of transferring information and learning. To successfully engage with a patient, communication must be designed to reach patients on their level, which can sometimes involve challenging them on higher-order processes, such as troubleshooting, prioritization, and adaptation. Bloom [2] introduced three domains by which individuals interact:

- Cognitive: Involves intellect—the understanding of information from basic recall to knowledge, application, analysis, synthesis, and evaluation

- Affective: Involves the emotions from a low-order process, such as listening, to a higher-order process, such as resolving an issue. It involves the development of attitudes, emotions, motivations, character development, engagement, and values toward a particular subject or learning experience.

- Psychomotor: Involves physicality and how that develops from basic motor skills to intricate performance

Of the three domains, the affective tends to influence all professional skills strongly, yet it is the most difficult to teach. However, all three domains are involved in verbal communication. The reasons for verbal communication may include the following [3]:

- To establish a rapport with the patient/client and/or the patient's/client's family/caregiver
- To enhance the relationship among the patient/client, their family/caregiver, and the PT/PTA
- To obtain information concerning the patient's/client's condition and progress
- To transmit pertinent information to other healthcare professionals and providers and support personnel

---

1 https://www.apta.org/siteassets/pdfs/policies/direction-supervision-pta.pdf

- To provide education and instructions to the patient/client and the patient's/client's family/caregiver
- To increase the patient's/client's adherence to education and the continuum of care at home
- To decrease the patient's/client's health risks

## Cultural Diversity and Verbal Communication

From a cultural diversity perspective, problems in verbal communication may arise when the PT or the PTA and the patient/client bring two completely different worldviews, languages, or backgrounds to the interactions. As the clinician interacts with patients/clients from diverse cultures, the clinician's norms of verbal communication may differ and clash with theirs. The clinician may form inappropriate judgments about the patient/client, creating barriers to communication and effective patient/client care. The clinician's ethnocentrism and decreased cultural competence may cause verbal communication problems. For example, some people are uncomfortable with periods of silence and tend to associate it with a person being inarticulate or ineffectual. However, African Americans often value silence and nonverbal communication. They also are often very spiritual. When in the company of strangers, they can be private about their family matters [3]. Navajo Indians often appreciate long periods of silence, understanding an attentive, silent listener to communicate interest. Asian Americans also can appreciate silence. They may verbally communicate with the clinician by agreeing with certain information to "save face" and not to be considered offensive [3].

PTs and PTAs must be knowledgeable about cultural issues, especially when interacting with patients/clients and their families/caregivers with different cultural backgrounds and/or limited English proficiency (see **Table 8-2**). A patient's/client's English limitations do not reflect the patient's/client's intellectual functioning level or ability to communicate in the native language.

Familial colloquialisms, such as specific informal expressions, used by the patients/clients or their families/caregivers can also affect verbal communication in the physical therapy examination, evaluation, assessment, and interventions. Some patients/clients from other cultures prefer to use verbal communication as an alternative to written communication when receiving information about a home exercise program (HEP) or certain treatment precautions. Considering linguistic cultural competence, PTs and PTAs must attempt to learn and use keywords in the language of their patients/clients to better communicate with them in

clinical settings. Presenting verbal communication differently is necessary for it to be effective in different situations. In addition, consideration must be given to the following aspects of each patient/client [3]:

- Health beliefs
- Health perceptions
- Attitudes
- Level of education

Healthcare professionals tend to use family members, friends, or volunteers to communicate with patients/clients from other cultures. Doing so may present a risk of breaching patient privacy and confidentiality and not receiving the necessary information from the patient/client (especially if it is sensitive). Also, filtering information through family, friends, or volunteers can be clinically detrimental to patients/clients and lead to malpractice problems for the PT/PTA. For example, a PT asked a patient from Russia (who was being treated for back pain), as a contraindication of treatment, if she was pregnant or trying to become pregnant. The patient stated to her American cousin in her native language: "No, no, I cannot become pregnant since I am not married." In reality, the patient was over 2 months pregnant, but she did not want her cousin to know the truth. Ultimately, this presented a negative clinical outcome for the patient and a malpractice liability for the PT. A trained medical interpreter could have circumvented such a problem. Professional interpreters are a better solution than family, friends, or volunteers.

Professional interpreters can provide culturally sensitive and high-quality language assistance services to ensure understanding on both sides of the medical equation. In physical therapy, the same as in other areas of health care, top-quality interventions cannot be provided without effective communication. Optimal communication enhances patient satisfaction, improves outcomes, and provides greater patient/client safety. Addressing language barriers in health care must be integral to physical therapy efforts.

## Verbal Communication Success

For healthcare providers, the success of verbal communication depends on the following factors [5]:

- The way the material is presented, including the provider's vocabulary, the clarity of voice and purpose, and the organization of the material
- The attitude of the provider
- The tone and the volume of the provider's voice
- The degree to which the patient/client listens, including the patient's mental status

**Table 8-2** Cultural Communication Guidelines [4]

| Culture | Verbal Guidelines | Nonverbal Guidelines |
| --- | --- | --- |
| People of Arab Heritage | Take time to get acquainted.<br>Good manners are important.<br>The patient may speak loudly and expressively.<br>Privacy is important.<br>Use titles unless told to do otherwise. | Expect to shake hands upon arrival and departure, although some Muslim men may not shake a woman's hand.<br>Modesty is valued.<br>They may stand close during a conversation, and eye contact is expected. |
| People of Chinese Heritage | Speak in a quieter voice.<br>Do not ask closed questions.<br>Ask for repeat demonstrations to ensure understanding.<br>Ask the patient what they prefer to be called, as surnames are often used first, and some Chinese use Westernized English names. | Explain what you are doing before touching the patient.<br>Some may prefer to avoid eye contact as a sign of respect. |
| People of Cuban Heritage | Voices may be loud and speech fast.<br>Address the patient with their title unless directed to do so otherwise. | Lively facial expressions and gestures are common.<br>Gratitude may be expressed via handshakes and hugs. |
| People of Hmong Heritage | There are several dialects of Hmong language, so use an appropriate interpreter.<br>The person may say "yes" to indicate that they heard you rather than understood.<br>Ask for a demonstration to indicate understanding.<br>The head of the family may make health decisions. | Do not use direct eye contact; instead, use occasional short glances. |
| People of Japanese Heritage | Most can speak, read, or write English to some extent.<br>Saying "no" is considered to be impolite.<br>Use their family name with a formal greeting. | They often do not show overly emotional behaviors but may use smiles and laughter to cover for embarrassment or anxiety.<br>Body space should be respected.<br>Greet them with a handshake.<br>Do not hold eye contact for long periods. |
| People of Jewish Heritage | Speak clearly if English is not their first language.<br>Use formal names. | Hasidic men are not permitted to touch women, including shaking hands. They may avoid talking or looking at women.<br>Only touch them when providing care.<br>Non-Hasidic Jews may not follow these traditions. |
| People of Mexican Heritage | Conversing is important.<br>Use formal names.<br>Ask who makes decisions for the family.<br>Listen to the patient's ideas. | Traditionally, eye contact may be avoided.<br>Explain the purpose of touching. |
| People of American Indian Heritage | There may be variations from tribe to tribe.<br>Use moderate voice tones.<br>They are often comfortable with silence and may not share thoughts until a relationship has been built.<br>They may disregard directions if trust has not been developed.<br>Family beliefs and traditions are highly valued.<br>The opinions of elders are very important. | Touching should be explained as part of the intervention.<br>Pointing a finger is considered rude, as is direct eye contact. |

Data from Purnell L: Guide to Culturally Competent Health Care. Philadelphia, PA, F.A. Davis, 2005.

During the verbal interaction, the healthcare provider must ensure an understanding of the patient's goals immediately after meeting the patient by focusing on the patient's information and asking questions. The material provided to the patient must be presented, considering the patient's age, the presence of a language barrier, the degree of the patient's anxiety, and the level of the patient's understanding.

The healthcare provider's vocabulary should be precise and accurate and contain terms understandable to the patient. For example, if the provider uses technical jargon, the technical terms can confuse the patient. Also, the patient may feel that the provider is disinterested and does not empathize with them. The healthcare provider must speak clearly and concisely in a normal tone of voice. Healthcare providers must constantly be aware of the tone and volume of voice, especially when delivering unpleasant news to a patient. Any procedure or intervention has to be verbally explained to the patient logically, step by step, accompanied by written instructions, diagrams, or nonverbal demonstrations.

## Delivery of Verbal Communication

Verbal communication can be delivered to a patient/client through the following channels:

- Face-to-face discussions in which the PT/PTA imparts the desired meaning to the patient/client and the patient/client can also ask questions. It is considered the best delivery method of verbal communication in health care.
- Telephone discussions in which the PT/PTA can interact with the patient/client; however, confidential patient/client medical information should not be discussed over the telephone.
- In group discussions, the PT/PTA can communicate the same messages to a group of patients/clients; however, the message is not personalized because the patient's/client's medical information is confidential. Group discussion can be used in physical therapy for group exercise programs.
- Third-party discussions where the PT/PTA can communicate with the patient/client through another person (such as a family member or a caregiver). This method is limited in delivering the intended

Recommendations for verbal communication:

- The PTA's verbal commands should focus on the most important aspects of the desired action for treatment.
- The PTA's instruction should remain as simple as possible and must never incorporate confusing medical terminology.
- The PTA should emphasize the person who is a patient by utilizing patient-first language. An example of patient-first language is "the patient with a total knee arthroplasty" rather than "the total knee arthroplasty patient."
- The PTA should detail the general sequence of events to the patient/client before initiating treatment.
- The PTA should ask the patient/client questions before and during treatment to establish a rapport with the patient and to provide feedback on the current status of the treatment.
- The PTA should speak clearly in moderate tones and vary their tone of voice as required by the situation. PTAs should show enthusiasm but not be too energized to sound or appear distractible.
- The PTA should pause to allow the patient to understand what the message is trying to convey. Speaking too quickly may make it difficult for the patient to comprehend the information.

- The PTA should be sensitive to the patient's/client's level of understanding and cultural background.
- The PTA should explain and repeat directions as needed by the patient. The tone of voice may reveal signs of irritation or frustration. Responding with patience and smiling will help decrease patient anxiety and assist the patient in understanding more fully.
- PTAs should ask patients to repeat instructions or demonstrate exercises to determine if true understanding has occurred. It is common practice to have a patient perform a return demonstration of a home exercise plan after the initial instruction or upon a return visit to therapy to ensure patient understanding and correct errors. A patient may think that they understand or are performing the tasks correctly, so asking if they understand may not illuminate any problems with comprehension.
- The PTA should be aware that when a person feels uncomfortable or unsure, they add word fillers such as "um" or "ok."
- If the PTA repeatedly says the same thing to a patient, while it may be intended to be encouraging, it may sound insincere. An example is repeatedly praising, such as "good job," after every activity the patient completes.

meaning and by medical information confidentiality status (unless the family member is legally a personal representative of the patient/client).

## Effective and Ineffective Listening and Questioning

### Effective Questioning Strategies

To understand a patient, the PT/PTA must learn to ask questions to get the information needed for clinical decision-making. There are two common types of questioning strategies: closed and open. **Closed questioning** asks for short factual answers. An example of a closed question would be, "Do you have pain today?" The answer could be a simple yes or no. **Open questioning** asks the person to give a more detailed answer. An example of an open question would be, "What activities are difficult because of your pain?" The patient could give short answers, but the question lends itself to a more lengthy answer that will provide the PT/PTA with clearer information on which to make clinical decisions. Many times, a PT/PTA will use closed questions that lead them to more open questions that allow them to increase their understanding. However, the PT/PTA should avoid leading the patient. An example of a leading question would be "Does that hurt?" rather than "How does that feel?" The patient might not have considered that they may feel pain and should not have been asked if that was a possibility. Appropriate questioning will allow the PT/PTA to gain the necessary information for effective patient interaction.

### Effective Listening in Verbal Communication

Effective listening is meaningful in health care for a variety of reasons, including:

- To focus on the patient's verbal and nonverbal communication while remaining nonjudgmental
- To clarify information that the patient just explained to the provider. This is often referred to as restatement and is used to assure the patient that you have understood what they intended to say.

- To reflect on the patient's message in terms of the content and the implied feelings
- To summarize the message the patient said to the provider. This is used to clarify the listener's understanding.

There are several kinds of listening in general:

- Analytical listening: Used for a specific type of information and arranging the information in categories; an example in physical therapy would be listening to the patient's description of pain.
- Directed listening: Used for the patient's answers to specific questions; an example in physical therapy would be listening to their answers about the activities and positions that increase or decrease their pain.
- Comprehensive listening: Used to clarify what the patient said; an example in physical therapy would be listening to the patient explain why a task is difficult to perform and then the PTA repeating their understanding of what they heard to clarify that they understand the patient.
- Exploratory listening: Used when a person's interest in the subject is being discussed; an example in physical therapy would be the patient listening to the PT's recommendations of positioning techniques in sleeping to decrease the pain or the PT asking the patient specific questions about the patient's pain.
- Attentive listening: Used for general information to get the overall picture of the patient; an example in physical therapy would be a PTA listening to the PT's specific recommendations for a patient's treatment.
- Courteous listening: Used when feeling obligated to listen; an example would be listening to a story the patient is describing, even if it is irrelevant to the patient's examination and treatment.
- Selective listening: Used when not being attentive to the matter discussed but overhearing the conversation; an example would be a patient in a hospital bed listening to another patient's conversation in the next bed.

Generally, analytical, directed, and attentive listening can provide relevant information about the patient to be included in the patient's documentation. Exploratory listening can provide the most relevant information about the patient (see **Figure 8-3**).

### The Purposes of Effective Listening

Effective listening is the primary skill used in health care when interacting with the patient/client. It is also

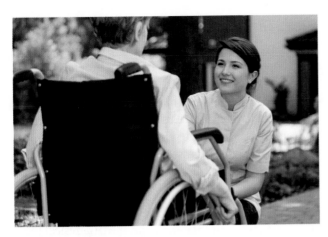

**Figure 8-3** Listening to the patient.
© Photographee.eu/Shutterstock

a pathway for engaging in a therapeutic relationship with the patient/client, building trust, and fostering the patient's/client's cooperation for treatment. In physical therapy, effective listening as a communication tool can help with the following:

- To gain better knowledge about the patient's problem(s)
- To receive better cooperation from the patient and the patient's family
- To solve problems concerning the patient's plan of care and interventions
- To encourage trust and build a therapeutic alliance between the patient and the clinician
- To improve the patient's treatment by encouraging continuous feedback from the patient

In addition, the healthcare provider's effective listening skills help gain higher-quality patient information, save time, solve problems, and reduce and prevent medical errors. Contrarily, poor listening creates misunderstandings, wastes time, and allows for mistakes. In the healthcare profession, mistakes can endanger a patient's life.

Effective listening is a skill that a healthcare provider can learn and practice. Effective listening requires effort, honesty, commitment, and perhaps changing one's behavior and becoming more compassionate and empathetic.

### Ineffective Listening Habits

The following are ineffective listeners' habits that need to be changed, particularly when working in the healthcare field:

- Ineffective listeners typically listen on and off. Most people think four times faster than someone can speak, and they have too much time to think

Methods of effective listening:

- The PT/PTA focuses their attention on the patient.
- The PT/PTA helps the patient to feel free to talk by smiling and looking at the patient.
- The PT/PTA pays attention to the patient's nonverbal communication, such as gestures, facial expressions, tone of voice, and body posture.
- The PT/PTA asks the patient to clarify the meaning of words and the feelings involved or to enlarge the statement.
- The PT/PTA repeats the patient's message to understand the meaning and content. Reflective listening allows the PTA to clarify what the patient has stated, and the patient can then correct any misperceptions.
- The PT/PTA takes notes as necessary to help remember or document what was said.
- The PT/PTA uses body language, such as nonverbal gestures (leaning forward, nodding the head, keeping eye contact, or keeping hands at their side), to show involvement in the patient's message.
- The PT/PTA does not abruptly interrupt the patient and thus gives adequate time to present the full message.
- The PT/PTA empathizes with the patient.

about their affairs and concerns. To overcome listening on and off, a PT/PTA must pay attention to a patient's nonverbal communication, such as gestures, eye contact, hesitation, or tone of voice.

- Ineffective listeners typically listen to words, ideas, or opinions. They prejudge the message being conveyed and respond with an emotional reaction rather than listening to all of the information and then making a response. When the PTA effectively listens, they can respond calmly and with empathy.
- Ineffective listeners consider the patient boring (and not saying anything new). They may not listen if the patient describes their symptoms or problems in detailed accounts. Often, patients can express the same message over and over concerning their health. This message can be significant in the patient's examination, assessment, and treatment. Also, some patients may need to explain detailed accounts of their symptoms or the effects of their treatments. To overcome wrong assumptions about the patient, a PT/PTA should listen intently to the patient's entire message (even if it is the same). If the message is too complicated, they should ask clarifying questions.

- Ineffective listeners are absorbed in their thoughts and often daydream when another person speaks. Daydreaming is usually a sign of tiredness and loss of concentration. To overcome daydreaming, a PT/PTA must try to take a short break from work, rest a few minutes, go back to the task, concentrate again on their work, and continue to listen carefully and intently to the patient.

- Ineffective listeners have favorite ideas, prejudices, and points of view that the patient can challenge or overturn. When that happens, the PT/PTA becomes defensive with the patient. To overcome this, the PT/PTA must respond to the patient constructively and respect the patient's point of view to maintain the therapeutic relationship between the PT/PTA and the patient.

Ineffective listening skills may cause ineffective treatment of the patient, which can lead to fewer referrals, poor documentation that can lead to denial of payment, and poor customer satisfaction that can lead to a poor reputation of care. Appropriate listening skills must be practiced, becoming as important to effective care as hands-on physical therapy skills.

## Defining Nonverbal Communication

Nonverbal communication is through body language, facial expressions, gestures, and eye contact. Other types of nonverbal communication are a person's physical characteristics, including clothing and grooming. Regarding physical characteristics, people sometimes inadvertently stereotype others, showing preferences for attractive people who are well dressed and well groomed. Clean clothing that fits well and good grooming can make a proper impression on a prospective employer and a new patient/client. The newly hired PT should use the other employees in the department as a guide for the expectations of the employer and the patient population. How a PTA presents themselves can contribute to their success relating to a patient/client and an employer.

The PT and the PTA should also consider that nonverbal communication varies and holds different meanings in different cultures. The receiver of nonverbal communication brings their cultural understandings and expectations to the interaction. In addition, the cultural perspective complicates the interaction and opens the potential for miscommunication and misunderstanding.

### Body Language

Body language includes a person's postures and gestures that convey messages from a sender to the receiver and from a receiver to the sender. The sender sends the message, and the receiver receives the message. Body language reveals a person's inner character and emotions. Open postures convey a person's willingness to receive a message.

Open postures can be any of the following:

- A person's standing or sitting with arms at their sides and legs uncrossed
- A person's standing or sitting straight
- A person's standing or sitting positioned at the same eye level as the receiver
- A person as a receiver facing the sender

Closed postures convey a person's unwillingness to receive a message (see **Figure 8-4**). Closed postures can be a person standing or sitting with arms and legs crossed, being slumped over, or as a receiver turned away from the sender. Crossed arms in front of the body and crossed legs convey a closed posture that does not allow others to send messages or indicate superiority. Arms crossed in front of the body also display a defensive posture, and the listener is not ready to receive messages. If the receiver is turned away

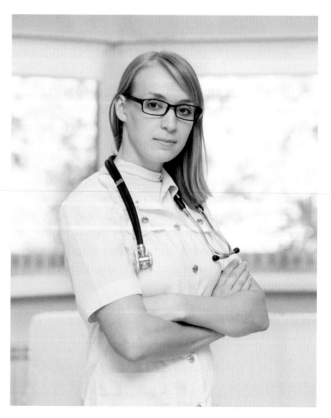

**Figure 8-4** Closed posture.
© Ermolaev Alexander/Shutterstock

from the sender, this shows that the receiver is avoiding communication by trying to distance themselves from the sender.

Facial expressions, including gestures and eye contact, can convey the acceptance or rejection of the presented thoughts and ideas. A smile, nodding, or direct eye contact can convey acceptance of thoughts and ideas. People can convey rejection of thoughts and ideas by rolling their eyes, looking up or down or away from the sender, shaking their head, or frowning.

Eye contact generally communicates a positive message. If two people want to communicate well, they will position themselves to look into each other's eyes (depending on the person's culture). If one person stands while the other sits, the one who stands has subconsciously placed themselves in a position of authority. As healthcare providers, when communicating with patients, it is crucial to be at the same eye level as the patient. For example, if the patient sits in a wheelchair, the healthcare provider should stoop down when communicating with the patient (see **Figure 8-3**).

A person's body language, especially facial expressions, can communicate a genuine interest in the patient and the patient's goals, concerns, ideas, and needs. Eye contact is also significant, especially while listening to a patient/client. Looking directly into someone's eyes (without staring) can also convey honesty and decision-making capability. However, prolonged eye contact (such as staring) communicates disagreement and anger.

Healthcare providers may use gestures, such as a comforting touch, to relax a patient and to show caring and dedication to the patient. In physical therapy, touch is significant when guiding the patient in performing physical therapy activities and exercises correctly.

Physical touch communicates a diversity of meanings across cultures. It can also be a powerful communicator of respect or disrespect and can hurt or heal. For example, a homeless patient may not have been physically touched in a long time or have experienced harmful contact rather than a loving or respectful touch. In addition, physical touch requires special considerations across genders and diverse cultures. For example, Arab-Muslim cultures place a high value on female modesty, and it would be inappropriate for a male PT to touch the patient or even to begin an initial examination without asking permission from the patient, the patient's husband, or the patient's family. Healthcare providers, including PTs and PTAs, must remember how important nonverbal communication is, especially when interacting with patients/clients from other cultures.

## Emotional Intelligence

Emotional intelligence refers to one's understanding of their own emotions and the emotions of others. This skill refers to being able not only to recognize emotion in the patient but also to respond accordingly. To do this well, healthcare workers should recognize and be conscious of their emotions when working with patients. Self-awareness requires introspection and deliberate self-assessment. According to science journalist Daniel Goleman, emotional intelligence involves empathy and social skills, such as influence, communication, leadership, collaboration, and cooperation. These are all skills that can be practiced and developed. Self-regulation or learning to respond to a patient's behaviors and emotions with calmness and awareness will allow for a better outcome for the patient [6].

### KNOWLEDGE CHECK

What is the difference between open and closed questions?

What type of listening is used to gather specific information to help assess a patient's symptoms?

What are the methods of effective listening?

What are the barriers to effective listening?

What postures are most useful when creating a therapeutic relationship?

How might cultural differences change how you verbally and nonverbally interact with a patient/client?

## Defining Written Communication

Written communication represents communication using messages conveyed in writing from a sender to a receiver. Healthcare providers use written communication to convey messages to patients/clients and provide information in medical records.

### Written Communication Given to the Patient/Client

In physical therapy, written messages to patients/clients can reinforce verbal instructions to perform activities or exercises by including additional information, informed consent documents, or surveys to obtain data about the quality of physical therapy services rendered to the patient. Written communication allows the reader to control their pace of understanding the material. For patients/clients from other cultural backgrounds, all written communication must be in their language of origin.

Specific guidelines for written communication given to the patient/client include the following [3]:

- Write the information the same way you talk to the patient/client.
- Use an active voice.
- Use short sentences and common words.
- For complicated words, give examples.
- Include interaction by adding a short question and asking the patient/client to write their answer; this adds to the patient's/client's active involvement in their treatment (and helps with adherence).

Examples of interaction methods for the information given to the patient/client include the following [3]:

- Writing a short question and asking the patient/client to write their answer
- Asking the patient/client to circle their best choice of one or two exercises from three or four pictures of exercises
- Asking the patient a few questions verbally about their exercises after the patient/client has read their written HEP handout

### HEP Handouts

The content of the written communication must be well organized, concise, and in layperson's terms. For example, in physical therapy, written handouts for exercises or activities, called HEP handouts, must be specific about the number of repetitions, the amount of exercise resistance (such as 1- or 2-pound weights), and the positions for performing the exercises or the activities. Physical therapy written handouts must have diagrams or pictures and the contact information of the PT or the PTA.

The primary purpose of a HEP handout is to impart useful, actionable information to the patient/client or the patient's/client's family. The words on the paper have to make complete sense to the patient. Also, the information should be consistent with the clinician's verbal explanations and demonstrations to the patient or caregiver. The handout must represent an extension of the treatment plan of care.

The HEP starts on the first day of treatment and continues to the day of discharge. If a caregiver is involved in the patient's treatment, the caregiver must participate early in the program to allow an easier transition when going home. The written materials should be short and developed in the patient's primary language. Technical terms and jargon must be avoided, and short sentences should be used as

much as possible. For example, complex words, such as achieve, utilization, inflammation, or indication, could be replaced with simple ones, such as do, use, redness, or sign.

Concerning the written form, each sentence should present only one idea and contain no more than one three-syllable word. Lines of the copy are suggested to be no more than 5 inches wide, and the type size should be 12 points or larger. The handouts should have a high contrast between the foreground and background and include large amounts of blank space on the page to accommodate patients with visual deficits.

The HEP handouts should be written at the fifth-grade reading level. The HEP handouts should sort the exercises logically and sequentially so that the patient does not have to change positions too much, such as transitioning from lying face up to sitting in a chair and then lying face up again.

The exercises have to be simple and very clear. Writing in a conversational style implies that the material was written directly to the patient. Uncomplicated drawings may supplement the written instructions, indicating frequency, duration, number of repetitions, and the method for progressing through the exercises.

Lengthy and complicated exercise routines will discourage a patient's continuing participation. Providing the least number of necessary exercises increases the chance of patient compliance. The clinician's presentation of the information constitutes another important element for the success of a HEP. For example, showing enthusiasm and interest when presenting the instructional material demonstrates concern for the patient and a degree of sensitivity to their needs. The element of verbal instruction and a good relationship with the patient could substantially enhance the effectiveness of a home program. A teaching aid, such as the HEP handout, is useless if not presented within the context of the total process of patient education and rehabilitation.

### KNOWLEDGE CHECK

What is the value of giving information to a patient in writing?

What are some good practices to employ when providing a HEP?

### Written Communication to Healthcare Professionals or Payer Sources

Communication intended for other healthcare professionals or payer sources must be written more formally than with patients. It should avoid using informal language, abbreviations, and slang and be more declarative. When communicating with other healthcare professionals or payer sources, it is important to use medical language and refrain from oversimplifying terminology. The communication should be straightforward with its purpose, and any reader requests should be clearly stated. If the purpose is information sharing or points are to be made, the writer should organize the data and not embellish the communication with unnecessary information.

An example of formal written communication with another healthcare professional:

June 15, 2015

Dear Dr. Jones,

Your patient, John Smith, has received physical therapy for low back pain. A trial of mechanical traction has proven to benefit his pain and radiculopathy in the left lower extremity. He has returned to work; however, his pain has returned after 2 days. Continued use of traction will allow the patient to self-manage his pain and functional abilities. We are requesting a prescription for a home lumbar traction unit. Please contact me for any additional information.

Sincerely,

Mary Brown, PTA

# Communicating with People with Disabilities

PTs/PTAs frequently interact with people with disabilities (PWDs). When writing or speaking about PWDs, it is important to put the person first. Group designations, such as "the blind" or "the disabled," are insensitive because they do not indicate the equality, individuality, or dignity of PWDs. Similarly, a "normal person" infers that the person with a disability is not normal, whereas a "person without a disability" is descriptive without being negative. Appropriate etiquette when interacting with PWDs is based on respect and courtesy. Tips to help when communicating with PWDs are as follows:

*General Tips.* When introduced to a person with a disability, it is appropriate to offer to shake hands. People with limited hand use or a prosthetic hand can usually shake hands (shaking hands with the left hand is an acceptable greeting). If you offer assistance to PWDs, wait until your offer is accepted, then listen to or ask for instructions. Address PWDs by their first names only when extending the same familiarity to all others.

*Communicating with Individuals Who Are Blind or Visually Impaired.* The clinician should speak to the individual when approaching and speak in a normal voice tone. When speaking in a group, remember to identify yourself and the person you are speaking to. It would be best not to attempt to lead the individual without first asking; allow the person to hold your arm and control their movements. Use descriptive words that provide verbal information that is visually obvious to sighted individuals when giving guidance. For example, if you approach a series of steps, mention how many. If you are offering a seat, gently place the individual's hand on the back or arm of the chair so that they can locate the seat. At the end of the session, the clinician should tell the individual that they are leaving.

*Communicating with Individuals Who Are Deaf or Hard of Hearing.* The clinician should gain the patient's attention before starting a conversation (e.g., tap the person gently on the shoulder or arm), and then look at the individual directly, face the light, speak clearly, in a normal voice tone, and keep hands or objects from obstructing the mouth. Short, simple sentences should be used. If the patient uses a sign language interpreter, speak directly to the person, not the interpreter. If you place a phone call to the patient, let the phone ring longer than usual. If a text telephone (TTY) is unavailable, the clinician should dial 711 to reach the national telecommunications relay service to facilitate the call.

*Communicating with Individuals with Mobility Impairments.* Whenever possible, the clinician should position themselves at the eye level of the wheelchair user without leaning on the wheelchair or any other assistive device. Never patronize people who use wheelchairs by patting them on the head or shoulder. Do not assume that an individual wants to be pushed—ask first.

*Communicating with Individuals with Speech Impairments.* If the clinician does not understand something the patient said, they should not pretend that they did but ask the individual to repeat what was said and then repeat it back. To help the patient, ask questions requiring only short answers or a head nod. It would be best if you did not speak for the individual or attempt to finish their sentences. If the clinician has difficulty understanding the individual, writing should be considered an alternative communication method, but only after asking if this is acceptable.

***Communicating with Individuals with Cognitive Disabilities.*** Whenever possible, the clinician and patient should communicate in a quiet or private location and be prepared to repeat what is said, orally or in writing. You must be patient, flexible, and supportive and should wait for the individual to accept an offer of assistance; do not "over-assist" or be patronizing.

# Social Networking in the Workplace

While social media can be a free promotional tool for an organization, the lines between "personal" and "professional" have become increasingly imprecise, introducing the need to regulate these communications. For example, the APTA has several recommendations for using social media in the workplace.[2] Based on

these recommendations and others, the clinician should adhere to the following recommendations:

- Strictly adhere to what is and is not permitted by the company's social media policies and regulations.
- Be professional and accurate in any communication.
- Avoid interacting with patients and supervisors on social media. Such familiarity may create not only awkward situations but also the potential for liability.
- Avoid creating separate personal and professional social media profiles.
- Do not misrepresent the APTA, other organizations, educational institutions, clinical sites, or employers.
- Avoid posting comments or photos on an account that identifies you as an employee of a company.
- Do not post any confidential information, trade secrets, or customer data that is not public knowledge.
- Demonstrate appropriate conduct following the Code of Ethics for the Physical Therapist and Standards of Ethical Conduct for the Physical Therapist Assistant.
- Do not use social media (Facebook, Twitter, Instagram, etc.) at work. Many employers block any access to unnecessary sites from computers.

## Discussion Questions

1. Discuss personal experiences with healthcare workers and create a list of attributes or behaviors that are positive and negative.
2. Create a list of communication strengths and weaknesses that you have.
3. Create three closed questions and then convert them to open questions. Create three leading questions and then convert them to exploratory questions.

## Learning Opportunities

1. Using the following skits, practice effective listening skills and reflective communication that conveys the PTA's understanding of what the patient stated.
   a. The patient explains how she fell down the stairs and broke her leg.
   b. The patient is describing where his pain is and what makes it better or worse.
   c. The patient explains her difficulty caring for her child after hurting her back.
   d. The patient describes what he did over the weekend that worsened his shoulder pain.
2. With a partner, create a paper airplane. After completing the task, analyze how you communicated during the task. Identify the attributes of a team you displayed and if one or more partners became the leader. Compare this to how you might interact within a physical therapy team.
3. Interview a PT/PTA team and identify strategies that they employ to help them work cohesively.

2 https://www.apta.org/social-media/succeeding-on-social-media

# References

1. Davis CM: Patient Practitioner Interaction: An Experiential Manual for Developing the Art of Health Care. Thorofare, NJ, SLACK Incorporated, 1994
2. Bloom BS: Taxonomy of Educational Objectives, Handbook I: The Cognitive Domain. New York, David McKay Co Inc., 1956
3. Dreeben O: Patient Education in Rehabilitation. Sudbury, MA, Jones & Bartlett Learning, 2010
4. Purnell L: Guide to Culturally Competent Health Care. Philadelphia, PA, F.A. Davis, 2005
5. Purtilo R, Haddad A: Health Professional and Patient Interaction. Philadelphia, PA, W.B. Saunders Company, 1996
6. Goleman D: Emotional Intelligence: Why It Can Matter more than IQ. New York, NY, Random House Publishing Group, 2006

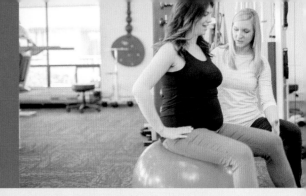

# CHAPTER 9

# Teaching and Learning

## OBJECTIVES

- Discuss the teaching and learning aspects of physical therapy.
- Describe patient education methods for people with difficulty reading, older adults, patients with visual and hearing impairments, patients who cannot speak English, and patients from other cultures.

## KEY TERMS

learning                    teaching

## Communication Methods for Teaching and Learning

Teaching and learning are important patient education processes during physical therapy interventions. Patient education or patient instruction is an essential aspect of healthcare delivery. Physical therapists (PTs) and physical therapist assistants (PTAs) must be able to assess the patient/client as the learner, understand their learning needs, and also provide a suitable teaching and learning environment. **Teaching** involves planning the process of imparting information and then implementing the plan. **Learning** involves a change in the learner that creates an understanding of information, changes in behavior and attitude, and the desire to use the information to help make life decisions.

### Teaching

In general, teaching means explaining and supplying information to the learner. Teaching also involves building the learning environment to help make it conducive to learning.

PTs and PTAs may be involved with academic teaching at colleges, universities, and other technical institutions, as well as clinical teaching. Clinical teaching or clinical instructional activities can occur with patients/clients, the patients'/clients' families and caregivers, and PT/PTA students. Teaching opportunities involving healthcare teaching are important to provide communities with information on specific conditions and interventions or health prevention topics. Examples might include speaking about appropriate exercise to members of a local chapter of the Multiple Sclerosis Society or providing a training session for certified nursing assistants on appropriate patient transfers to protect their backs.

For learning to occur, good teaching attributes should be present. First, the teacher should be enthusiastic about the topic. Teaching and learning should be fun, so the teacher must show that they enjoy discussing the topic. Secondly, the teacher should know about their topic. For clinical instruction, PTs and PTAs generally know the information well enough that they do not need to prepare; however, when creating in-services for other healthcare providers or presentations for the public, it is best to perform research

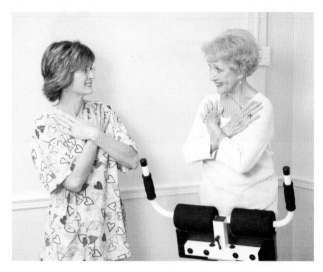

**Figure 9-1** Teaching proper form.
© Lisa F. Young/Shutterstock

to organize and present the information well. Lastly, the teacher should employ appropriate feedback and cueing to the learner. Initially, the teacher should encourage the learner with appropriate praise, such as "You're doing great!" or "Keep going, you're getting it!" While the PT/PTA often acts as the patient's cheerleader at this stage, it is important to be aware that not every patient action requires praise, and repeating the same phrase over and over loses its motivating power. Likewise, if the teacher attempts to cue a mistake or refinement of movement, they should use words that encourage and correct.

An example would be, "If you contract your trunk muscles before you squat, you will get better control of your leg movements," or "Look in the mirror as you lift your arm in the air. What do you see?" These statements do not focus on the patient making a mistake but allow the patient to move correctly and assist in self-awareness and self-correction (see **Figure 9-1**).

## Clinical Instructional Activities

In physical therapy, PTs and PTAs teach patients/clients the following:

- Information to help improve the patient's/client's ability to manage acute and chronic conditions
- Information for prevention, wellness, and opportunities for healthier lifestyles
- Material regarding exercises for reducing the effects of impairments/functional limitations
- Methods for active involvement in the patient's/client's physical therapy plan of care
- Material regarding adherence to home exercise, activities, and/or wellness programs

- Methods to maximize and promote independence in patients'/clients' activities of daily living and continuity of care

In addition, the clinical instructional activities must provide information to increase the patient's/client's understanding of their diagnosis and the specific rationales for interventions. The patient/client can use the information to manage their condition and to adapt to the home or work environment.

The healthcare professional also directs the clinical instructional activities at the patients'/clients' families and caregivers. Family and caregiver instructional activities may include training in specific techniques that increase, promote, and produce the identified patient/client outcomes. Most of the instruction focuses on the safety of the patient/client and the patient's/client's family and caregivers.

While teaching generally means that the professional is imparting information to the patient, it is important to recognize that the goal is for the patient to learn new attitudes and behaviors to improve their health and well-being.

Before teaching a patient, the PT or PTA must assess the learner to determine their current understanding and personal needs. Patient-centered teaching involves learning who the patient is and tailoring the teaching experience to the patient. Ask the patient how they learn best—via demonstration, written information, video, or audio. People can learn in multiple ways, and varying the teaching style may help the patient remain engaged in the learning process. Most patient teaching occurs over several treatment sessions, so developing a rapport of trust and understanding will help the PT/PTA create a teaching style that the patient will be more likely to accept.

Clinical instruction modes for patients/clients can take the following formats:

- Discussions
- Demonstrations
- Presentations
- Lectures
- Audiovisual materials or web-based learning methods
- Written demonstrations
- Illustrations of written information

When making demonstrations or presentations, the PTA should demonstrate or present the most important information first, keep the content brief and concise, emphasize the most important points, and be specific. The PTA should present the demonstrations and presentations at the level of the learner. The PTA should avoid technical terms when patients/clients are involved and limit extraneous information that may distract the learner.

When delivering lectures to the patient/client (and family/caregiver), the PTA should be concise, building on the information the learner has already processed and adding visual aids, such as illustrations, diagrams, or models. For example, before displaying audiovisual materials, the PTA should review the information, explain any technical terms used, or identify any equipment or intervention the patient/client may need. The PTA should also stop the video at appropriate times to explain critical aspects of the performance the patient/client may have to perform. After viewing the video, return demonstrations allow the PTA to assess how well the patient/client grasped the concepts presented. The PTA should observe the patient's/client's task performance, and then critique, praise, or help refine it.

Clinical instruction activities require that the clinician teacher provide the following things for the learner [1]:

- Respect for the patient's values, preferences, and expressed needs
- An overview of the objectives and purpose of the learning activity
- A description of how the learning activity fits with the patient's personal goals
- An environment that is quiet and appropriate for learning
- Reduction of conditions that negatively impact learning, such as pain or discomfort; anxiety; fear; frustration; feelings of failure, humiliation, embarrassment, boredom; or time pressures
- A teaching plan that is logical and sequential, uses patient-friendly language, and is understandable for the patient given their traits (e.g., culture, age, intellect, and educational level)
- Ample time for practice and answering questions
- Specific instructions to ensure that the clinician and patient have the same perceptions
- Appropriate assessment of learning immediately following the teaching and in subsequent treatment sessions
- Involvement of family members or friends to provide a support system for the patient

Other types of clinical instructional activities are clinical in-service and clinical education. Clinical in-service is an activity in which PTs, PTAs, or PT/PTA students prepare short educational programs to impart specific knowledge to peers. This tool can be an excellent way to teach others about topics from

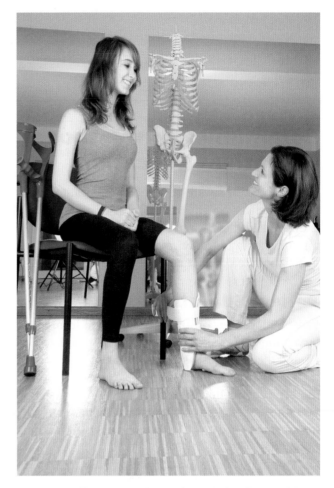

**Figure 9-2** Teaching patients about their injury and how to use crutches.
© RioPatuca/Shutterstock

continuing education courses that the professionals have attended. Presentation skills and topic organization will help the learner absorb and assimilate information quickly. Whenever possible, engage the learners by asking open-ended questions or having them participate in an activity (see **Figure 9-2**). When reviewing hands-on skills that the learner may already know, it may be useful to have the participants perform peer assessments to actively engage them in the learning process and tap into their skills. An example where this may be appropriate could be a review of safe transfer training with certified nursing assistants in a skilled nursing facility.

Clinical education involves activities in which the PT or PTA guides a student's learning experiences in the clinical environment. The American Physical Therapy Association (APTA) has a program to help clinical instructors learn strategies for teaching students—the Credentialed Clinical Instructor Courses. These courses help with organizational development and the implementation of teaching within the clinical environment.

# Communication Methods for Patient Education

PTAs should be aware of the communication skills used to deliver patient education. Each patient/client is different and has various learning requirements. As a result, communication modes may need to be adjusted to match each patient's/client's learning needs.

## Patient Education

Patient education constitutes a significant form of intervention in physical therapy clinical practice. The PT and the PTA must assess the patient's/client's abilities and learning styles and identify obstacles to learning. The instructional method of patient education needs to be adapted to the patient/client, especially for a patient/client with cognitive deficits or learning disabilities.

During patient education, the PT's or PTA's communication skills are critical. The therapist should communicate clearly and simply by using everyday words, rephrasing as necessary, and explaining new words. To ensure the message gets to the patient, besides speaking and writing, the therapist can use other materials, such as audiotapes, videotapes/DVDs, support groups, hotlines, and websites, for online information. In addition, the patient's understanding of information can be verified by asking open-ended questions and asking the patient to demonstrate how they will accomplish the instructions.

## Barriers to Learning

Sometimes, PTs and PTAs must adjust their teaching methods to accommodate a patient's learning ability. Patients who have learning, visual, or auditory impairments; who lack concentration; or who lack the motivation to learn will need other accommodations for learning to occur. Several learning styles and learning strategies are outlined in Chapter 1.

The following ideas may help to reduce barriers to learning:

- By adjusting the teaching method, therapists can adjust to a patient's learning style and special needs or by determining the patient's learning preference, such as reading, listening, watching, or doing.

- The teacher should focus on the patient's concerns and relate the importance of the topic being taught to those concerns. Avoid using fear tactics to gain the patient's attention. Instead, focus on the positive importance of learning and using the learned information. Especially when teaching a patient who appears unmotivated, it is important to utilize a factor important to the patient as motivation.

- The patient should be encouraged to bring a family member or a friend to the teaching session for support and to reinforce and clarify information.

- The teacher should break up information into logical "bits of information" so the patient can process what is being taught.

- Allow for practice. Many learners learn best kinesthetically, so "hands-on" practice will improve learning. Do not rely on closed questioning to verify learning for more didactic learning. "Do you understand?" or "Do you have any questions?" may be answered "yes" or "no" without ever allowing the teacher to substantiate understanding of the material taught.

- Ensure the materials are written in plain language for those with difficulty reading, consistently using the same words. When using new terms, define them and use repetition to reinforce the information. Sentences should be short and simple, each marked with a bullet point. Only five or six bullet points should be on each list. Attention can be drawn to essential information by making circles or arrows or adding dividers or tabs to the material.

- For individuals with learning impairments, successful instruction often includes using multisensory instruction, such as giving written directions, providing verbal instructions, and leading the patient through the physical activity you teach. The PTA may utilize different communication modes, such as videos with closed captioning or audio instructions. When providing written instructions, it may be helpful to highlight the most important information. Diagrams, graphics, and pictures may be more useful for patients with difficulty reading.

- For patients with an autism spectrum disorder, the PTA must consider strategies for communication. Autism spectrum disorders vary in the severity of the person's ability to communicate and perceive social interactions. Milder disorders may limit the person's understanding of nonverbal communication, while more severe forms can render the person nonverbal. The intellect of these patients also can range from very intelligent to impaired. Due to the wide variability in skill levels, visual and verbal instruction can be helpful due to the inability to identify a preferred learning tool. Repetition of information and use of demonstration may also be appropriate teaching strategies. People with an autism spectrum disorder usually respond better to routines that change very little and will have more difficulty with variety and changing from one activity to another. The PTA should also be aware that some individuals with this disorder may not tolerate physical touch.

- For older adults, the therapist needs to assess how and when the patient is ready to learn by finding out the patient's interest, determining their motivation to learn, and tying new information to past experiences. An environment conducive to learning can enhance the learning process, such as a quiet place, sitting near the patient, speaking clearly, and teaching in brief sessions (instead of long ones). Instructions can be taught one step at a time by demonstrating and describing the procedure and encouraging the patient to practice each step.

- For patients with visual impairments, therapists can introduce themselves and other people in the room, asking if the patient wants assistance and providing directions. When writing for a patient with visual impairments, the best method is to write the material in large print size (16-point font), use simple fonts, avoid italics, and write clearly and concisely (or print information in Braille).

- When speaking with patients with hearing impairments, the therapist can move a chair closer to face the patient, get their attention by touching them, and speak clearly and distinctly (not loudly). Pronunciation does not need to be exaggerated, but distracting and interfering sounds must be reduced. The room's light must be adequate because many patients with hearing impairments read lip movements and look at gestures, expressions, and pantomime actions.

- For patients who cannot speak English, the therapist can use certified interpreters to communicate key information to the patient. The patient must be comfortable with the interpreter, especially when discussing potentially embarrassing topics. Patients who cannot speak English will be very happy to be greeted in their native language and to have their names pronounced correctly. The therapist should speak clearly and concentrate on each patient's most important message(s).

- For patients from other cultures, the therapist needs to understand the patient's values and beliefs and pay attention to nonverbal communication, such as voice volume, postures, gestures, and eye contact. Working with the family decision-maker, who may be different from the patient, is essential for the success of an intervention. The treatment must be creative and may involve a spiritual advisor.

PTs and PTAs are teachers who need to recognize their strengths and weaknesses as teachers and pay close attention to their learners' needs. The PT/PTA will effectively teach and improve the patient's status by utilizing knowledge, enthusiasm, and encouragement.

### KNOWLEDGE CHECK

What should the PTA do to communicate during patient education effectively?
What obstacles to learning may be present when teaching a patient?
What strategies should a PTA employ to decrease obstacles to learning?

## Discussion Questions

1. The PTA is teaching a patient about good posture. Describe specific strategies that could be used to perform this task.

2. A patient with osteoporosis of the knee has come to physical therapy to manage their pain and in hopes of prolonging the need for a total knee replacement. The patient is morbidly obese and does not exercise regularly. The PTA recognizes that the patient's weight is part of the issue in resolving the knee pain and achieving the patient's goal of delaying surgery. Discuss methods of teaching this patient about their condition while respectfully understanding their obstacles.

3. Discuss the pros and cons of the different instructional modes (discussions, demonstrations, presentations, lectures, audiovisual material, web-based materials, return demonstrations, and illustrations of written information).

## Learning Opportunities

1. Utilizing one of the teaching strategies (demonstration, written communication, lecture, or discussion), prepare a plan to teach a patient how to move from supine to sitting.
2. Create an educational brochure about a topic relevant to physical therapy that could be used as a learning tool. An example might be safety in the home.
3. Explore the internet to find technology to assist in teaching hearing or visually impaired patients.

## Reference

1. Falvo DR: Effective Patient Education. A Guide to Increased Adherence, 4th ed. Sudbury, MA, Jones & Bartlett Learning, 2011

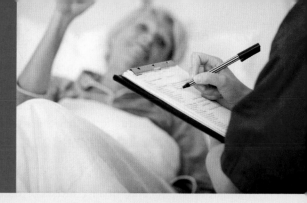

# CHAPTER 10

# Introduction to Documentation and the Medical Record

## OBJECTIVES

- Describe the significance and purpose of the physical therapy medical record.
- Identify the American Physical Therapy Association's guidelines for physical therapy documentation.
- Discuss documentation elements of the initial examination (including the patient history), visit/encounter reports, progress reports, and discharge reports.
- Define the SOAP mnemonic and its meaning.
- List the standardized titles and names used in physical therapy.
- Describe the emergence and importance of the electronic medical record.

## KEY TERMS

assessment data

electronic medical/health record (EMR/EHR)

functional outcome report (FOR)

objective data

point-of-service documentation

problem-oriented medical record (POMR)

sign

SOAP format

source-oriented medical record (SOMR)

subjective data

symptom

## Medical Records

Healthcare providers use written communication in medical records, including medical documentation. In physical therapy, documentation is the primary method for communication between third-party payers and the providers of physical therapy services.

### Documentation for Reimbursement

Documentation provides the basis for coverage decisions by third-party payers. Documentation of the

### Why do we need physical therapy documentation?

- For reimbursement
- For assurance of quality care
- For assurance of continuity of care
- For legal reasons
- For research and education
- For marketing

clinical intervention must show the physical therapy clinical decision-making involved and provide the necessary rationale to support the interventions. The documentation must describe physical therapy effectiveness, showing evidence of the patient's improving functional abilities to ensure reimbursement. When reading the documentation, the third-party payer is assured that physical therapy services were cost-effective and carried out by a skilled practitioner. In recent years, documentation of outcomes has become mandatory via specific quality indicator data reporting. Led by the Centers for Medicare and Medicaid Services, electronic documentation systems have increasingly been used to prove outcomes and will soon be used to process payment incentives or penalties.

## Documentation for Assurance of Quality Care

Documentation of physical therapy services provided to the patient and the patient's response to interventions is important for communicating with the physical therapy team to ensure quality care. Through documentation, the physical therapy team members can define a patient's problems, outline the plan of care (POC), identify barriers to recovery, and describe goals for efficient and skilled physical therapy interventions. A review of medical records can also be used to analyze the quality of care offered to the patient (also called quality assurance). Quality of care ensures a therapist's compliance, a department's efficiency and effectiveness, and a patient's accomplishment of functional outcomes.

## Documentation for Continuity of Care

Physical therapy documentation also guides physical therapists (PTs) and physical therapist assistants (PTAs) in the intervention's outcomes and goals and establishes a communication tool among PTs, PTAs, and other healthcare providers who are members of the rehabilitation team. The continuity of care is reflected in the documentation by describing the patient's responses to an intervention and any necessary modifications to the intervention.

## Documentation for Legal Reasons and Research/Education

Healthcare professionals consider legal aspects of documentation in case of a lawsuit or malpractice issue

to provide objective evidence of the care they performed. Documentation also provides useful information to researchers and educators. Objective analysis of the effectiveness of physical therapy services can be conducted using accurate data from clinical practice. Evidence-based research through clinical practice is a significant tool used in advancing physical therapy education and the progress of the physical therapy profession.

## Documentation for Marketing

Documentation can also be an important marketing tool because it includes descriptions of successful functional outcomes the patient achieves and the skilled and efficient quality of care offered to the patient.

## The American Physical Therapy Association's Documentation Guidelines

The American Physical Therapy Association (APTA) has several documentation guidelines[1]:

- Documentation is critical to ensure that individuals receive appropriate, comprehensive, efficient, person-centered, and high-quality healthcare services throughout the episode of care.
- Documentation elements for the initial examination and evaluation include the following: examination, evaluation, diagnosis, prognosis, intervention, and outcomes.
- All documentation must be legible, written in black or blue ink, and use medically approved abbreviations or symbols. The PT/PTA must cross mistakes out with a single line through the error, initial and date them.
- Documentation of a visit, often called a daily note or treatment note, documents the sequential implementation of the PT's POC and includes changes in the individual's status, a description, and progressions of specific interventions used. For example, do not use "patient tolerated the treatment well" but describe the response, such as "heart rate increased to 90 beats/minute; blood pressure (BP) response; movement exhibited decreased endurance and increased pain."
- Each intervention session must be documented; the patient's name and identification number must be on each page of the documentation record.

---

1 https://www.apta.org/your-practice/documentation/defensible-documentation/elements-within-the-patientclient-management
-model/documentation-of-a-visit

- The PT or PTA may provide documentation, depending on who provided the services. Administrative or support personnel can also document administrative information (schedule changes or authorization updates) in a record or chart and may assist a PT in recording information in a patient's or client's record as directed.
- A competent adult must sign informed consent for the interventions. If the adult is not competent, the consent must be signed by the patient's/client's legal guardian. The parent or an appointed guardian must sign the consent if the patient is a minor.
- Each document must be dated and signed by the PT/PTA, using their first and last names and professional designation. A professional license number may be included, but it is optional.
- All communications with other healthcare providers or healthcare professionals must be recorded.
- Depending on the practice setting, check with the policies and procedures of the clinic or facility, state practice act, and payer requirements to determine if there are any procedures for documenting verbal orders in a patient's or client's record.
- Documentation of referral sources or self-referral should occur within the initial documentation.
- Cancelations and no-shows should be documented.

---

**KNOWLEDGE CHECK**

What are the purposes of documentation?
What are the recommendations for effective documentation?

---

# Types of Medical Records

Physical therapy documentation can be written in different types of medical records. The most used include **problem-oriented medical records (POMRs)** and source-oriented medical records (SOMRs).

## Problem-Oriented Medical Records

The POMR is a method of organizing and documenting patient information systematically and comprehensively, focusing on the patient's health problems. The POMR lists problems in order of importance and provides a coherent plan for dealing with each.

---

The sections of the POMR may include the following:
- Clinical findings (data)
- Problem list
- Intervention plan
- Progress notes
- Discharge notes

---

Each section contains the appropriate information from each discipline. The data included in the POMR is kept at the front of the chart and evaluated as frequently as indicated concerning recording changes in the patient's status and progress made in solving the problems. Using the POMR, healthcare facilities can create comprehensive medical records containing information from each discipline. This method enhances communication among healthcare providers, ultimately helping with the patient's care.

The advantages of POMR include the provision of organization and structure of the medical information, chronological description of interventions, a specific plan for managing the patient's problems, and improved communication among healthcare providers.

## Source-Oriented Medical Records

The **SOMR**, arranged by the medical services offered in the clinical facility, is another organizational method for medical records. Some hospitals use SOMRs by labeling each discipline's section in the chart with a tab marker. The first section of the SOMR is the physician's section, followed by sections for the other disciplines, such as nursing, pharmacy, dietary, social services, physical therapy, occupational therapy, speech and language pathology, and laboratory results. The healthcare providers from each discipline document their content in the section designated for their discipline. Some healthcare providers criticize the SOMR format because reading each section for information is difficult.

## SOAP Records

SOAP is an acronym for an organized structure to keep the progress notes in the chart. Each entry contains the date, the patient's identification number, and the title of the patient's particular problem, followed by the SOAP headings.

The beginning of a SOAP-organized note can identify the discipline's diagnosis or problem and should be placed in the problem list section of the POMR.

The SOAP headings represent the following:

- Subjective findings: Information provided by the patient (symptoms) or the patient's family/caregiver
- Objective findings: Results of the signs found in the examination
- Assessment: Overall response to interventions and the effects of interventions, changes in patient status, and the healthcare provider's opinion about the patient's progress
- Plan: The plan for further diagnostic or therapeutic action or the next intervention session

## Electronic Medical Records

**Electronic medical records (EMRs)**, or **electronic health records (EHRs)**, are digital versions of medical records that allow healthcare providers to store, manage, and access patient health information electronically. These electronic records offer several advantages over paper records, such as:

- Improved accuracy and completeness of patient information
- Easier and quicker access to patient information
- Improved patient safety through reduced medical errors
- Increased efficiency and productivity for healthcare providers
- Improved communication and collaboration among healthcare providers
- Enhanced support for clinical decision-making and research

However, EMRs also present challenges, such as the need for strong cybersecurity measures to protect sensitive patient information. From a payer perspective, access to a limited set of Health Insurance Portability and Accountability Act (HIPAA)-compliant EHR data provides real-time direct access to the information they need to approve the payment. Finally, from a patient's perspective, EMRs can be used to validate their health insurance coverage, which can help them maintain insurance benefits and enhance continuity of care.

### KNOWLEDGE CHECK

What is the difference between POMRs and SOMRs? What are the four sections of the SOAP format, and what does each heading represent?

# Types of Physical Therapy Documentation Reports

Physical therapy uses four types of documentation reports:

- Initial evaluation report
- Visit/encounter treatment notes
- Progress reports
- Discharge reports

## Initial Examination/Evaluation Report

The initial examination and evaluation reports form the foundation of all other reports, such as visit/encounter notes, progress reports, and discharge reports. Through the initial evaluation report, the PT establishes the primary purpose for intervention and outlines the expectations for progress (**Figure 10-1**).

The initial examination and evaluation report can be written in the SOAP format, a narrative format, or another format. Because the POMR format does not focus on the patient's functional limitations but mostly on the patient's impairments, some PTs prefer a different format called the **functional outcome report (FOR)** in the initial examination report.

The FOR format follows a sequence of information different from the SOAP format. The FOR format is more appropriate in an initial examination report because it includes the reason for referral, the patient's functional limitations, physical therapy assessment, therapy problems, functional outcome goals, and intervention plan and rationale. The FOR format is

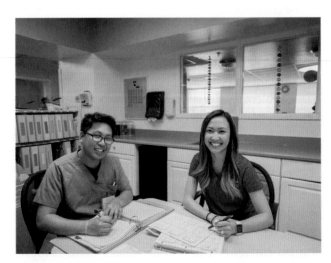

**Figure 10-1** Accurate and timely documentation is part of the PT's and PTA's job.

becoming popular in physical therapy because it can easily demonstrate the effect of impairments on functional limitations, and it is relatively uncomplicated for reviewers.

## Initial Examination and Evaluation Report Elements

The initial examination and evaluation report may contain the following elements:

- Referral, including the reason for referral and the specific treatment requested by the referral source
- Data accompanying the referral, including the primary diagnosis (or onset date), secondary diagnoses, medical history, medications, and other complications or precautions
- Physical therapy history, including the patient's date of birth, age, gender, the start of care, and the primary complaint
- Referral diagnosis, including the mechanism of injury and the prior diagnostic imaging (or testing)
- Prior therapy history
- Evaluation data, including the patient's cognition, vision, hearing, vital signs, vascular signs, sensation and proprioception, coordination, balance, posture, pain, edema, active range of motion (AROM), passive range of motion (PROM), strength, bed mobility, transfers, ambulation (level and stairs), wheelchair uses, orthotic/prosthetic devices, durable medical equipment used or needed, activity tolerance, special tests, architectural considerations, requirements to return to prior activity level (including work, school, or home), outcome measures data, and wound description (for wound care, including the incision status)
- Prior level of function, including mobility at home and in the community, employment, or school
- Treatment diagnosis
- Assessment, including the reason for skilled care
- Problems
- POC, including specific intervention strategies, frequency, duration, patient instruction/home program, caregiver training, short-term goals and dates of achievement, long-term goals and dates of achievement, and patient's rehabilitation potential

## Patient History

Patient history is part of the initial examination and evaluation. Patient history refers to a complete medical history of the patient's chief complaints, present illness, past history, allergies, current medications,

lifestyle and habits, social history, vocational and economic history, and family history. The healthcare provider takes the history in an orderly manner, keeping the patient focused and discouraging irrelevant information. Patient history can include the following documentation elements:

- Personal information, including the patient's age, gender, and occupation
- Medical diagnosis and any precautions related to physical therapy
- Patient's chief complaint, including the patient's description of their condition, the reason for seeking assistance, and identification of the patient's primary problem
- Patient's present illness, including the symptoms associated with the patient's primary problem, such as the location of the problem (may use a body chart), severity, nature (such as aching, burning, or tingling), persistence (constant versus intermittent), and aggravated by activity versus relieved by rest
- The onset of the patient's primary problem, including mechanism of injury (if traumatic), sequence and progression of symptoms, date of the initial onset and status up to the current visit, prior treatments and results, and associated disability
- Patient's past history, including prior episodes of the same problem; prior treatments and responses; other affected areas (or body parts); familial, developmental, and congenital disorders; general health status; medications; and X-rays or other pertinent tests
- Patient's lifestyle, including the patient's profession or occupation, assistance from family or friends, occupational and family demands (spouse, children, job expectations), activities of daily living (ADLs, such as hobbies, sports), and the patient's concept of the impact of functional (including cosmetic) and socioeconomic factors

## Treatment Notes

Treatment, or progress, notes (written by the PTs and/or PTAs) are generally short, depending on the format and frequency of the report, the practice setting, the patient type, and the payer involved. As with the initial evaluation report, these notes must include the patient's full name, date of birth, medical records number, and room number. The information can be written as a SOAP note or in a narrative format.

The **SOAP** notes also follow the sequence of data organization corresponding to subjective, objective, assessment, and plan. The narrative format notes vary.

However, the narrative format notes must be organized properly and consistently describe treatment comparisons. The SOAP notes are used the most in physical therapy for treatment notes.

## Progress Reports

The PTs write progress reports and provide documentation of the continuum of care to provide reasons for skilled physical therapy services. The focus of progress reports is on the reevaluation of problems identified in the initial evaluation or any other new problem that has developed since the last formal reevaluation. The progress reports need documentation describing the skilled interventions, the complicating factors that affected the duration of skilled care, and the comparative data from the initial evaluation or the last reevaluation. The format of a progress report varies; however, it must contain the following general elements:

- Attendance
- Current baseline data, including patient's cognition, vision, hearing, vital signs, vascular signs, sensation and proprioception, coordination, balance (sit and stand), posture, pain, edema, AROM and PROM, strength, bed mobility, transfers, ambulation (level and stairs), wheelchair utilization, orthotic/prosthetic devices, durable medical equipment used or needed, activity tolerance, special tests, architectural considerations, requirements to return to prior activity level (including work, school, or home), and wound description (for wound care and including the incision status)
- Treatment diagnosis
- Assessment, including the reason for skilled care
- Problems
- POC, including specific treatment strategies, frequency of treatment, duration of treatment, patient instruction/home program, caregiver training, short-term goals and dates of achievement, long-term goals and dates of achievement, and the patient's rehabilitation potential

## Discharge Reports

Discharge reports are the last of the four reports used in physical therapy. Per APTA requirements, they are written by the PT and describe the outcome of physical therapy services. The essential elements of a discharge report include the following:

- Attendance
- Current baseline data, including patient's cognition, vision, hearing, vital signs, vascular signs, sensation and proprioception, coordination,

balance (sit and stand), posture, pain, edema, AROM and PROM, strength, bed mobility, transfers, ambulation (level and stairs), wheelchair use, orthotic/prosthetic devices, durable medical equipment used or needed, activity tolerance, special tests, architectural considerations, requirements to return to prior activity level (including work, school, or home), outcome measures data, and wound description (for wound care, including the incision status)
- Treatment diagnosis
- Assessment, including the reason for skilled care
- Problems
- POC, including specific intervention strategies, frequency of treatment, duration of treatment, patient instruction/home program, caregiver training, short-term goals and dates of achievement, long-term goals and dates of achievement, and discharge prognosis

### KNOWLEDGE CHECK

What information is found in the initial evaluation? What are the differences between a treatment note, a progress report, and a discharge report?

## SOAP Writing Format

The SOAP format reports are used the most in physical therapy practice. They can be written daily or weekly.

## Visit/Encounter SOAP Format Reports

The PT or the PTA can write the daily or weekly SOAP format reports.

The SOAP format data can be used as follows:

- By the PT to write the initial examination and evaluation reports
- By the PT to write the reexamination and reevaluation progress reports
- By the PT and the PTA to write their visit/encounter progress notes

The PT writes the SOAP initial examination and evaluation reports during the initial examination and evaluation. The SOAP reexamination and reevaluation reports, called progress reports, are written by the PT periodically throughout the time the patient receives physical therapy. The PT or the PTA writes the visit/encounter SOAP progress notes daily. The PT is also responsible for the discharge examination and the discharge evaluation reports, which are the patient's/client's final examination and evaluation. The APTA considers establishing the discharge plan and documenting the discharge summary/status the responsibility of the PT, not the PTA. However, the laws in various states may differ. The PTA can write a SOAP note (called a discharge summary) summarizing the patient's care in their last physical therapy intervention, without any reexamination and reevaluation (interpretation of the data) and write the postdischarge POC.

## Subjective Data in SOAP Format Reports

As stated earlier, the SOAP mnemonic stands for **s**ubjective, **o**bjective, **a**ssessment, and **p**lan. The S section at the beginning of the SOAP note contains the subjective data and includes information provided by the patient or the patient's family. The subjective data also includes any pertinent information regarding physical therapy offered by the patient's family and caregiver. Every time patients are seen in physical therapy, they are asked about their chief complaint(s). The complaints causing the patient to seek medical help are symptoms included in the SOAP note's subjective part.

Patient's Symptoms

- A **symptom** is any change in the body or its functions perceived by the patient.
- A symptom represents the subjective experience of a disease. Some frequent examples of patients' symptoms in physical therapy are pain, stiffness, weakness, numbness, and loss of equilibrium.
- Elements of the patient's symptoms (in the SOAP note) may include the date when the symptoms occurred, the location of the symptoms, how they occurred, aggravating or relieving factors, the severity, and any associated symptoms.

## Physical Therapy Diagnosis versus Medical Diagnosis

When using the POMR format, the patient's problems are listed (and numbered in certain facilities) before the subjective section of the SOAP note. The patient's medical diagnosis differs from their physical therapy diagnosis.

The patient's medical diagnosis identifies the cause of the patient's illness or discomfort. A medical diagnosis is determined by a physician's evaluation and diagnostic tests. The medical diagnosis is equivalent to the patient's pathology.

As per the Guide to Physical Therapist Practice, physical therapy diagnosis is the clinical classification by a PT of a patient's impairments, functional limitations, and disabilities [1]. Using the International Classification of Impairments, Disabilities, and Handicaps (ICIDH) developed by the World Health Organization, physical therapy diagnosis also represents the data obtained by physical therapy examination and other relevant information to determine the cause and nature of a patient's impairments, functional limitations, and disabilities [1]. For example, for a musculoskeletal problem, a patient's medical diagnosis could be a "right hip fracture." The physical therapy diagnosis, in contrast, could be "transfer and gait dependency." A patient's difficulties with transfers and dependency on assistive devices while walking represent the patient's impairments and functional limitations. For a neurologic problem, a medical diagnosis could be "multiple sclerosis," while the physical therapy diagnosis could be "ataxic gait and frequent falling." A patient's difficulties, such as lack of muscular coordination while walking and frequent falling, represent patient impairments and functional limitations.

## Subjective Data in Progress SOAP Format Notes

The **subjective data** in the progress SOAP note includes information about the patient and the patient's condition that is described to the PT or the PTA by the patient or a representative of the patient. A symptom is a subjective experience the patient reports, such as fatigue or pain. Subjective information must be relevant to the patient's physical therapy diagnosis and treatment plan. As a result, the subjective information must not include all the patient's complaints, only the condition(s) relevant to the physical therapy diagnosis/prognosis and intervention plan.

The PT/PTA must use active, directed, attentive, and exploratory listening to include relevant information in the subjective section. For example, the PT/PTA can use verbs, such as states, reports, and says, to write about subjective data. Also, the patient can be directly quoted, especially concerning a patient's attitude about physical therapy or descriptions of activities that the patient can or cannot perform. When the subjective information is provided by someone other than the patient, the PT/PTA must document the name of the person who provided the information and the person's relationship with the patient.

Pain information can be located in the subjective or objective part of the SOAP note. As the patient describes the pain to the PT/PTA, it would be reported in the S section. If a standardized tool, such as the McGill Pain Questionnaire, is used, the information may be more appropriately documented in the O section. The documentation location should be consistent within the practice so that all personnel working can locate the information easily. The patient must illustrate the description of pain in some form of a pain profile using pain scales, a checklist of descriptive words, or body drawings.

The subjective data may include the following:
- Patient's complaints of pain
- Patient's response to the previous intervention
- Patient's description of functional improvements, such as being able to do ADLs
- Patient's lifestyle situation, such as being able to go out to dinner or entertain friends like they used to do before this condition
- Patient's goals, such as to be able to drive their car in 2–3 weeks
- Patient's compliance or difficulties with the home exercise program (HEP)

The SOAP examination note written by the PT in the initial examination and evaluation (or reexamination) is much more detailed than the visit/encounter progress SOAP note written by the PT and the PTA during physical therapy interventions. The initial examination SOAP note includes, in addition to the patient's complaints, information about the patient's medical history, environment, emotions and attitudes, level of functioning, and goals.

An example of a subjective part of the progress SOAP note for a patient who had a right total knee replacement 4 weeks ago might be:

**S.** Patient reports that for the past weekend, she could walk (using the cane) in her home up and down five stairs, three times/day, without her right knee buckling.

Other examples of subjective information in the progress note may include the following:
- The patient described having numbness and tingling in the back of her left leg down to her calf.
- She said she was diagnosed with a herniated disk in her back last year.

- On an ascending scale of 0–10, the patient rates his right arm and shoulder pain at 6/10 with movement and 2/10 without movement.
- She said: "I need to get better fast and be able to go to work as a secretary."
- He denies any discomfort in his back while sitting at his desk.
- The patient said he had a car accident on February 15, 2019.

## KNOWLEDGE CHECK

What information is found in the objective section of the SOAP format?

## Objective Data in SOAP Format Notes

The O section of the SOAP note contains the objective data. The **objective data** can be reproduced or confirmed by another healthcare provider with the same training as the one gathering the objective information.

### Patient's Signs

Data in the objective section of the SOAP note contains the signs of the patient's disease or dysfunction. A **sign** is a disease manifestation that can be seen or measured objectively by someone other than the involved, such as a rash or a high temperature.

The diagnostician can see, hear, measure, or feel a sign. Finding such signs can be used to confirm or deny the diagnostician's impressions of the disease suspected of being present. An example of a sign in physical therapy would be the patient's gait pattern, such as flexed posture and shuffling gait (as in Parkinson's disease).

In physical therapy, the objective part of the SOAP note also contains the patient's treatment session.

## Objective Data in Progress SOAP Format Notes

The PTA should write the objective data of the progress SOAP note so that another PTA may reproduce or continue the intervention or that a reader untrained in physical therapy (such as an insurance representative or a lawyer) may determine the effectiveness of the treatment session.

Data about visual or tactile observations, such as posture or palpation reassessments performed by the

The objective section in the progress SOAP note may contain the following:

- The results of the physical therapy measurements and tests, such as manual muscle testing (MMT), goniometry, gait assessment, and specific neurologic assessments (such as balance, sensation, or proprioception)
- The description of the interventions provided to the patient, such as physical agents and modalities, therapeutic exercises, wound care, functional training (such as gait using assistive devices), patient education/instruction (such as postsurgery precautions), and discussion and coordination with other disciplines (such as occupational therapy practitioners who want to give the patient a shoehorn to be able to put their shoes on)
- The description of the patient's function, such as performing transfers, gait (with or without assistive devices, on even or uneven surfaces and stairs), or bed mobility (such as turning from supine to side-lying to sitting)
- The PTA's objective observations of the patient during interventions (such as the increase in the number of exercise repetitions), tests and measurements (such as compensating for muscular weakness), and patient education/instruction (such as understanding the HEP on the first performance)

PT or the PTA, is also included in the objective part of the SOAP note. The SOAP note's objective section also includes other data, such as written copies of the HEP.

The objective information of the progress SOAP note must include the following:

- Description of the reason(s) for intervention and the intervention provided to the patient. The data must include enough detail that another PT or PTA could read the description and replicate the intervention. Documentation of the previous treatment note should not be repetitive but should include a rationale for changing the intervention. For example, descriptions of why therapeutic exercise was progressed, a modality was discontinued, or observable changes in the patient's functional status indicate patient progress.
- Description of the patient's response to each intervention. This data is important for the PT/PTA to be able to replicate or change the intervention to obtain the most effective patient response. The PT/PTA should not write what they did regarding the intervention (such as "Applied moist hot pack to the patient's lower back"). Instead, the PT/PTA should write the patient's response to the moist hot pack (such as "Patient had decreased muscular spasm of right erector spinae at L2–L4 level after application of moist hot pack to the muscles for 20 minutes while the patient was in the prone position").

- Description of tests/measurements after interventions. This data is significant because by repeating tests and measurements performed in the initial examination, the PT/PTA can describe the results by relating them with the initial examination findings. Outcome measures are standardized assessments that identify functional outcomes and help establish the progress toward the outcomes established during the evaluation. A periodic assessment of the patient's progress will help to determine if the physical therapy is successful.

- Utilization of words that describe the patient performing a function. Descriptions of the quality of a patient's movement define the patient's true ability to complete functional tasks and develop the reader's visualization of the patient's functional status.

- Logical organization of information. This data can give the reader a clear image of the patient's interventions and progress.

- Utilization of words that portray skilled physical therapy services. Documentation should include a specific decision-making rationale that relates the impairment and functional limitation to the intervention that no one other than the PT or PTA could provide.

- Copies of any additional written information (such as exercises and/or patient education material) given to the patient for home use

The objective data of the initial examination and evaluation (or reexamination) (written by the PT) is more complex than the objective information of the progress SOAP note (written by the PT and the PTA). The data in the initial examination may contain the following information:

- Patient's cognitive status, communication, and judgment
- Patient's musculoskeletal findings, such as range of motion, strength, or posture
- Patient's neurologic findings, such as pain, reflexes, or sensation
- Patient's cardiovascular findings, such as BP, pulse, respiration, or endurance
- Patient's functional status, such as transfers, mobility, ADLs, or work/school activities
- Patient's outcome measure data

## *Example of Objective Information in Progress SOAP Notes*

An example of an objective part of the progress SOAP note for a patient who had a right total knee replacement 4 weeks ago might be:

**O.** Patient performed: 10 minutes stationary bicycle; closed kinetic chain (CKC) strengthening exercises standing at the wall and bending right knee 10 times, 3 sets with 1-minute rest between sets; sitting in a chair, strengthening exercises for right knee extension, using a 3-pound weight around the right ankle, 10 repetitions, 3 sets with 1-minute rest between the sets; standing and holding onto the back of the chair, strengthening exercises for right knee flexion, using a 3-pound weight around the right ankle, 10 repetitions, 3 sets with 1-minute rest between the sets; long sitting ice pack for 10 minutes to right knee; patient sitting reassessed for right quadriceps strength using MMT: is 4/5.

Other examples of objective information in the progress note may include the following:

- The patient transferred partial weight bearing (PWB) on the right lower extremity (RLE) from bed to w/c and back with a maximum assist of one for strength and balance and with verbal cueing for PWB status.
- BP 140/90; pulse 95 beats per minute (BPM), irregular.
- AROM of right shoulder flexion 0°–115°.
- The patient performed self-stretching exercises, three repetitions, to increase right shoulder flexion and abduction with elevation, sitting, and sliding the right arm on the table.
- The diameter of the wound from the right to the left outer edge is 5 cm today compared to 6.2 cm on 9-27-19.

### KNOWLEDGE CHECK

What information is found in the objective section of the SOAP format?

## Assessment Data in SOAP Format Notes

The A section of the SOAP note contains the assessment data, which represents a summary of the information from the subjective and objective sections of the SOAP note. The assessment is one of the most important sections of the SOAP note because it tells the reader whether physical therapy is helping the patient.

In the assessment section, the PT/PTA discusses the patient's response to the intervention, the effectiveness of the intervention, and the patient's progress/lack of progress toward the goals established by the PT in the initial examination and evaluation. Also, in the assessment section, the PT/PTA remarks about the patient's progress toward the patient's goals as expressed by the patient in the subjective section of the SOAP note. (These goals are tied in with the intervention and the reassessment data from the objective section of the SOAP note.)

All comments in the assessment section of the progress SOAP note must be supported by evidence from the subjective and objective sections' data. During the interventions, the patient's reassessments are conducted by the PT or the PTA regularly and are documented in the objective assessment section of the SOAP note to determine the effectiveness or lack of effectiveness of the interventions.

The assessment section may contain the following:

- Patient's overall response to intervention, such as decreased pain, improved range of motion, or improved gait pattern
- Patient's progress toward short- and long-term goals (from the PT's initial evaluation)
- Explanations as to why the interventions are necessary
- Effects of interventions on the patient's impairments and functional limitations
- Comparison of patient's abilities from the previous date to the current date

When interpreting the data in the assessment section of the SOAP report, the PTA (or the PT) should avoid the following documentation errors:

- Making undetermined general comments about the patient's condition or progress, such as "patient is walking better today" or "patient tolerated treatment well"
- Describing the patient's progress without showing evidence in the subjective and objective sections of the SOAP note
- Overlooking meeting the patient's short- and long-term goals (from the initial examination and evaluation)

The **assessment data** in the initial examination and evaluation (or reexamination) (written by the PT) is more complex than the assessment information in the progress SOAP note. The data may contain the following:

- Analysis of the problems and plan of action (including a summary of impairments, functional limitations, and disabilities)
- Short-term goals that can be accomplished in 2–3 weeks from the start of the intervention
- Long-term goals that are functional goals (written in functional terms) that can be accomplished in 4–5 weeks (or longer) from the start of the intervention

## *Example of Assessment Information in Progress SOAP Notes*

An example of the assessment part of the progress SOAP note tying in information from the subjective and the objective sections of the SOAP note for a patient who had a right total knee replacement 6 weeks ago might be:

**S.** Patient reports that for the past weekend, she could walk (using the cane) in her home up and down five stairs, three times/day, without her right knee buckling.

**O.** Patient performed: 15 minutes stationary bicycle; CKC strengthening exercises included wall squats 10 times, 3 sets with 1-minute rest between sets, short-arc quad strengthening exercises for the right knee using a 5-pound weight around the right ankle, 10 repetitions, 3 sets with 1-minute rest between the sets, hamstring curl strengthening exercises for the right knee, using an 8-pound weight around the right ankle, 10 repetitions, 3 sets with 1-minute rest between the sets; long sitting ice pack for 10 minutes to right knee; patient sitting, reassessed for right quadriceps strength using MMT: is 4+/5.

**A.** Patient is progressing in physical therapy: tolerated increased weight to 3 pounds with strengthening exercises; patient met short-term goal #1 to ascend and descend five steps independently; right knee scar is red and healing.

Other examples of assessment information in the progress note may include the following:

- Strengthening exercises effectively increased the patient's strength by 1/2 of the MMT grade. The patient met his short-term goal #1 to transfer from sit to stand independently.
- The patient consistently used proper body mechanics and leg muscles while lifting.

- The patient needed frequent verbal cues for total hip replacement (THR) precautions to maintain the RLE in abduction while transferring from bed to w/c.
- The patient is not progressing toward the goal of independence in ambulation for 50 feet with a standard walker (SW).

All the data needs to be supported by the subjective and objective information in the note.

### KNOWLEDGE CHECK

How does the SOAP format's assessment section differ from the subjective and objective sections?

## Plan Data of SOAP Format Notes

The P section of the SOAP note contains the plan. The plan data of the progress SOAP note contains information that the PTA may need to apply regarding the patient's interventions before and during the treatment session(s) or between the sessions. They also indicate when the next session will occur or how many sessions will be scheduled. The plan section of the progress SOAP note uses verbs in the future tense. PTAs should avoid meaningless and nonspecific documentation, such as "continue with the current plan of care."

The plan section may contain the following:

- Plan for the next treatment session, including a justification for the continuation of care
- Plan for consultation with another discipline as necessary
- Frequency of the treatment
- Plan for reevaluation or discharge by the PT
- Plan to discuss with the PT changes in the patient's condition, the introduction of new exercises, specific patient complaints, suggested modifications to the POC

The plan data of the initial examination and evaluation (or reexamination) SOAP note written by the PT is more complex than the plan information in the progress SOAP note written by the PT and the PTA. The examination SOAP note contains information about the specific intervention plan for the patient's identified problem(s) and the frequency and duration of the interventions.

An example of the *plan* part of the progress SOAP note for a patient who had a right total knee replacement 4 weeks ago could be:

**P.** Will continue with therapeutic exercise and increase repetitions and weights next session to improve the patient's ability to transfer in and out of her bed independently; will start neuromuscular reeducation using proprioception exercises next session to improve balance during transfers.

Other examples of plan information in the progress note may include the following:

- Will discuss with the PT the possibility of adding self-stretching exercises as a HEP.
- The PT will see the patient next visit for reassessment.
- Will order a rolling walker to be available for the next treatment session on 10-25-19.
- Will do gait training on stairs next visit to allow the patient to return home.
- At the next visit, will increase the weights to 5 pounds in Progressive Resistance Exercise (PRE)-strengthening exercises to allow the patient to lift objects above his head at work.

### KNOWLEDGE CHECK

What components should be present in the plan section of the SOAP format?

## Legal Issues in Documentation

In physical therapy, documentation guidelines should specifically comply with jurisdictional, regulatory, and insurance company (including Medicare/Medicaid) requirements.

General guidelines for physical therapy documentation are as follows:

- The patient's right to privacy should be respected regarding documentation of the examination and evaluation, reexamination and reevaluation, and the SOAP note.
- Only the patient can authorize the release of medical information, including written physical therapy documentation in writing.
- All inquiries for medical information to the PTA should be directed to the supervising PT or physician.
- Written physical therapy records should be maintained safely and securely for 7 years.

In physical therapy documentation, verbal communication is used in telephone conversations regarding the following:

- Verbal referrals for physical therapy treatment from other healthcare providers
- Receiving information about the patient from the patient (or the patient's representative)
- Receiving inquiries about the patient's medical condition or treatment from different persons

When a PTA verbally takes a telephone referral from another healthcare provider, the PTA needs to document the following in writing:

- The date and time of the call
- The name of the person calling
- The name of the PTA who took the referral
- The name of the patient and all other details regarding the referral
- The date when a written copy of the referral will be sent to the physical therapy office/department
- The name of the PT who will be responsible for the referred patient

In addition, PTs/PTAs may receive calls about changes in a patient's condition. These calls also need to be documented in writing regarding the date and time of the call, the name of the person calling, the name of the PT/PTA taking the call, and a summary of the conversation. The PT/PTA should direct the caller to call 911 or the nearest hospital's emergency department if it is an emergency.

## Standardized Titles and Names Used in Physical Therapy

The physical therapy profession has created a standardized terminology for consistency in titles identifying professionals' areas of expertise, which the APTA recognizes. The following paragraphs define the uniform terminology that should be used for physical therapy:

- The acronym APTA in public relations and marketing should be used in conjunction with the APTA title.
- The APTA supports the use of PT as the regulatory designation of a physical therapist. Other letter designations, such as RPT, LPT, or academic and professional degrees, should not be substituted for the regulatory designation of PT. PTA is the preferred regulatory designation of a physical therapist assistant.

- The APTA supports the recognition of the regulatory designation of a PT or a PTA as taking precedence over other credentials or letter designations. To promote consistent communication of the presentation of credentials and letter designations, the APTA recognizes the following preferred order:
  - PT/PTA
  - Highest-earned physical therapy–related degree
  - Other earned academic degree(s)
  - Specialist certification credentials in alphabetical order (specific to the American Board of Physical Therapy specialties)
  - Other credentials external to the APTA
  - Other certifications or professional honors (e.g., FAPTA)
- The APTA supports the designations of SPT and SPTA for PT and PTA students, respectively, up to the time of graduation. Graduates should be designated per state law after graduation and before licensure. If state law does not stipulate a specific designation, graduates should be designated in a way that clearly identifies that they are not licensed PTs or licensed or regulated PTAs.
- The APTA is committed to promoting the PT as the professional physical therapy practitioner and the PTA as the only individual who assists the PT in providing selected physical therapy interventions. The PT is responsible for the patient and patient/client management. The PTA changes selected interventions only to progress the patient as directed by the PT and promote patient safety and comfort. The APTA is further committed to incorporating this concept into all Association policies, positions, and program activities, wherever applicable.
- When used with physical therapy services, the term *professional* denotes the PT. The PT conducts the practice of physical therapy.
- The PTA is a technically educated healthcare provider who assists the PT in providing physical therapy.
- The PTA is educated and works under the PT's direction and at least general supervision. The PTA is the only individual who assists the PT per the APTA's policies and positions in delivering selected physical therapy interventions. The PTA is a graduate of a PTA education program accredited by the Commission on Accreditation in Physical Therapy Education (CAPTE).

- The APTA uses the term *physical therapist professional education* to refer to the basic education of the PT to qualify them to practice physical therapy, and the term *physical therapist postprofessional education* to refer to the advanced physical therapy educational studies undertaken by a PT to enhance their professional skills and/or knowledge. When used in physical therapy services, "professional" denotes the PT.
- Only PTs may use or include the initials PT or DPT, and only PTAs may use or include the initials PTA in their technical or regulatory designation. Additionally, the APTA supports including language to protect the exclusive use of these terms, titles, and designations in statutes and regulations.

### KNOWLEDGE CHECK

What is the regulatory designation of a PTA?

# Defensible Documentation

PTs and PTAs should know that defensible documentation is intrinsic to contemporary physical therapy clinical practice. PTs have been continuously seeking to integrate the latest evidence into their practices. The evidence can include better tests and measures, new and improved equipment, new theories of disease pathology, and more efficient interventions. Consequently, evidence-based practice needs to be documented using researched clinical guidelines and approved physical therapy protocols. Third-party payers, other healthcare providers, and consumers expect this documentation from physical therapy providers.

PTs have a large role in creating effective defensible documentation. They should include documentation that achieves the following[2]:

- Reflects the PT's decision-making process
- Indicates evidence of the PT's unique body of knowledge and skill
- Provides the PT's verification of their professional judgment

PTAs should work closely with PTs to help facilitate the patient's/client's functional outcomes using evidence-based interventions. This can be accomplished by evaluating and discussing current

---

research from journal articles and reviews regarding evidence-based interventions. The APTA's website, PT Now Article Search, Hooked on Evidence, and the Physical Therapy Outcomes Registry provide a literature review for evidence-based interventions.

The APTA recommends the following tips for documentation that reflects evidence-based care:

- PTs should incorporate valid and reliable tests and measures as appropriate.
- PTs and PTAs should keep current with research through journal articles, reviews, and the APTA's PT Now and Open Door websites.
- PTs should include standardized tests and measures in the clinical documentation.
- PTs and PTAs should review and incorporate evidence-based interventions into clinical physical therapy.

Data from American Physical Therapy Association. Physical Therapy Documentation of Patient and Client Management. n.d. https://www.apta.org/your-practice/documentation

# Computerized Documentation

Computer-based documentation is rapidly becoming the norm in physical therapy facilities. While not compelled to utilize EHRs, regulations are changing that may require physical therapy to utilize computerized systems in the next few years. Documentation systems can run on desktop computers, notebook or laptop computers, touchscreen computers, and personal digital assistants (PDAs) (see **Figure 10-2**).

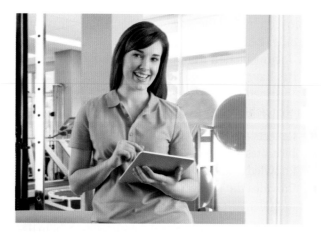

**Figure 10-2** Electronic records are becoming commonplace in health care.
© DNY59/E+/Getty Images

Notebook computers and PDAs allow the PT/PTA to enter information while performing examinations/evaluations, assessments, or interventions with the patient. This practice is known as **point-of-service documentation**. It requires that the PT and PTA be adept at communicating with and attending to the patient while documenting patient responses, collecting objective data, monitoring exercises, or assessing progress. This type of documentation requires practice and thoughtfulness from the PT or PTA. Being overly concerned with documentation activities can take away from the interaction with the patient, and the PTA should mindfully monitor their behavior to prevent inadequate therapeutic interactions. Another advantage of wireless communication is that it allows the PT/PTA to instantly retrieve the patient's record electronically. The benefits of computerized documentation include the following:

- Submitting information to insurance companies electronically
- Monitoring the clinician's productivity
- Tracking patients' visits
- Easing patient scheduling
- Minimizing documentation paperwork
- Integrating billing
- Maximizing efficiency
- Increasing reimbursement
- Improved communication between healthcare teams

The negative consequences of using electronic records include the following:

- Distractions by documentation while working with the patient
- Concerns about safeguarding the information from malicious entities
- Cost of upgrading hardware and software to maintain an operational system
- Need for a backup system of documentation if the electronic system fails

### KNOWLEDGE CHECK

What information should be included in the documentation to verify professional judgment?
What are the advantages and disadvantages of EMRs?

## Discussion Questions

1. Describe the six reasons documentation is required and discuss how those are related.
2. Locate the Defensible Documentation for Patient/Client Management webpage using the APTA website. Discuss the components of appropriate documentation and the common errors that can lead to payment issues.

3. Watch a classmate complete a functional task, such as picking up an object from the floor or putting on their coat. Write a descriptive paragraph about the activity. Within a group, analyze how effectively the information would fit into the observation section of a SOAP note.

## Learning Opportunities

1. Create a reference sheet for what information goes into each section of the SOAP note.
2. Interview a PTA in clinical practice about the challenges of documentation in today's reimbursement environment.
3. Utilizing the following poorly written SOAP note, rewrite the note using best practice guidelines.

John Doe                        Mar 19, 2019

S. Patient complained of R knee pain 5/10. c/o pain with walking.

O: tx- 4/10. IFC applied to R knee @ 80bps for 15 mins.
Scan 90%, intensity 8mA.
4 electrodes placed encompassing anterior patella.
No change in parameters at 5 min. check.

A: Patient tolerated treatment well.

P: 6/10 tx left. PT will re-evaluate patient at next visit.
Will add home exercise program at next visit.

Jane Doe, SPTA   3/21/19

## Reference

1. American Physical Therapy Association: Guide to Physical Therapist Practice 3.0. Alexandria, VA, American Physical Therapy Association, 2014

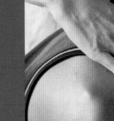

# CHAPTER 11

# Reimbursement and Research

## OBJECTIVES

- Define commonly used terminology in reimbursement.
- Describe Current Procedural Terminology (CPT) codes and the 8-minute rule.
- Describe reimbursement for Medicare, Medicaid, private insurance companies, and health maintenance organizations.
- Compare and contrast the value of the different types of research to provide evidence for clinical physical therapy practice.
- Describe the value of validity and reliability in research.
- Discuss the main elements of a research study.
- Describe how to read a research report.

## KEY TERMS

abuse
capitation
case mix
case studies
Centers for Medicare and Medicaid Services (CMS)
Children's Health Insurance Program (CHIP)
Children's Health Insurance Program Reauthorization Act (CHIPRA)
claims
clinical practice guidelines
coinsurance

consumer-driven healthcare plans
copayment
Current Procedural Terminology (CPT)
deductible
diagnosis-related groups (DRGs)
durable medical equipment (DME)
fee-for-service (FFS)
fraud
gatekeeper
health maintenance organization (HMO)
levels of evidence
Medicaid

Medicare
Medicare Advantage
Medicare Part A—hospital insurance
Medicare Part B—supplementary medical insurance
Medicare Part D—Prescription Drug Coverage
Merit-Based Incentive Payment System (MIPS)
observational studies
preferred provider organization (PPO)
randomized controlled trials
systematic reviews

## Overview

Reimbursement is the payment of funds by a patient or an insurer to a healthcare provider for services rendered. While the need for health care has not changed, healthcare reimbursement has frustrated providers over the past five decades as insurance companies have tried to solve the problem of unaffordable health care for certain groups while also trying to control the costs. Healthcare spending can be a significant portion of a country's gross domestic product (GDP) and is a key factor affecting the overall cost of health care. In the United States, healthcare spending accounts for a significant portion of the federal budget and is a major driver of the national debt. Factors that impact healthcare spending include advancements in medical technology, an aging population, the prevalence of chronic diseases, and the cost of drugs and medical services. To help control the costs, the government and health insurance companies have initiated limitations on what and how they reimburse for healthcare services and supplies. Some of these limitations include the need for more detailed documentation; frequent changes in guidelines, regulations, and policies; and the introduction of patient copayments to cover expenses not covered by the insurance industry.

As future employees, physical therapist (PT) and physical therapist assistant (PTA) students must be familiar with insurance and reimbursement limitations, concepts, and terminology. As reimbursement rates continue to change, there must be a balance between the high cost of health care and sufficient reimbursement for professional services.

Clinicians and scientists undergo research to provide answers to questions, improve patient outcomes, and create knowledge and understanding of physical therapy activities. Research determines the effectiveness or lack of effectiveness of various physical therapy services for patients/clients. PTs/PTAs must become comfortable with the various **levels of evidence** used in research to make accurate determinations about which treatments and methods are the most efficacious.

# Reimbursement

Healthcare reimbursement, which refers to the payment process for patient health services, is complex and constantly changing and encompasses the methods used by insurance companies, government programs, and other payers to determine the amount that will be paid to healthcare providers for the services they deliver. Initially, the United States followed a retrospective reimbursement model in which healthcare providers were paid after the services were rendered by submitting a **claim**. The payer then determined the amount to be paid based on the terms of the payer's contract with the provider and the information included in the claim. In contrast to retrospective reimbursement, health insurance companies shifted to a prospective reimbursement model, where the payer and the provider agree on a predetermined payment

amount before the service is provided. For example, capitation and managed care arrangements often utilize this reimbursement method, where a provider receives a fixed amount per patient per month, regardless of the specific services provided. Some of the more common terms used in reimbursement are described as follows:

- Health insurance refers to various purchased policies that cover an individual for health-related services and supplies. Health insurance companies offer policies paid for by individuals, employers, and the government.
- Health insurance policy. An annual contract between an individual or a group and an insurance company that provides financial protection against medical and healthcare expenses (e.g., inpatient hospital services, outpatient surgery, physical therapy, medical tests, imaging studies, and prescription drugs). It occasionally covers some supplies, such as **durable medical equipment (DME)** (e.g., crutches, walkers, wheelchairs), but in most cases, the patient is responsible for the full payment.
- The patient, or policyholder, purchases a health insurance policy and is considered the first party. The policyholder pays a premium to the insurance company in exchange for coverage, which may include the cost of preventative care, diagnostic services, treatments, and hospitalization (covered services). The PT, as the healthcare professional delivering physical therapy services, is considered the second party. The insurer is the third party and makes the payment for services under the insurance coverage policy.
- Health insurance premium. The monthly fee paid to a health insurance company, or health plan, to provide health coverage. Other health insurance costs can include deductibles (the amount that the policyholder pays before a health insurer reimburses for all or part of the remaining cost of the covered services), **coinsurance** (the policyholder is required to assume responsibility for a percentage of the cost of the covered services), and **copayments** (a fee that the policyholder is required to pay for specific health services at the time of service).
- Employer-sponsored health insurance (group insurance). A type of health insurance coverage provided by an employer to its employees as a benefit of employment. The employer typically pays a portion of the premium, and the employee is responsible for the remaining portion (deductible).

Employer-sponsored health insurance can offer access to a wider network of healthcare providers, lower out-of-pocket costs, and the ability to enroll dependents, such as a spouse or children.

- Deductible. A **deductible** is a predetermined dollar amount a policyholder must pay out of pocket before their health insurance coverage begins. Deductibles serve as a way for insurance companies to share the cost of health expenses with policyholders. In general, the higher the deductible, the lower the monthly premium, and vice versa. For example, if an individual has a $2,500 deductible, they are responsible for paying the first $2,500 of eligible medical expenses, and their insurance covers the remaining costs. After the deductible is met, the policyholder may still be responsible for copayments (also known as a copay, a fixed dollar amount that an insured individual pays out of pocket for a specific medical service or prescription drug, regardless of the actual cost. The copay is in addition to the deductible and is typically paid at the time of service) and coinsurance (a cost-sharing arrangement typically used with a deductible in which the policyholder and the insurance company each pay a certain percentage of the covered medical expenses. For example, if the policyholder has a 20% coinsurance rate and the medical expenses total $1,000, the policyholder would pay $200, and the insurance company would pay $800).

- Open enrollment. A period of time each year during which individuals who are eligible for health insurance can enroll in a new plan, change their existing coverage, or enroll for the first time. During this period, individuals can compare different health insurance plans and choose the one that best fits their needs and budget. Open enrollment periods are usually set by government health insurance programs, such as Medicare and the Affordable Care Act (ACA) marketplace, or private employers offering group health insurance plans.

- The term *capitation* means a reimbursement method that pays the provider a monthly fee based on the number of patients enrolled in the insurance plan. A capitated payment is a form of reimbursement for healthcare services in which a healthcare provider is paid a predetermined (fixed) amount for each patient enrolled in their care. *Capitation* and *capitated payment* are terms used mostly by managed care organizations.

- **Fee-for-service** payment is a payment for specific healthcare services provided to a patient. The

## Box 11-1 A Deductible, Copayment, and Insurance Example

A patient covered under their health insurance policy requiring a $1,500 deductible, $25 copayment, and 80/20 coinsurance sustained an ankle fracture. The patient is now coming for physical therapy, so at the time of each visit and each subsequent visit, the patient must pay a $25 copayment. In addition, for the physical therapy treatment during each session, the patient's health insurance company is responsible for paying 80% of the expenses, and the individual is obligated to pay the remaining 20% until the $1,500 deductible is met. It is important to remember that the detectable applies to all medical expenses incurred during the policy period (except pharmacy expenses) and not just for the physical therapy visits.

payment can be made by the patient or by an insurance carrier. Unlike the capitated payment, a fee-for-service payment means that when a procedure is performed, a fee is charged, and the insurance company pays the fee. PTs were reimbursed for 100% of the billed procedures in the past. The current healthcare market has caused insurance companies to reimburse only a percentage of the total bill. Medicare uses the resource-based relative value scale (RBRVS) to determine the payment for physician services. Each healthcare service is assigned a relative value unit (RVU) based on the resources required to provide the service (the physician's time and effort, the cost of any supplies or equipment used during the service, and the overhead costs associated with providing the service). The RVU is used to calculate the payment amount for the service. This system formed the foundation for the Medicare Fee Schedule.

- Value-based reimbursement is where providers are paid based on the quality and outcomes of the care they deliver rather than the volume of services they provide.

- Managed care means various methods of financing and organizing healthcare delivery in which costs are contained by controlling the provision of benefits and services. Physicians, hospitals, and other healthcare agencies contract with the managed care system to accept a predetermined monthly payment for providing services to patients enrolled in a managed care plan. The enrollee's access to health care is limited to the physicians and other healthcare providers affiliated with the plan. Various administrative incentives and constraints (specific rules and regulations influence clinical decision-making) influence clinic decision making.

- A **health maintenance organization (HMO)** is a prepaid healthcare program of a group practice that provides comprehensive medical care, especially preventative care, whose main goal is to control healthcare expenditures.
- A **preferred provider organization (PPO)** is similar to an HMO; however, it will allow patients to choose out-of-network providers but will not pay 100% of those charges.
- A point-of-service (POS) plan is a type of healthcare insurance plan that allows patients to choose using between in-network and out-of-network healthcare providers for their medical needs. In a POS plan, the patient pays less for using in-network providers and may be required to pay more for using out-of-network providers.

- Copayment is a monetary amount the patient pays to healthcare professionals each time a service is provided. Deductibles are portions of healthcare costs the patient must pay before getting benefits from the insurance company. For example, a deductible of $1,000 means that the patient will pay the first $1,000 of healthcare costs, and the insurance company will then begin assisting with healthcare bills.
- Healthcare professionals dislike the term *denial* because it means an insurer refuses to reimburse for services rendered.
- Eligibility determines whether a patient qualifies for benefits based on enrollment date, preexisting conditions, and valid referrals.
- Prior authorization is a procedure required by some healthcare insurers requiring the patient or healthcare provider to contact them to approve procedures or health care. Examples of activities that require preauthorization are surgical procedures or physical therapy services. In addition, some insurers limit the number of visits that can be provided in a calendar year or per diagnosis.
- National Provider Identification (NPI) is a unique number that identifies individual healthcare providers and healthcare organizations when they perform such activities as billing. There are two categories of healthcare providers for NPI: Type 1 (individual) and Type 2 (organization).
  - Type 1 entities include PTs, physicians, chiropractors, dentists, nurses, and pharmacists.

- Type 2 entities include hospitals, home health agencies, ambulance companies, clinics, group practices, HMOs, laboratories, nursing homes, pharmacies, and DME suppliers.
- ICD-10-CM refers to the International Classification of Diseases, Tenth Revision (ICD-10), devised by the World Health Organization (WHO). WHO's ICD-10 classification system was designed for diagnosis codes only and contained no procedural codes. ICD-10-CM (Clinical Modification) is a U.S. clinical modification of WHO's ICD-10, developed to support U.S. health information needs, and is used to classify and code diseases, symptoms, injuries, and other health conditions for insurance billing and medical recordkeeping. The **Centers for Medicare and Medicaid Services (CMS)** developed a new Procedure Coding System (ICD-10-PCS) for inpatient procedures. Some common ICD-10-CM codes used in physical therapy include:
  - M54.5—low back pain
  - M25.51—pain in joint, shoulder
  - M79.7—myalgia
  - S33.0—sprain of the lumbar spine
  - M54.30—radiculopathy, site unspecified
  - M47.812—spondylosis with myelopathy, cervical region
  - G89.29—chronic pain syndrome, unspecified site
  - M62.83—muscle weakness (generalized)
  - M19.9—arthrosis, unspecified
  - G57.00—sciatica, unspecified side
- The term *CPT* stands for **Current Procedural Terminology**. CPT is a list of descriptive terms that contain five-character numeric codes assigned to nearly every healthcare service. When billing occurs, healthcare providers must choose a CPT code that identifies the services provided. Annually, the American Medical Association, the organization that creates codes, reviews the codes allowing for additions and deletions. CPT codes are broken down into different types. Physical therapy providers utilize the procedural codes found primarily in the 97000 range. Each code identifies a procedure. Some examples of frequently utilized codes include the following:
  - 97110 therapeutic exercise
  - 97112 neuromuscular reeducation
  - 97530 therapeutic activities

These are considered timed codes. When billing for a timed activity, it is important to record the exact number of minutes that the procedure was performed. Billing is done in units, with each unit being 15 minutes. When billing for Medicare, the number of units billed will be based on the 8-minute rule. This rule states that timed code procedures must last at least 8 minutes to bill 1 unit. Thus, any procedure lasting between 8 and 22 minutes is deemed 1 unit. Therefore, a unit equals 15 minutes plus or minus 7 minutes. This rule holds even when multiple units of a single CPT code exist, so that 2 units equals 23–37 minutes, 3 units equals 38–52 minutes, etc. To determine the total number of units allowable, the PTA divides the total treatment time by 15. While the 8-minute rule is specific to Medicare, some insurance companies also follow this rule. The PTA should consult the physical therapy department manager to ensure consistent and accurate billing is performed according to the department's policies.

Other CPT codes are considered untimed. The provider utilizes untimed codes for procedures that do not require constant supervision. Some examples of untimed codes include the following:

- 97012 mechanical traction
- 97014 electrical stimulation (unattended)

These codes are billed as 1 unit and do not fall under the 8-minute rule.

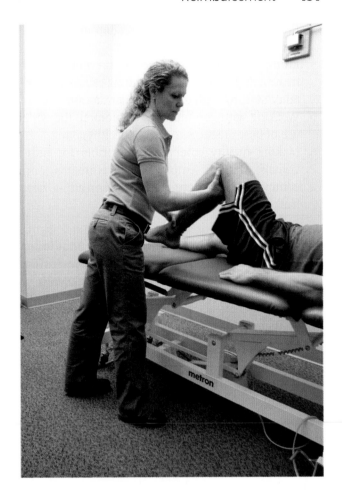

## KNOWLEDGE CHECK

What is the term for money paid by the patient to the healthcare professional each time a service is provided?

What is the difference between eligibility and prior authorization?

What are CPT codes and ICD-10 codes?

## Reimbursement Organizations

Medicare, Medicaid, private health insurance companies, and HMOs can reimburse physical therapy services.

### Medicare

**Medicare** is the largest provider of healthcare services in the United States. The Social Security Amendments, established in 1965 by the U.S. Congress as Title XVIII of the Social Security Act, contained the groundwork for the Medicare program, a federally subsidized health insurance program for people aged 65 years and older, and Medicaid, jointly funded by the state and federal governments to provide healthcare services to people experiencing poverty. Over the years, changes to Medicare have been made regarding program eligibility, coverage, and reimbursement. Currently, Medicare is for the following persons:

- People aged 65 or older. Medicare is an entitlement program for Americans aged 65 and older who have contributed to Medicare through taxes or have met other eligibility requirements to become a beneficiary. The various types of Medicare are described further.
- People younger than 65 years with certain disabilities
- People of all ages with end-stage renal disease (permanent kidney failure requiring dialysis or a kidney transplant)

The CMS administers the Medicare program and, in partnership with the states, the Medicaid program. CMS has developed Quality Strategies to assist the agency in improving patient care, containing healthcare costs, and promoting the overall health of individuals. The Quality Strategies have developed six initiatives to meet their goals:

1. Making care safer by reducing the harm caused in the delivery of care
2. Ensuring that each person and family is engaged as partners in their care

3. Promoting effective communication and coordination of care

4. Promoting the most effective prevention and treatment practices for the leading causes of mortality, starting with cardiovascular disease

5. Working with communities to promote the wide use of best practices to enable healthy living

6. Making quality care more affordable for individuals, families, employers, governments, and communities by developing and spreading new healthcare delivery models

Medicare has four parts: Part A, hospital insurance; Part B, medical insurance; Part C, **Medicare Advantage**; and **Part D, Medicare Prescription Drug Coverage**. Most people do not pay a premium for Part A because they or a spouse already paid it through their payroll taxes while working. However, most people pay a monthly premium for Part B. Part C, Medicare Advantage, is an optional health plan that replaced Medicare + Choice (Medicare Part C, created by the Balanced Budget Act of 1997—see Chapter 2) that includes health plans offered by private companies but approved by Medicare. These plans are required to provide at least the same level of coverage as Original Medicare, but many offer additional benefits, such as dental, vision, and hearing coverage, as well as coordinated care for chronic conditions. Medicare Advantage plans require individuals on Medicare to pay additional monthly premiums and may have other cost-sharing requirements, such as copays, deductibles, and coinsurance. Part D, Medicare Prescription Drug Coverage, is an optional benefit available to individuals enrolled in Medicare Part A (hospital insurance) and/or Medicare Part B (medical insurance). Private insurance companies offer Part D plans and are approved by Medicare. The plan covers a wide range of prescription drugs and offers different levels of coverage and cost-sharing, such as deductibles, copays, and coinsurance. The cost of a Part D plan can vary depending on the specific plan and the drugs an individual takes.

Medicare payments for physical therapy services vary based on where the services are provided.

---

**Medicare Part A (hospital insurance)** helps cover:

- Inpatient care in hospitals, including critical access hospitals and skilled nursing facilities (SNFs; not custodial or long-term care)
- Hospice care and some home health care (beneficiaries must meet certain conditions to get these benefits)

---

**Medicare Part B (medical insurance)** helps cover the following:

- Doctors' services and outpatient care
- Medically necessary services to diagnose or treat a medical condition
- Part A claims for patients whose claim limit has been exhausted or denied due to ineligibility of claims. For example, a patient does not meet the qualifications for a hospital stay but is in the hospital for observation.
- Some other medical services that Part A does not cover, such as some of the services of physical and occupational therapists and some home health care. Part B helps pay for these covered services and supplies when they are medically necessary.

---

- The prospective payment system (PPS) is a fixed payment method established in advance matched to diagnosis classifications known as **diagnosis-related groups (DRGs)** in the acute care setting. The amount is based on various factors, such as the cost of providing the service, the complexity of the service (**case mix**), and the expected outcome. PPS is also utilized in inpatient rehabilitation hospitals, SNFs, long-term care hospitals, home health care, hospice, hospital outpatient departments, and inpatient psychiatric facilities. There are several types of PPS, including per-case payments, per-diem (daily rate) payments, and bundled (a group of related services is bundled into a single payment) payments.

- Within the SNF, Medicare pays for therapy via Part A or B. Each patient entering the SNF receives an assessment known as the minimum dataset, which looks at functional skills, hearing, vision, cognitive skills, and so on. This information determines the skilled care the resident will require from the staff (nursing, physical therapy, occupational therapy, speech-language therapy). Before October 2019, the resource utilization group (RUG) classification was used to determine what amount of reimbursement Medicare Part A would pay for the resident's SNF stay. RUG levels were determined by totaling the amount of nursing care and the number of minutes a patient receives physical therapy, occupational therapy, and speech-language therapy. Examples of levels include ultra, very high, high, medium, and low. Beginning in October 2019, CMS is shifting away from the number of therapy minutes used by the residents and will begin classifying residents by their characteristics. The new payment system,

Patient-Driven Payment Model (PDPM), will look at individual residents in the SNF and score them in each of the five categories:

1. Physical Therapy Case Mix
2. Occupational Therapy Case Mix
3. Speech-Language Pathology Case Mix
4. Nursing Case Mix
5. Non-Ancillary Case Mix (relates to medications and medical supplies)

SNFs are reimbursed for residents on Medicare Part A based upon the resident's case mix components during their qualified stay in the SNF.

- When a patient enters an inpatient rehabilitation facility, a system similar to that in an SNF is used. The patient will be assessed using inpatient rehabilitation facility assessment instruments to classify and identify the predetermined payment amount.

- The Outcome and Assessment Information Set (OASIS) is the assessment tool used for home health care. This tool shows patient improvement over time and is also used to classify patients for payment groups. In a continued revamp of the PPSs, CMS has a newly proposed Home Health Patient-Driven Groupings Model (PDGM) that will most likely be adopted for implementation in 2020. This system will look at patients' case mix factors and place them into one of 432 case mix groups. This system will be similar to the SNF system and will continue to move the payment process from fee-for-service to a quality payment system.

In addition to the predetermined groupings to determine payment, Medicare does allow healthcare providers to identify when services are being provided to patients with multiple health problems and adjusts the amount of payment based on geographic location.

- Medicare Part B outpatient therapy services changed with the passage of the Bipartisan Budget Act of 2018. Therapy services were subject to a cap that would not allow more than $2,010 to be billed for combined physical therapy and speech-language pathology services and $2,010 for occupational therapy services. As of 2018, the former Medicare therapy caps are now annual thresholds that PTs can exceed. This legislation has changed the billing to a soft cap of $2,230 for PT and speech-language pathology services combined and $2,230 for occupational therapy services in 2023. If a patient exceeds this dollar amount, the provider can apply a modifier of KX to the billing code to indicate the medical necessity for continued services, allowing the

---

### Box 11-2 KX Modifier

The KX modifier must be included in claim lines to indicate that services at and above the physical therapy thresholds are medically necessary and that documentation in the patient's medical record justifies the services. Based on their condition, this includes documentation that patients require continued skilled physical therapy (beyond the amount payable under the threshold to achieve their prior functional status or maximum expected functional status within a reasonable amount of time).

Modified from American Physical Therapy Association. Medicare Payment Thresholds for Outpatient Therapy Services. n.d. https://www.apta.org/your-practice/payment/medicare-payment/coding-billing/therapy-cap

---

### Box 11-3 Children's Health Insurance Program Reauthorization Act

CHIPRA is a federal law enacted in 2009 to reauthorize the **Children's Health Insurance Program (CHIP)**. The law provided funding for CHIP and made changes to the program to improve access to health care for low-income children and pregnant women. CHIP provides health coverage to children in families who earn too much to qualify for Medicaid but cannot afford private insurance. The reauthorization of CHIP under CHIPRA helped ensure continued funding for the program and support for children's access to health care.

---

continued provision of services (up to $3,000) before a medical review occurs to confirm the necessity of these services. The Medicare patient with a complicated medical history needing extended services can continue receiving therapy with appropriate documentation.

- Outpatient services for Medicare Part B have seen a shift in payment programs. The **Merit-Based Incentive Payment System (MIPS)** was established by the Medicare Access and the **Children's Health Insurance Program Reauthorization Act (CHIPRA)** of 2015 (MACRA). MACRA was intended to accelerate the transition to a healthcare system that rewards quality and value rather than volume to improve health outcomes. Under MACRA, healthcare providers are paid through one of two pathways that link payments to the quality of care (Quality Payment Program—QPP) provided. Providers began reporting performance data for the QPP in 2017, with payment adjustments beginning in 2019. Services in clinics not associated with SNFs, hospitals, and rehabilitation facilities are subject to the QPP. The QPP is divided into two programs:

- Merit-Based Incentive Payment System. MIPS builds on the traditional fee-for-service architecture in Medicare. A MIPS-eligible clinician is subject to a performance-based payment adjustment through MIPS so that payment rewards providers for delivering high-quality care and achieving better health outcomes. While most Medicare providers began in MIPS when the program started, the law intended for providers to transition into advanced alternative payment models (APMs).

- Advanced APMs. A payment system that gives added incentive payments to provide high-quality and cost-efficient care. APMs can apply to a specific clinical condition, a care episode, or a population. Providers can participate in an eligible advanced APM and be excluded from the MIPS payment adjustments.

Each system aims at moving away from a fee-for-service and toward payment for quality services. Within each system, individual PTs will be required to submit information related to patient outcome measures and other standards of quality services. The submitted data will create a rating for the PT. For example, the data collected in 2019 was utilized to provide incentive payments or penalties in 2021. PTs with high percentage ratings will receive a bonus payment from CMS, those with low percentage ratings will receive penalties, and those with midrange percentages will receive neither incentives nor penalties.

Participation in the program is based on the number of Medicare beneficiaries seen, the amount billed to CMS annually, and the number of services provided annually. While PTAs are not considered MIPS eligible, the services they bill using the PT's NPI will affect their supervising PT's MIPS rating. Thus, the PTA needs to provide quality services as part of the PT/PTA team.

**Medicare Fraud and Abuse.** Medicare and other insurance companies can be targets for fraud and abuse.

- **Fraud** is the intentional deception or misrepresentation of fact that can cause unauthorized benefit or payment, for example, a provider that bills Medicare for services or supplies they did not perform.

- **Abuse** refers to actions that are improper, inappropriate, outside acceptable standards of professional conduct, or medically unnecessary. For example, a provider performs and bills for an unnecessary treatment.

PTs and PTAs must always comply with state and federal laws concerning fraud and abuse.

---

**KNOWLEDGE CHECK**

What benefits are paid for by Medicare Part A and Medicare Part B?

What is the PPS?

What new payment models are implemented in skilled nursing, outpatient, and home health agencies?

---

### Medicaid

**Medicaid** was enacted in 1965 as a jointly funded program in which the federal government matched state spending to provide medical and health-related services. The U.S. Congress originally established Medicaid as Title XIX of the Social Security Act. Medicaid is funded jointly by state and federal governments. Although there are specific federal requirements for Medicaid concerning eligibility, benefits, and provider payments, states have a wide degree of flexibility in designing their programs. Medicaid services are designed for children, nonelderly low-income parents, other caretaker relatives, pregnant women, nonelderly individuals with disabilities, and low-income older adults. CMS requires that states provide the following services:

- Inpatient hospital services
- Outpatient hospital services
- Early and Periodic Screening, Diagnostic, and Treatment (EPSDT) services
- Nursing facility services
- Home health services
- Physician services
- Rural health clinic services
- Federally qualified health center services
- Laboratory and X-ray services
- Family planning services
- Nurse–midwife services
- Certified pediatric and family nurse practitioner services
- Freestanding birth center services (when licensed or otherwise recognized by the state)
- Transportation to medical care
- Tobacco cessation counseling for pregnant women

Other services are considered optional and are determined on a state-by-state basis, including physical therapy services.

Additionally, some states have regulations that do not allow PTAs to provide services to Medicaid patients to contain costs. Other notable state regulations may include a small premium or a copayment for services the Medicaid enrollee must pay.

The ACA requires that states expand the services of Medicaid to provide coverage to nonelderly, nondisabled adults with incomes at or below 138% of the federal poverty level (FPL). The health plans must cover the following benefits: (1) ambulatory patient services; (2) emergency services; (3) hospitalization; (4) maternity and newborn care; (5) mental health and substance use disorder services, including behavioral health treatment; (6) prescription drugs; (7) rehabilitative and habilitative services and devices; (8) laboratory services; (9) preventative and wellness services and chronic disease management; and (10) pediatric services, including oral and vision care. A Supreme Court ruling determined that states can choose or decline Medicaid expansion. States that choose the expansion receive federal government subsidies. As of 2021, 36 states and the District of Columbia have chosen to expand their Medicaid programs, while 14 states have not. States that refuse the expansion retain the right to create various optional benefit services. PTs and PTAs must be aware of the regulations within their state. The Medicaid.gov website and the American Physical Therapy Association (APTA) website offer up-to-date information and webpage links that can provide valuable information about regulations and requirements for providing care to patients with Medicaid coverage.

For up-to-date information about Medicare and Medicaid, its rules, and current application, students should refer to the Medicare website at http://www.cms.gov.

### Private Insurance

Employers primarily fund private health insurance through benefits plans.

**Private Insurance Companies.** Private insurance companies, such as Blue Cross Blue Shield, Humana, and Coventry, provide insurance to individuals and employees through employer-provided plans. Each plan purchased may have various benefits, require copayments, and require authorization for services. The patient and the healthcare provider need to understand the requirements for the physical therapy episode. The APTA has developed the Physical Therapy Model Benefit Plan Design as a resource to help insurance companies understand the purpose and benefits of physical therapy to their policyholders.

**Patient Protection and Affordable Care Act.** In 2010, Congress passed the Patient Protection and Affordable Care Act, commonly called the

---

**Box 11-4 Consolidated Omnibus Budget Reconciliation Act**

COBRA generally requires that group health plans sponsored by employers with 20 or more employees in the prior year allow employees to continue their group coverage after leaving a job or otherwise lose access to their employer-sponsored coverage. Since the mid-1980s, COBRA has provided a realistic way for people to maintain coverage between jobs if they had a preexisting condition and could not qualify for medically underwritten individual health coverage.

---

ACA or Obamacare. The law requires that uninsured Americans gain access to insurance and that CMS and states create Health Insurance Marketplaces, expand Medicaid, and regulate private health insurance plans to improve healthcare access and move to an outcome-based healthcare system. ACA provides consumers with subsidies (premium tax credits) that lower costs for households with incomes between 100% and 400% of the FPL and expands the Medicaid program to cover all adults with income below 138% of the FPL, although not all states have expanded their Medicaid programs. Also, the ACA added a new alternative to the Consolidated Omnibus Budget Reconciliation Act (COBRA) (see **Box 11-4**). Originally, individuals who did not receive insurance through their employer (or a government program) but could afford to pay for it had to purchase insurance that met federal requirements or pay a financial penalty. However, in 2017, opponents of the ACA managed to pass a statute in Congress to eliminate the financial penalty. The ACA requires each state to provide a health insurance marketplace, also called the "Marketplace" or "Exchange," where individuals can browse various healthcare plans available under the ACA.

Before and after its enactment, the ACA faced strong political opposition and legal challenges, but in June 2021, the Supreme Court upheld it for the third time.

**Workers' Compensation.** Workers' compensation is employer-purchased insurance to cover medical costs when an employee is injured while performing their job. This insurance is purchased from the state; employers in almost every state must purchase this for their employees. As with other insurances, various requirements and cost-containment practices must be known to provide cost-effective physical therapy.

## Health Maintenance Organizations

An HMO is a form of managed care. Managed care provides services by a limited number of healthcare professionals for a fixed prepaid fee. A managed care company is a third-party payer that directs patients to providers contracted with the managed care company. Managed care monitors healthcare services to the patient to avoid excessive and inappropriate treatment. The goals of managed care are to ensure favorable patient outcomes and to contain medical expenses. For example, in managed care services, a patient has access first to the primary care physician (PCP). The patient cannot see a specialist before the PCP determines whether the patient needs to see the specialist. The PCP also determines if an outpatient (less costly) intervention is necessary instead of an inpatient (more costly) intervention. Also, patients needing health care must have an office visit first instead of an emergency department visit and use less expensive (older) medications instead of more expensive (newer) medications. As a rule, the managed care system may not pay for the treatments or procedures if they are outside managed care guidelines.

An HMO is a managed care option requiring enrollees to visit only providers within the HMO network. Managed care and HMOs were created to curb the enormous expense of healthcare costs that arose in the 1960s and 1970s. The initial role of HMOs was to decrease healthcare costs by providing preventative health care. Instead of treating individuals as they become ill, HMOs aim to keep individuals healthy by providing preventative medicine. Healthcare providers who are members of an HMO receive a fixed annual fee for each member. In general, HMOs and managed care organizations are under financial pressure to limit the spending on every patient. This demand, in many situations, may cause (from the healthcare providers' perspectives) inequitable healthcare decisions regarding patients' interventions.

HMOs can be divided into four groups:

- Staff HMOs, in which the healthcare providers are employees of the HMO, providing care only for HMO members
- A separate group of physicians provides group HMOs, (not employees of the HMO) having contracts with the HMO to treat only members of the HMO
- Individual practice associations (IPAs), in which there are contracts between the HMO and the individual physicians stipulating that the physicians can use their own offices to treat HMO and non-HMO patients

- Network HMOs that are like IPA HMOs, except that instead of contracts with individual physicians, the HMO has contracts with several large physician groups who treat HMO as well as non-HMO patients

There are also different HMO plans: the prepaid group plan, PPO, and IPA. Typically, employers contract with managed care or HMO services to benefit their employees. Employees may have to pay a small fee for each visit as a copayment.

The PCP is the **gatekeeper** who authorizes other medical services, such as diagnostic testing or rehabilitation services. In managed care, the gatekeeper or the PCP refers the patient to the provider designated as the one who directs an individual patient's care. In practical terms, the gatekeeper or the PCP is the one who refers patients to specialists or subspecialists for care.

PTs must obtain a provider number to treat patients within a specific HMO. Also, HMOs require authorization for physical therapy services even if the PCP made the referral. The HMO may deny physical therapy payment for services even though authorization for physical therapy was granted. PTAs may not be authorized to treat HMO patients in outpatient or home care settings.

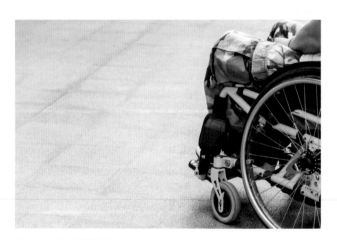

© panumas nikhomkhai/Shutterstock

## Tricare and the Veterans Health Administration System

Tricare is a health program for members of the armed services and their families. It acts as an insurance company providing services to these eligible candidates only. Just as with private insurance, benefits, copayments, and authorization for services will vary with the member's plan. As of 2020, Tricare permits PTAs to provide physical therapy when supervised by a licensed registered PT.

The Veterans Health Administration is the healthcare system for active and retired military personnel who qualify. Services available at inpatient hospitals and outpatient clinics include preventative care and diagnostic and treatment services.

### Consumer-Driven Healthcare Plans

**Consumer-driven healthcare plans**, designed to encourage patients to become more involved in their health care, are a type of healthcare insurance plan that places more responsibility on the patient to manage their healthcare expenses. These plans typically have lower monthly premiums but higher deductibles and out-of-pocket costs. Patients are responsible for paying for much of their medical expenses, including routine healthcare services and diagnostic tests. The people most likely to benefit from these plans are the young and healthy, as the plans can be more expensive for patients who need a lot of medical care or those who experience unexpected health problems.

## Reimbursement in Physical Therapy

The switch from a retrospective to a PPS reimbursement system significantly impacted the reimbursement and delivery of physical therapy. The advent of managed care entities had a similar effect. More recently, the Balanced Budget Act of 1997, a federal law in the United States that aimed to balance the federal budget by limiting spending and increasing revenues through its changes to Medicare and Medicaid programs, has brought its challenges (see Chapter 2).

The reimbursement amount for physical therapy services varies depending on the patient's insurance coverage, the type of therapy provided, and the location of the therapy services. From a PT's perspective, changes in the mechanisms to obtain reimbursement frequently occur in bill coding (CPT, modifiers, etc.), the collection of copays, visit limits, and documentation.

Perhaps the most contentious issue is the introduction of copays, designed to help discourage the overutilization of healthcare services and to help control costs. Some insurance plans require a copay for each visit, while others require a copay only after a certain number of visits or when a certain dollar amount has been reached. For example, it is not unusual for a patient to pay $50 per physical therapy visit, which exceeds the reimbursement paid by the plan to the care provider. Also, many individuals have

had to make difficult financial decisions about decreasing the frequency of their physical therapy visits and spending the money on other living costs.

Despite the advent of direct access, which allows for evaluation and some forms of treatment without a physician referral in all 50 states and DC, full autonomy for physical therapy has yet to be attained as many insurance companies continue to place restrictions on reimbursement with time or visit limits. To counteract these restrictions, some PT practices have initiated first-party payment policies, where the patient pays the provider directly for covered services instead of the patient seeking reimbursement from their insurance company. Given the increasing popularity of consumer-driven healthcare plans, more and more patients are deciding to pay for what they deem valuable.

The ever-increasing difficulties with reimbursement reinforce the importance of evidence-based methods to clinicians and for them to provide a high-quality experience for their patients.

---

**KNOWLEDGE CHECK**

Who is eligible for Medicaid services?
What is the difference between private insurance and HMOs?
Explain the differences between retrospective and prospective reimbursement.

---

## Basic Research Elements

Research is critical to understanding the what, how, and why in physical therapy intervention and management. Physical therapy research provides evidence that can guide clinical practice. Sometimes, the results of the research may support current clinical practice. Other times, research results may point to areas of clinical practice that need to be modified. Reading research articles, analyzing research outcomes, and discussing relevance to physical therapy practice are important tasks for practicing PTs and PTAs.

The body of knowledge rationale for physical therapy research concerns characteristics of the physical therapy profession, such as identity and performance. Because physical therapy, as with other applied medical professions, encompasses a combination of arts and sciences in its body of knowledge, its identity and performance can be discovered and enhanced only through research. Research can demonstrate the efficacy of physical therapy in health care by augmenting

## Box 11-5 Research Types

There are several types of research, each with its unique methods, design, and purpose. Some of the most common types of research include:

- Quantitative Research: This type involves collecting and analyzing numerical data through surveys, experiments, or observational studies. The goal of quantitative research is to test hypotheses and establish cause-and-effect relationships between variables.
- Qualitative Research: This type focuses on the subjective experiences and perspectives of individuals and seeks to understand the meaning and context of their experiences. Qualitative research methods include in-depth interviews, focus groups, and observation.
- Experimental Research: This type involves manipulating one or more independent variables to observe the effects on a dependent variable. Experimental research is often used to establish cause-and-effect relationships.
- Correlational Research: This type examines the relationship between two or more variables without manipulating any variables. Correlational research can be used to identify patterns and associations between variables but cannot establish cause-and-effect relationships.
- Survey Research: This type involves collecting data through self-administered questionnaires or interviews. Survey research is often used to gather information about the attitudes, opinions, or behaviors of a large sample of individuals.
- Longitudinal Research: This type involves collecting data from the same individuals over an extended period. Longitudinal research is often used to study changes in variables over time and to identify trends or patterns of change.
- Case Study Research: This type involves an in-depth examination of a single individual, group, or organization. Case study research is often used to gain a deeper understanding of a specific phenomenon or to provide insight into a unique or complex issue.

## Box 11-6 Research Concepts

Several fundamental concepts in research are important to understand when designing and conducting research studies. Some of the most important research concepts include the following:

- Research Question: A clear and well-defined research question is the foundation of any successful research study. The research question should be specific and focused and should guide the entire research process.
- Hypothesis: A hypothesis is a tentative explanation or prediction about the relationship between variables. Hypotheses are often used in experimental research to guide the design and interpretation of results.
- Variable: A variable is any factor that can change or be manipulated in a research study. There are several types of variables, including independent variables, dependent variables, and confounding variables.
- Sampling: Sampling refers to selecting a subset of individuals from a larger population to conduct a study. The choice of sampling method will depend on the research question, the resources available, and the study's goals.
- Validity: Validity refers to the accuracy and reliability of the results of a study. There are several types of validity, including construct validity, internal validity, and external validity.
- Reliability: Reliability refers to the consistency and stability of the results of a study. Reliability is important to ensure that the results of a study can be replicated and that the findings are not influenced by random error.
- Bias: Bias refers to systematic errors in a study's design, conduct, or interpretation that can influence the results. Bias can occur at several stages of the research process, including sampling, data collection, and data analysis.
- Confound: A confound is a variable associated with a study's independent and dependent variables and can influence the results. Confounds can make determining the true relationship between variables difficult and lead to incorrect conclusions.
- Power: Power refers to the ability of a study to detect a difference or effect if it exists. Power is important to ensure a study has enough statistical power to detect a meaningful difference or effect.

## The Significance of Physical Therapy Research

Healthcare students are often asked to review research as a learning task. The task may be to teach them about research or immerse them in professional practice

established interventions and perhaps discovering new ones. However, the most important reason for research in physical therapy, as well as in health care in general, is improving patient care. Through clinical research, PTs and PTAs (under the supervision of PTs) can apply the obtained information to their patients. Therefore, PTAs, as members of the physical therapy clinical team, need at least a basic knowledge of research elements to understand and evaluate the physical therapy research literature.

topics. However, as healthcare professionals, PTs and PTAs may choose to do a specific reading because of a specific need. Quality improvement (QI) may be one of these motivations. QI is a practice that measures a specific practice quality, implements practice changes, and monitors outcomes to determine the effect. When considering QI issues, PTs and PTAs may need to review current research to determine appropriate change strategies that show merit for improving the process.

An example of a QI issue may be monitoring how many days the average patient with a total knee arthroplasty remains in acute care and what factors accelerate or slow a patient's discharge. Researching the factors others have monitored may assist the QI inquiry in accurately accounting for all important factors related to the problem. A second type of research is when PTs and PTAs have a specific question about their practice. For example, they are interested in understanding if isometric quadriceps exercises are appropriate for strengthening during a patient's acute phase with a meniscus repair. This type of research is used to inform evidence-based practice.

During this inquiry, the PT or PTA has a specific question and looks for the best evidence. After determining the findings to be both supportive and of good quality, they will implement a practice change. Evidence-based practice is a common theme throughout health care because it confirms the effectiveness and dissuades a trial-and-error intervention method. The last type of research activity may be to stay informed. The practice of health care is constantly changing. Physical therapy researchers publish their research to inform and promote further questioning of current and future practice ideas. To stay current and relevant in practice, it is important to understand what is found in professional journals. This, in turn, may lead the practicing PT or PTA to begin a research project.

## Search Strategies

Those inexperienced in searching for information in research archives are often overwhelmed by the terminology, the number of databases available, and the sheer volume of articles that can come up in a query. A basic understanding of search strategies can help to improve the process, making it less daunting and time-consuming.

The first step is to be clear about how the learner intends to use the information [1]. For students, the professor has often laid out the purpose of the assignment with specific objectives and requirements to assist in answering this question. Understanding the question is being answered is a critical step because it assists the student in their choice of database and their choice of words or phrases to search.

The second step is to create a basis of understanding of the topic so that the learner can understand the terminology and have a foundation of information [1]. This activity may be best completed by looking at textbooks and trusted websites. Learners should be cautious about typing their topic into a search engine to locate credible information. An internet search engine will pick all sites with the search words; the reader must then discern which are credible and which should be avoided. Trusted websites are often associated with hospitals (.com or .org), educational institutions (.edu), or the government (.gov). However, one should not overlook organizational sites with credible research-based information, such as the American Heart Association or The Michael J. Fox Foundation for Parkinson's Research. Once the learner understands the topic, they can use the relevant terminology to perform database searches.

Common databases that are used in healthcare searches include:

- Cochrane Library: A collection of databases that contain independent evidence on which to base clinical treatment decisions
- Cumulative Index to Nursing and Allied Health (CINAHL) Plus: A database of current nursing and allied health journals
- EBSCOhost: A database of journals, magazines, and newspaper articles on almost any topic
- Gale Virtual Reference Library: Used to locate online reference books for basic information on a topic
- Health Reference Center Academic: Has up-to-date information on a wide range of healthcare topics, including periodicals, reference books, pamphlets, and videos
- Health Source, Nursing, and Allied Health Collection: Provides nearly 600 scholarly full-text journals, including nearly 450 peer-reviewed journals
- MedlinePlus: Produced by the National Library of Medicine and gives accurate and up-to-date information about diseases and conditions
- ProQuest: Includes journal, magazine, and newspaper articles on a topic
- PubMed: Another National Library of Medicine resource that provides access from the mid-1960s to the present
- Rehabilitation & Sports Medicine Source: An index of over 200 sports medicine and rehabilitation journals
- Rehabilitation Reference Center: An EBSCOhost product that provides evidence-based clinical references

Choosing the correct database to search can prevent the learner from experiencing undue frustration and spending a great deal of time with few useful results [1]. Healthcare databases house thousands of research topics, and an ineffective search using the wrong words or database can lead to an overwhelming number of hits or no hits. Students should use the library resources and the librarian at their institution to make this process more effective.

After choosing the database, the learner should utilize several strategies to gain the best search information [1]. Using keywords or phrases from the background learning should guide the search word choices. The PICO format (Patient + Intervention + Comparison + Outcome) can help identify the keywords to search.

Additionally, the search can be improved by placing quotation marks ("") around the phrase or using the word AND or OR to improve the results. Some databases offer an advanced search tab that guides the learner through the search keyword process. The advanced search also allows you to search for the keywords in specific article areas, such as in the title or abstract. The learner should know synonyms often end in different results, and using the same keywords in different databases may yield more results.

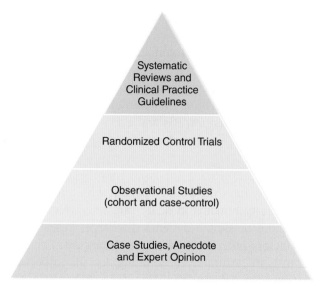

**Figure 11-1** Levels of evidence.

## KNOWLEDGE CHECK

What are the three reasons for reading research?
What are the steps to a successful search strategy?

## Evaluating the Evidence

Within research, there are a variety of different types of studies. Each study has its purpose and can be evaluated for its levels of evidence. The term *level of evidence* refers to the degree of confidence the reader can place in the research, which is based on the study design. It is helpful to consider the levels as a pyramid (**Figure 11-1**) [2]. Each level is useful in finding the best evidence to answer the research question. For example, lower levels of evidence research should not be dismissed as irrelevant.

**Systematic reviews** are created by systematically searching for, evaluating, and summarizing all the medical research about a particular topic. The research is ranked and can be combined with other studies to produce more statistically significant findings using meta-analysis. The value of a systematic review is that it can give useful information

and may provide reliability. Reliability in research refers to the ability of the research activity to show the same results when repeated by another researcher [2].

**Clinical practice guidelines** (CPGs) are systematically designed recommendations based on a review of clinical research to assist the healthcare provider in making patient care decisions.

**Randomized controlled trials** are created when test subjects are randomly placed into experimental and control groups. The experimental group receives the treatment variable, while the control group is the group that does not receive the treatment variable. The control group allows the researcher to have a baseline to compare with the experimental group's result. Variables are certain characteristics that take different forms in a randomized controlled study. Examples of variables include physical therapy treatments, such as electrical stimulation, gait training, or ultrasound. Other variables can be patients' signs and symptoms, such as pain, tingling, weakness, strength, or range of motion. The term *independent variable* applies mostly to experimental research in which the researcher manipulates or observes the variable so that its value can be related to the dependent variable. Although the researcher often manipulates the independent variable, it can also be a classification where subjects are assigned to groups. In a study where one variable causes the other, the independent variable is the cause. In a study in which groups are being compared, the independent variable is the group classification. In a research study, the independent variable defines a principal focus of research interest, and the dependent variable is the research outcome. In an experiment, the dependent variable may be what was caused or what changed due to the study. In comparing groups, the dependent variable is what the groups differ on.

**Observational studies** include cohort studies and case-control studies. Cohort studies identify two groups of patients—one that received an intervention and one that did not—and watch them for the anticipated outcome over a period. Similarly, the case-control study uses patients with and without a particular outcome and looks for a similar intervention variable.

**Case studies** are investigations of a single individual or group for which the researcher provides an in-depth description of their disorder, interventions, and outcomes. Anecdotes and expert opinions are also placed into this level of evidence, as they can be useful clinically but do not have unbiased research to support their claims.

### KNOWLEDGE CHECK

What are the levels of evidence?
Why is it important to assess the levels of evidence?

## Reading a Research Article

When reading and evaluating a research article, the PTA can consider the following questions:

- What problems are the researchers solving? Why are these problems important?
- What did they do (as opposed to what the researchers said or implied they did)?
- What methods are they using?
- What is the contribution of their work (such as what is interesting or new in their work)?
- Would you, as a researcher, solve the problem differently?
- What were the results? Did the researchers do what they set out to do?
- Are the results reliable and valid?
- Do all the pieces of the researchers' work fit together logically (**Figure 11-2**)?

Elements of a research study:
- Title and abstract
- Introduction
- Methods
- Results
- Discussion and conclusion

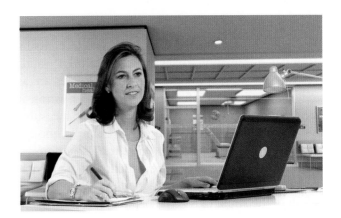

**Figure 11-2** Evidence-based practice requires PTs and PTAs to read the research critically.
© Monkey Business Images/Shutterstock

### Title and Abstract

The title of a research article should be informative so that the reader can learn enough about the research content. After reading the title, if the reader is interested in the topic, they read the abstract. Abstracts of research articles must contain specific information about the presented work's purpose, method, results, and major conclusions. The information reported in the abstract must be consistent with the information reported in the research article.

### Introduction

The introduction aims to acquaint the reader with the work's rationale and defend it. The introduction places the work in a theoretical context, enabling the reader to understand and appreciate the objectives. The introduction should allow the reader to distinguish between previous and current research. From the introduction, the reader can find out the type of study, hypothesis, specific purposes, pertinent research literature, and if the references are appropriate and comprehensive.

The following questions are the central points for evaluating the introduction section of a research article:

- Is the problem important? Has the problem been clearly stated?
- Did the researcher provide a theoretical context for the research study?
- Did the researcher utilize the research literature for the framework of their study?
- Did the researcher utilize the references appropriately and comprehensively?
- Is the type of study design clear (such as experimental or nonexperimental)?
- Are the purposes of the study and the hypothesis (or guiding questions) stated clearly?

## Methods

The methods section of a research article contains essential information to evaluate the study's validity. Validity means how meaningful test scores are as they are used for specific purposes. In other words, it means the degree to which an instrument measures what it is intended to measure. For example, the validity of the "special" stretch that the PTA performed on the patient to increase the patient's elbow flexion range of motion can be questioned regarding the position of the stretch, the type of stretch, and the PTA's experiences performing the stretch. In this example, the special stretch is the independent variable that may or may not cause a change in the dependent variable, the patient's elbow flexion range of motion. The experiment can be evaluated by looking at internal validity or external validity. Internal validity is the degree to which the observed differences in the dependent variable are the direct result of manipulating the independent variable, not some other variable. In the example, to establish internal validity for this study, it would have to be proven that the special stretch, not other variables, caused improvements in the patient's elbow flexion range of motion. To achieve internal validity, the relationship between the independent and dependent variables must be free from the effects of extraneous factors. External validity is the degree to which the results are generalizable to individuals (the general population) outside the experimental study. Achieving external validity is almost impossible because it depends on the experiment's interaction with the specific type of subjects tested, the specific setting in which the experiment was carried out, or the time in history when the study was performed.

The methods section includes information about the subjects, the study design (if experimental or nonexperimental), the instrumentation or the equipment used in the study, the research procedures reporting data collection, operational definitions, issues of validity, and the data analysis describing how the data was analyzed. The reader of the methods section can find out who the subjects were, what inclusion or exclusion criteria were used for these subjects, and how the subjects were selected. The type of research design specified in the methods section can tell the reader about control groups, the number of independent or dependent variables, and/or how often the treatments or measurements were applied. The instrumentation subsection of the methods section documents the reliability and validity of the instruments used in the study, and the data analysis subsection discusses statistical analysis or other appropriate procedures to analyze the data. The methods section gives the reader a clear picture of what was done in the study at each step.

The following questions are the central points for evaluating the methods section of a research article:

- How were the subjects selected, and how many subjects were researched?
- Was the design of the research study identified, and is it appropriate for the study?
- Was randomization used when the subjects were included in groups?
- Was a control group used?
- How many independent variables were used?
- How often were physical therapy treatments and measurements applied?
- Was the instrumentation described in enough detail?
- Were the reliability and validity of the instruments documented?
- Were data collection procedures described clearly and in enough detail to be replicated?
- Were operational definitions for all independent and dependent variables provided?
- Were statistical analyses appropriate? Did the researcher explain the reason for using the stated statistical analyses?
- Did the researcher address each research question in the data analysis?
- What was the alpha level?

The alpha level is the probability of concluding that the null hypothesis is false (when true). The researcher sets the alpha level before data analysis, which usually contrasts with the probability level generated by the data analysis. The statistical result using the acceptable alpha level (0.05) can allow rejection of the null hypothesis and acceptance of the research hypothesis. The alpha level as a probability can typically be between 0.05 and 0.01. The lower the alpha level, the better the experiment. Let us suppose the statistical alpha level is equal to or lower than the alpha level set by the researcher before data analysis. In that case, the results show that the expected difference is due to chance. The statistical results of an experiment due to chance typically indicate true differences in the measured dependent variable. For example, an alpha level of 0.05 means that the statistical results of the experiment can happen 5 times out of every 100.

## Results

The purpose of the results section of a research article is to present and illustrate the research findings. These findings should be presented objectively without interpretation or commentary. In this section, the reader can evaluate the study's major finding if the results were presented clearly, the tables and figures were presented accurately, the hypothesis was addressed, and the results were statistically significant.

The following questions are the central points for the evaluation of the results section of a research article:

- Did the researcher present the results clearly?
- Did the researcher present the figures and tables accurately?
- Are the results statistically significant?

### Discussion and Conclusion

The discussion and conclusion section of the research article provides an interpretation of the study's results and supports the conclusions using evidence from the experiment and generally accepted knowledge. The reader should be able to agree with the conclusions drawn from the data, examine if the conclusions were overgeneralized, and look for factors that could have influenced or accounted for the results.

The following questions are the central points for evaluating the discussion and conclusion section of a research article:

- How did the researcher interpret the results?
- Did the researcher clarify if the hypotheses were rejected or accepted?
- Did the researcher consider alternative explanations for the obtained findings?
- Are the discussions of the results supported by the research literature?
- Does the researcher provide the limitations of the study?
- Are the results of the study clinically important?
- Does the researcher mention how the results apply to clinical practice?
- Does the researcher provide suggestions for further study?
- Do the research conclusions flow logically from the obtained results?

Finally, at the end of the evaluation of the research article, the reader can reflect on the study by concentrating on particular questions and deciding whether the researcher's answers were true, appropriate, and justified. The reader can use the same approach to evaluate oral and poster presentations.

## KNOWLEDGE CHECK

What is found in each part of a research article?
What is validity?
What is reliability?

## Suggestions for How to Read a Research Paper

Some readers prefer to read a research paper sequentially from the beginning to the end; however, some readers prefer a different sequence, such as the following [3]:

- Read the title. What is the paper about?
- Read the abstract. It should give you a concise overview of the paper.
- Read the introduction. Look for motivations, relation to other work, and a more detailed overview.
- Read the structure of the paper. What do the remaining sections address? How do they fit together?
- Read the previous/related work section. How does this work relate? What is new or different about this work?
- Read the conclusions. What were the results?
- Read the body of the paper. Some people may want to skip the statistical analyses the first time through.

The references will only be important for the reader if the topic is important. The references can point the reader to related research and research upon which the current study builds.

## How to Write a Research Report

After reading a research article, a student may want to write a report about the published research literature. The written research report should have two main components:

- A concise summary of the research article, providing an overview of what the researcher did (and why), what methods the researcher used, and what the results were
- A brief critique of the research article, giving a technical (physical therapy) evaluation of the work, explaining what things were unclear or not addressed, and describing the merits of the work

The following are guidelines for writing a research report:

- The research article should be read critically and not superficially.
- The PTA student should use their understanding of the research article to write a cohesive summary, not a play-by-play account of the article.
- The PTA student should be concise but include some technical physical therapy details.
- The PTA student should understand the key points of the research article.
- The PTA student should not copy choice phrases from the research article.

## Discussion Questions

1. Utilizing the internet, discuss the issues surrounding the capitation of physical therapy services at $1,940 per year for Medicare patients.
2. Describe the differences between Medicare and Medicaid.
3. Identify what the following acronyms stand for and their relationship to reimbursement.
   a. CMS
   b. DRG
   c. PPS
   d. ACA
   e. CPT
   f. ICD-10-CM
   g. HMO
   h. SNF
   i. PDPM

## Learning Opportunities

1. Research the tenets of the ACA and describe how it affects physical therapy.
2. A PTA is working with a PT to develop an evidence-based assessment tool for new patients with total knee arthroplasty. Develop a plan for obtaining research that would help you with this task.
3. A PT is presenting an in-service for the physical therapy department where they are interning. They utilize case studies for evidence. Describe the value of levels of research that may assist them with their presentation.

## References

1. Domholdt E: Physical Therapy Research: Principles and Applications. Philadelphia, PA, W.B. Saunders, 2000
2. Dang D, Dearholt S: Johns Hopkins Nursing Evidence-Based Practice: Model and Guidelines, 3rd ed. Indianapolis, IN, Sigma Theta Tau International, 2018
3. Greenhalgh T: How to Read a Paper: The Basics of Evidence-based Medicine. West Sussex, Wiley Blackwell BMJ Books, 2019

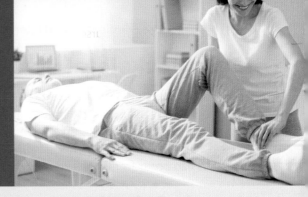

# CHAPTER 12

# Examination and Intervention of the Body Systems

## OBJECTIVES

- Describe specialized examinations for musculoskeletal, neurologic, cardiopulmonary, and integumentary systems.
- Describe the different components that one can use in a musculoskeletal intervention.
- Describe the various neurophysiologic approaches to improve motor control and motor learning.
- Name interventions used in cardiovascular and pulmonary physical therapy.
- Describe the various components that one can use as part of an integumentary intervention.

## KEY TERMS

| | | |
|---|---|---|
| congestive heart failure (CHF) | flaccidity | orthosis |
| dyspnea | flexibility exercises | proprioception |
| dystonia | hydrotherapy | prosthesis |
| edema | hypertonia | rigidity |
| evaluation | hypotonia | spasticity |
| examination | kinesthesia | therapeutic exercises |

## Overview

As described in Chapter 5, physical therapy examinations and interventions involve assessing and treating individuals with conditions that negatively affect the various body systems. The key aspects of physical therapy **examination** include a thorough examination to assess the patient's movement, strength, range of motion (ROM), balance, coordination, and functional abilities, which may also include findings from diagnostic tests, such as X-rays, magnetic resonance imaging (MRI), and ultrasound. Based on the examination findings, physical therapists (PTs) make a diagnosis and develop a plan of care (POC) tailored to the patient's specific needs and goals. Physical therapists establish the correct diagnosis and then use various interventions to help patients regain their functional abilities, improve their overall quality of life, and promote overall wellness.

# Musculoskeletal System

The musculoskeletal system includes bones, fascia, muscles with their related tendons and synovial sheaths, bursa, and joint structures, such as cartilage, menisci, capsules, and ligaments. Damage to these structures can occur from direct trauma or overuse.

## Musculoskeletal System Examination

The musculoskeletal system examination begins with the patient's/client's history and includes relevant questions about the patient's musculoskeletal condition.

A variety of tests and measures are used to assess the musculoskeletal system. The type and number of the tests and measures used are modified based on the history and the systems review, but may include the following [1]:

- Observation of the patient. Observational information is the foundation of the early clinical impression as the clinical search for patient consistency

and reliability begins. The observation begins when the patient enters the clinic, from when the clinician greets them to when they take them to the treatment room. This early observation can provide information including, but not limited to, how the patient protects the involved body part, whether the patient has an abnormal gait, and the level of discomfort the patient experiences. Other information includes [2]:

- Does the patient prefer to stand, sit, or move?
- How does the patient change positions to greet the clinician, easily or guardedly?
- Does the patient require assistance in ambulation, transferring, or changing clothing?
- Does the patient look directly into the clinician's eyes or look away? Is there nervousness or fear present?
- Is there an exaggerated pain response demonstrated by facial expressions and/or complaints?
- With an adult, is the spouse, or significant other, in attendance, and does their presence seem appropriate?

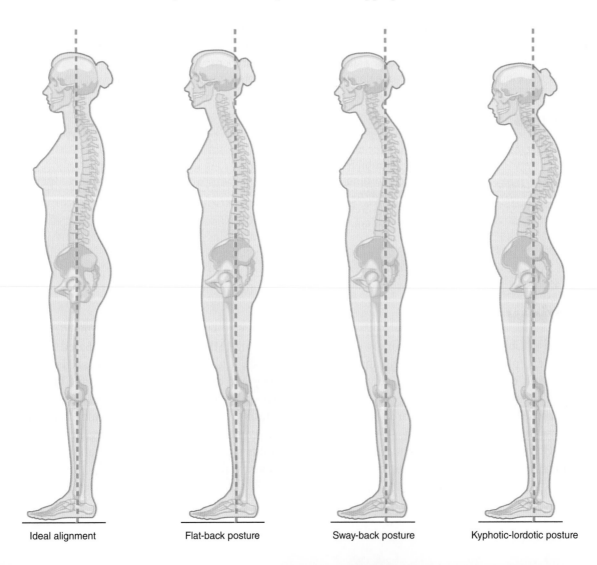

Ideal alignment                Flat-back posture                Sway-back posture                Kyphotic-lordotic posture

- With a child, is there any unexplained or excessive bruising, and does the parent or guardian appear to be answering for the child? These findings might indicate an abuse occurring at home.
- Do the observation findings match the patient history findings?

- Postural analysis. *Good posture* is a subjective term to describe what is correct based on ideal models. A posture must produce physical functional limitations or impairments to be classified as abnormal or dysfunctional. Many postures occur throughout the day in a multisegmented organism, such as the human body, and whether maintained statically or executed repetitively, abnormal alignment may result from alterations in muscle force transmission or joint load distribution. The postural examination evaluates the position maintained by the body when standing and sitting relative to space and other body parts. The clinician must assess the patient from all angles: the front, the back, and the sides.
- Palpation. There is disagreement about when the palpation assessment should occur in the examination, in the beginning, throughout, or at the end. The purposes of a palpation examination are to check for any vasomotor changes in the skin (temperature, moisture), localize specific sites of tenderness and/or swelling, identify specific anatomic structures and their relationship to one another, identify soft-tissue texture changes or myofascial restrictions, locate changes in muscle tone, checking pulses, and locate any deformity suggestive of a fracture, severe muscle or tendon lesion.
- Range of motion. ROM examination evaluates the available motion at a joint or a series of joints. A normal joint has an available range of active or physiologic motion, which is limited by a physiologic barrier as tension develops within the surrounding tissues. At the physiologic barrier, there is an additional passive ROM (PROM). Active ROM (AROM) refers to the extent to which contractions of a joint's muscles can move it actively without assistance or resistance from external forces. AROM testing gives the clinician information about the quantity of available physiologic motion, muscle substitutions, the willingness of the patient to move, the integrity of the contractile and the inert tissues, the quality of motion, symptom reproduction, and the motion restriction pattern. PROM refers to the extent to which a joint can be moved passively, with no effort from the muscles, and is performed by an external force, such as a therapist or a device, to move the joint to its fullest extent without resistance. ROM is measured in degrees of a circle using a goniometer (see **Figure 12-1**). It is not within the scope of this text to cover every aspect of goniometry, but typically, a joint compared with the uninvolved joint with less motion than is considered functional is hypomobile, and a joint with more motion than is considered functional is hypermobile.
- Flexibility. Flexibility depends on neuromuscular control and connective tissue extensibility. There are two primary types of flexibility: static and dynamic
  - Static. The available ROM to a joint or series of joints. Tests such as the straight leg raise,

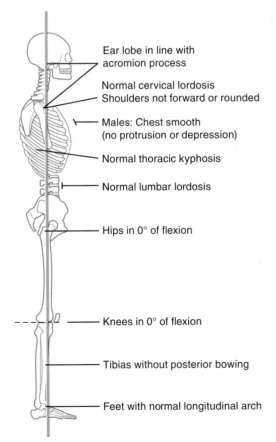

Ear lobe in line with acromion process

Normal cervical lordosis
Shoulders not forward or rounded

Males: Chest smooth (no protrusion or depression)

Normal thoracic kyphosis

Normal lumbar lordosis

Hips in 0° of flexion

Knees in 0° of flexion

Tibias without posterior bowing

Feet with normal longitudinal arch

**Ideal line of gravity**

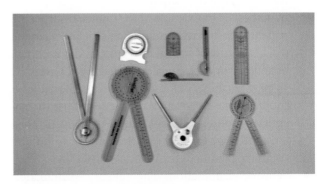

**Figure 12-1** Various goniometers.

the toe touch, and the sit and reach, which are valid and reliable, are used to measure static flexibility.

- Dynamic. The ability to perform moving stretches that use momentum to increase ROM. The measurement of dynamic flexibility involves active tests, such as the lunge, the squat, and leg/arm swings.

Decreased flexibility is usually the result of muscle imbalances because of various factors, including but not limited to aging, inactivity, injury, adaptive shortening of structures, and certain medical conditions. The hamstrings and the hip flexors are the most common muscle groups prone to decreased flexibility. Clinicians use stretching techniques to improve both contractile and non-contractile tissue extensibility when there is limited range of motion (ROM) due to scar tissue formation, adhesions, or contractures, resulting in a loss of tissue extensibility.

- Strength. Strength testing assesses the nerve supply to the muscle and measures the ability of a musculotendinous unit to act across a bone-joint lever arm system to generate or passively resist movement against gravity and variable resistance. Manual muscle testing (MMT) (see **Figure 12-2**) is used to evaluate the relative strength of specific muscles and identify muscle weakness patterns. Rating categories and values for the MMT include Normal (5), Good (4), Fair (3), Poor (2), Trace activity (1), and Absent activity (0).

- Joint integrity and mobility. The integrity of the joint surfaces is one of several anatomic factors that may limit a joint's ability to move through a full, unrestricted ROM. Joint play refers to the available motions (glide, spin, and roll) at the joint surfaces. The PT can assess the amount of joint play and use joint mobilization techniques to preserve or increase joint play.

- Special tests. Numerous special tests have been designed for each body area depending on the structure being tested to help rule in/rule out a diagnostic hypothesis. For example, if the clinician suspects a patient has suffered an anterior cruciate ligament (ACL) rupture, a special test, such as the Lachman or anterior drawer, can aid the diagnosis. Given the suspect reliability of most special tests, the clinician should avoid overreliance on them and use the patient's response to all provocative maneuvers (clustering results) to produce a framework to build a complete picture of the clinical entity [3].

- Sensory examination. The sensory examination in physical therapy includes tests for superficial,

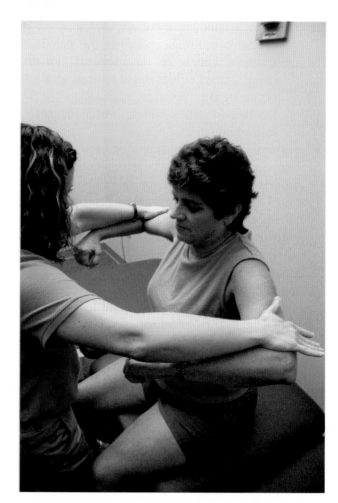

**Figure 12-2** Manual muscle testing.
© wavebreakmedia/Shutterstock

deep, and combined sensations. First, the superficial responses need to be assessed. Then, if there are impairments of the superficial responses, it is necessary to assess the deep and combined sensations. Superficial sensations include pain, temperature, light touch, and pressure. Deep sensations include **kinesthesia**, **proprioception**, and vibration. Combined sensations include tactile localization, two-point discrimination, barognosis, stereognosis, graphesthesia, and texture recognition. Other neurologic tests may include testing for spinal nerve integrity.

- A dermatome is a specific skin area supplied by a single spinal nerve. It is important to remember that there is no current, diagnostically accurate dermatome illustration—medical and allied health textbooks commonly contain multiple, conflicting dermatome maps, most of which rely on research from the 1940s [4].

- Key muscles are specific muscles that are innervated by a nerve root. Key muscle testing

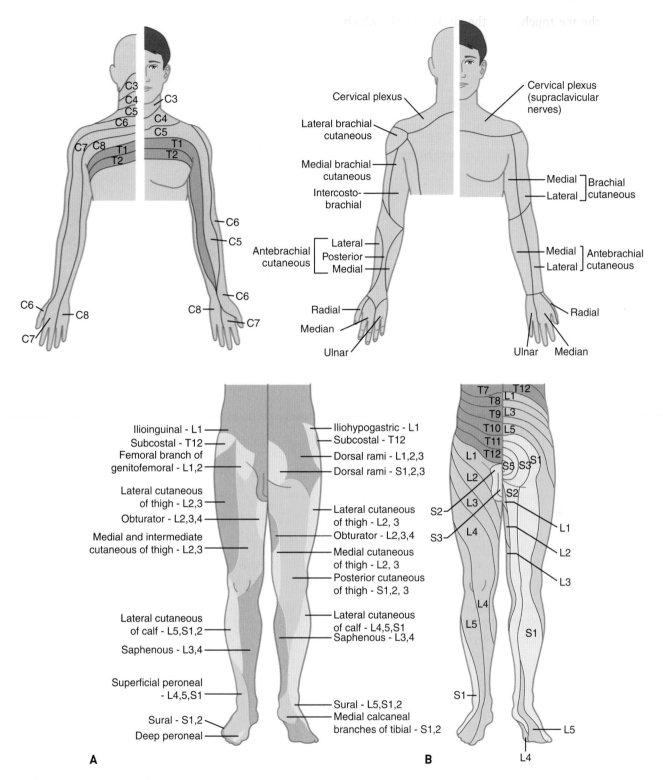

A

B

is the best method for any suspected nerve root and peripheral nerve lesion.

- Deep tendon reflexes (DTRs) indicate the ability of a nerve to respond to a stimulus. A reflex is a subconscious, programmed unit of behavior. The muscle stretch reflex (deep tendon) is one of the simplest known reflexes and depends on the health of the large motor neurons, the muscle spindles, and the small

anterior horn cells. The assessment of reflexes is extremely important in diagnosing and localizing neurologic lesions, as it provides a direct way of assessing the peripheral nervous system (PNS) and an indirect way of examining the central nervous system (CNS).

- Cranial and peripheral nerve integrity. A cranial nerve examination examines the function of the 12 cranial nerve pairs distributed to the head and

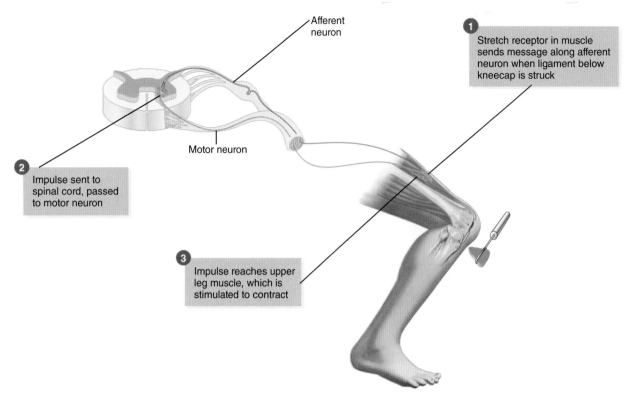

Afferent neuron

**1** Stretch receptor in muscle sends message along afferent neuron when ligament below kneecap is struck

Motor neuron

**2** Impulse sent to spinal cord, passed to motor neuron

**3** Impulse reaches upper leg muscle, which is stimulated to contract

neck, except for one nerve (cranial nerve 10, the vagus nerve) distributed to the thorax and abdomen. Cranial nerve examination is recommended for patients suspected of having a brain, brainstem, and/or cervical spine lesion.

- Vital signs. In addition to other neurologic examinations, an assessment of the cardiopulmonary system is essential, including examining the patient's vital signs (such as heart rate [HR], respiration, and blood pressure) and noting any sign of cardiac decompensation. Cardiopulmonary deficits found by examining vital signs can interfere with physical therapy interventions and recovery. Vital signs also can show the patient's aerobic capacity and endurance.

- Anthropometrics. The anthropometric examination includes measurements that give information about the length, girth, and volume of a patient's body. This information is important to identify the equality of a patient's legs or the **edema** a patient may have in a limb. The clinician also includes the assessment of the patient's height, weight, and body mass index (BMI).

- Aerobic capacity/endurance

- Mentation, hearing, and vision. The PT has to evaluate the patient's ability to concentrate and respond by examining the patient's attention, orientation, and cognition. The patient's attention is the patient's awareness of the environment or the ability to focus on a specific stimulus without

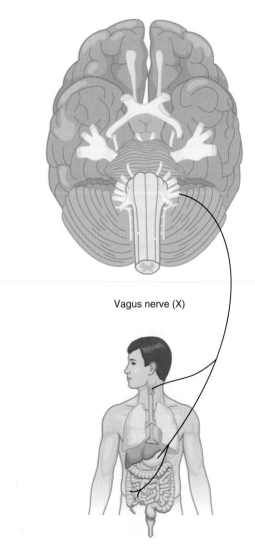

Vagus nerve (X)

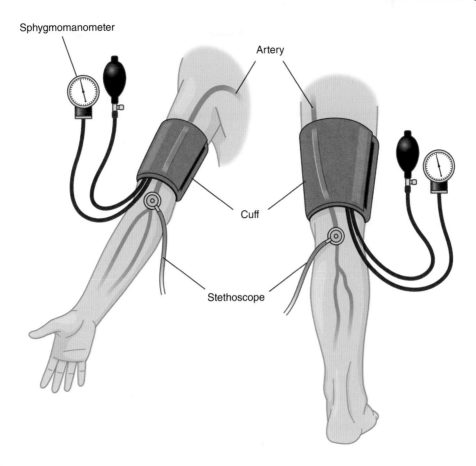

distraction. The patient's orientation refers to their time, person, and place awareness. A patient's cognition is a complex process that examines thinking skills, such as language use and calculation, perception, memory awareness, reasoning, judgment, learning, intellect, social skills, and imagination [5]. Three categories from the above cognition elements are typically used to test a patient. For example, a patient's long-term and short-term memory is assessed. Long-term memory is recalling experiences or information gained in the distant past, while short-term memory is recalling experiences or information gained in the immediate past. Neurologic diseases or injuries to any of the memory regions found in the brain impair an individual's ability to incorporate new memories or recall and use prior ones.

Hearing and vision impairments may be present with aging, diseases, or trauma, which can interfere with the patient's communication and quality of life. A gross hearing examination can be performed by observing the patient's response to normal conversation. A gross visual examination can assess the patient's visual acuity and peripheral field vision.

- Muscle tone. Abnormalities of muscular tone are common in neurologic disorders. These can range from **spasticity** to **rigidity** to flaccidity. Tone, in

general, is defined as the resistance of muscles to passive elongation or stretch. Additionally, one can consider tone as the level of tension a muscle possesses when resting. Three groups categorize tonal abnormalities: **hypertonia**, **hypotonia**, and **dystonia**. For example, patients can have flaccidity on the side of the body opposite the brain lesion immediately after a cerebrovascular accident (CVA). **Flaccidity** is a lack of tension when the muscle is at rest, so the patient has poor or no ability to create enough tension in the muscle to move. Patients also can have spasticity on the side of the body opposite to the brain lesion a few hours (or a few days or weeks) after the stroke. Spasticity is an excessive contraction in response to the stretch of a muscle that can occur when the patient is actively moving or being passively moved.

- Balance and control. Postural and balance examinations involve the patient's ability to control the body parts and position them in equilibrium using skeletal muscles against gravity. For example, a patient who has had a stroke may not maintain balance while sitting, standing, or walking. As a result, the patient's body may lean toward the affected side. Standardized balance examinations include the Berg Balance Test, the Timed Up and Go (TUG) test, and the Tinetti Performance Oriented Mobility Assessment.

- Motor function and mobility. A functional examination determines the effect of the condition or injury on the patient's daily life. Human functional activities are divided into basic activities of daily living (ADLs), such as bathing, dressing, hair combing, eating, transfer activities, walking, or bed mobility, and instrumental ADLs (IADLs), such as meal preparation, light housework, shopping, or driving the car. A functional examination uses different functional tools, such as the Barthel Index, which tests for self-care and patient mobility; the Katz Index of Independence in Activities of Daily Living; and the Functional Status Index.

- Gait. The PT or the physical therapist assistant (PTA) can assess the gait from the front, behind, and side, observing the patient's trunk and upper limbs, the pelvis and lumbar spine, and the lower extremities down to the ankle and foot. The PT/PTA must also observe the activities that occur in gait from when the patient's lower extremity touches the ground to when the same lower extremity contacts the ground again. The activities observed are called a gait cycle. Each portion of the gait cycle (see **Figure 12-3**) involves specific movements and control. The PT or PTA must understand the terminology and practice this examination and documentation process. During gait examination, it is also important to examine the patient's footwear and feet to observe any wearing down of the heels and socks and any callus formation, blisters, corns, and bunions. The clinician must also observe the patient walking with and without shoes, with and without assistive or prosthetic/orthotic devices, on level ground, on different surfaces, and stairs. If the patient cannot walk independently, the clinician must identify the required assistance (**Figure 12-4**).

- Outcomes measures. Outcome measures are healthcare metrics used to assess the effectiveness of a program or intervention to provide data that can be used to evaluate the success of a program, determine areas for improvement, and allocate resources more effectively. Using these standardized tests and measures regularly during a patient's physical therapy episode of care is an important way to objectify the patient's function and abilities. The measures look at the patient's functional abilities, identify if the physical therapy intervention is moving toward the predicted outcomes, and assist the PT in adjusting the POC. Some examples of outcome measures include the Oswestry Low Back Pain Disability Questionnaire, Lower Extremity Functional Scale, Quick DASH (Disability of the Arm, Shoulder, and Hand), and OPTIMAL (see **Figure 12-5**). It is also possible to integrate outcome measures with electronic health records for easy incorporation into documentation. Two examples of software that do this are the Outcome Registry, developed by the American

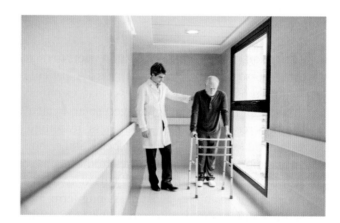

**Figure 12-4** Gait examination.
© alvarez/E+/Getty Images

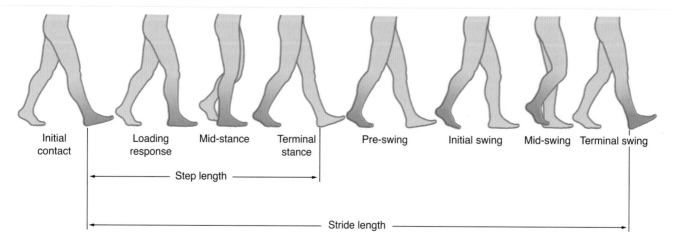

| Initial contact | Loading response | Mid-stance | Terminal stance | Pre-swing | Initial swing | Mid-swing | Terminal swing |

Step length

Stride length

**Figure 12-3** The various components of the gait cycle.

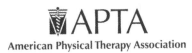

**American Physical Therapy Association**

## OPTIMAL INSTRUMENT
### Demographic Information

1. Date of Birth _____
   mm / dd / yyyy

2. Sex
   1) ____Male
   2) ____Female

3. Race
   1) ____Aleut/Eskimo
   2) ____American Indian
   3) ____Asian/Pacific Islander
   4) ____Black
   5) ____White
   6) ____Other

4. Ethnicity
   1) ____Hispanic or Latino
   2) ____Not Hispanic or Latino

5. Insurance (Please check all that apply)
   1) ____Workers' compensation
   2) ____Self-pay
   3) ____HMO/PPO/private insurance
   4) ____Medicare
   5) ____Medicaid
   6) ____Auto
   7) ____Other

6. Education (Please check one)
   1) ____Less than high school
   2) ____Some high school
   3) ____High school graduate
   4) ____Attended or graduated from technical school
   5) ____Attended college, did not graduate
   6) ____College graduate
   7) ____Completed graduate school/advanced degree

7. Please check the combined annual income of everyone in your house:
   1) ____Less than $10,000
   2) ____$10,000–$14,999
   3) ____$15,000–$24,999
   4) ____$25,000–$34,999
   5) ____$35,000–$49,999
   6) ____$50,000–$74,999
   7) ____$75,000–$99,999
   8) ____$100,000–$149,999
   9) ____$150,000 or more

8. Employment/Work (Check all that apply)
   1) ____Working full-time outside of home
   2) ____Working part-time outside of home
   3) ____Working full-time from home
   4) ____Working part-time from home
   5) ____Working with modification in job because of current illness/injury
   6) ____Not working because of current illness/injury
   7) ____Homemaker
   8) ____Student
   9) ____Retired
   10) ____Unemployed
   Occupation:_____

9. Do you use a: (Check all that apply)
   1) ____Cane?
   2) ____Walker, rolling walker, or rollator?
   3) ____Manual wheelchair?
   4) ____Motorized wheelchair?
   5) ____Other:_____

10. With whom do you live? (Check all that apply)
    1) ____Alone
    2) ____Spouse/significant other
    3) ____Child/children
    4) ____Other relative(s)
    5) ____Group setting
    6) ____Personal care attendant
    7) ____Other:_____

11. Where do you live?
    1) ____Private home
    2) ____Private apartment
    3) ____Rented room
    4) ____Board and care/assisted living/group home
    5) ____Homeless (with or without shelter)
    6) ____Long-term care facility (nursing home)
    7) ____Hospice
    8) ____Other

**Figure 12-5** OPTIMAL outcome measure.

# OPTIMAL INSTRUMENT

## Difficulty–Baseline

| Instructions: Please circle the level of difficulty you have for each activity today. | Able to do without any difficulty | Able to do with little difficulty | Able to do with moderate difficulty | Able to do with much difficulty | Unable to do | Not applicable |
|---|---|---|---|---|---|---|
| 1. Lying flat | 1 | 2 | 3 | 4 | 5 | 9 |
| 2. Rolling over | 1 | 2 | 3 | 4 | 5 | 9 |
| 3. Moving–lying to sitting | 1 | 2 | 3 | 4 | 5 | 9 |
| 4. Sitting | 1 | 2 | 3 | 4 | 5 | 9 |
| 5. Squatting | 1 | 2 | 3 | 4 | 5 | 9 |
| 6. Bending/stooping | 1 | 2 | 3 | 4 | 5 | 9 |
| 7. Balancing | 1 | 2 | 3 | 4 | 5 | 9 |
| 8. Kneeling | 1 | 2 | 3 | 4 | 5 | 9 |
| 9. Standing | 1 | 2 | 3 | 4 | 5 | 9 |
| 10. Walking–short distance | 1 | 2 | 3 | 4 | 5 | 9 |
| 11. Walking–long distance | 1 | 2 | 3 | 4 | 5 | 9 |
| 12. Walking–outdoors | 1 | 2 | 3 | 4 | 5 | 9 |
| 13. Climbing stairs | 1 | 2 | 3 | 4 | 5 | 9 |
| 14. Hopping | 1 | 2 | 3 | 4 | 5 | 9 |
| 15. Jumping | 1 | 2 | 3 | 4 | 5 | 9 |
| 16. Running | 1 | 2 | 3 | 4 | 5 | 9 |
| 17. Pushing | 1 | 2 | 3 | 4 | 5 | 9 |
| 18. Pulling | 1 | 2 | 3 | 4 | 5 | 9 |
| 19. Reaching | 1 | 2 | 3 | 4 | 5 | 9 |
| 20. Grasping | 1 | 2 | 3 | 4 | 5 | 9 |
| 21. Lifting | 1 | 2 | 3 | 4 | 5 | 9 |
| 22. Carrying | 1 | 2 | 3 | 4 | 5 | 9 |

23. From the above list, choose the 3 activities you would most like to be able to do without any difficulty (for example, if you would most like to be able to *climb stairs*, *kneel*, and *hop* without any difficulty, you would choose: *1.* _13_ *2.* _8_ *3.* _14_ )

1.____ 2.____ 3.____

24. From the above list of three activities, choose the primary activity you would most like to be able to do without any difficulty (for example, if you would most like to be able to *climb stairs* without any difficulty, you would choose: Primary goal. _13_)

Primary goal. ____

The OPTIMAL may be used without permission or restriction per our website, www.apta.org/optimal. Please note, however, that it remains the copyrighted intellectual property of *Physical Therapy* (PTJ) and the following citation must be included for all uses:

**Figure 12-5** (Continued)

## Confidence–Baseline

| Instructions: Please circle the level of confidence you have for doing each activity today. | Fully confident in my ability to perform | Very confident | Moderate confidence | Some confidence | Not confident in my ability to perform | Not applicable |
|---|---|---|---|---|---|---|
| 1. Lying flat | 1 | 2 | 3 | 4 | 5 | 9 |
| 2. Rolling over | 1 | 2 | 3 | 4 | 5 | 9 |
| 3. Moving–lying to sitting | 1 | 2 | 3 | 4 | 5 | 9 |
| 4. Sitting | 1 | 2 | 3 | 4 | 5 | 9 |
| 5. Squatting | 1 | 2 | 3 | 4 | 5 | 9 |
| 6. Bending/stooping | 1 | 2 | 3 | 4 | 5 | 9 |
| 7. Balancing | 1 | 2 | 3 | 4 | 5 | 9 |
| 8. Kneeling | 1 | 2 | 3 | 4 | 5 | 9 |
| 9. Standing | 1 | 2 | 3 | 4 | 5 | 9 |
| 10. Walking–short distance | 1 | 2 | 3 | 4 | 5 | 9 |
| 11. Walking–long distance | 1 | 2 | 3 | 4 | 5 | 9 |
| 12. Walking–outdoors | 1 | 2 | 3 | 4 | 5 | 9 |
| 13. Climbing stairs | 1 | 2 | 3 | 4 | 5 | 9 |
| 14. Hopping | 1 | 2 | 3 | 4 | 5 | 9 |
| 15. Jumping | 1 | 2 | 3 | 4 | 5 | 9 |
| 16. Running | 1 | 2 | 3 | 4 | 5 | 9 |
| 17. Pushing | 1 | 2 | 3 | 4 | 5 | 9 |
| 18. Pulling | 1 | 2 | 3 | 4 | 5 | 9 |
| 19. Reaching | 1 | 2 | 3 | 4 | 5 | 9 |
| 20. Grasping | 1 | 2 | 3 | 4 | 5 | 9 |
| 21. Lifting | 1 | 2 | 3 | 4 | 5 | 9 |
| 22. Carrying | 1 | 2 | 3 | 4 | 5 | 9 |

The OPTIMAL may be used without permission or restriction per our website, www.apta.org/optimal. Please note, however, that it remains the copyrighted intellectual property of Physical Therapy (PTJ) and the following citation must be included for all uses:

**Figure 12-5** (*Continued*)

### When can you use PROM exercises?

- When the patient cannot move a joint
- When an AROM exercise is prohibited
- After surgery or injury and in cases of complete bed rest, paralysis, or coma
- To maintain the mobility of joint connective tissue
- To maintain the elasticity of the muscle
- To increase the synovial fluid for joint nutrition
- To assist circulation
- To prevent joint contracture
- To decrease pain
- To help in the healing process

Physical Therapy Association (APTA), and Focus on Therapeutic Outcomes (FOTO), developed by Focus on Therapeutic Outcomes, Inc.

## ROM Exercises

ROM exercises are exercises that move a joint through the extent of its limitations. ROM exercises can be passive ROM exercises, active ROM exercises, and active assistive ROM exercises.

### PROM Exercises

PROM is a joint movement performed by a PT, PTA, family member/caregiver, or a mechanical

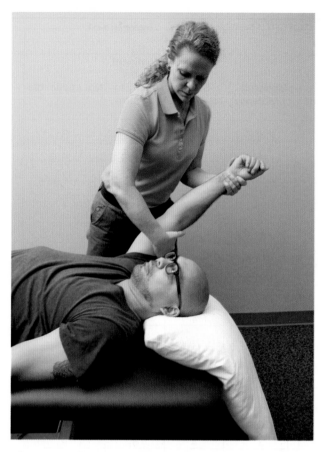

**Figure 12-6** Patient receiving PROM to his shoulder.

device without muscle contraction by the patient (see **Figure 12-6**). An example of a mechanical device that produces PROM is the continuous passive motion (CPM) device, which passively moves a desired joint continuously through a controlled ROM without patient effort for as long as 24 hours per day. Manual PROM exercises can be applied to the patient by the patient himself or herself using an involved extremity.

## AROM Exercises

AROM means the patient performs the ROM movement actively through muscular contraction. AROM exercises allow the patient to voluntarily contract the muscle(s) around a given joint to move the joint throughout its entire range or a specified range.

### When can you use AROM exercises?

- To increase muscular strength
- To promote bone and soft-tissue integrity
- To promote coordination and motor skills
- To prevent deep vein thrombosis (DVT) after surgery or immobilization
- To increase blood circulation
- To prepare for functional activities, such as ambulation or ADLs

## Active-Assisted ROM Exercises

Active-assisted ROM (AAROM) exercise is used when the patient needs assistance to complete the AROM—the patient cannot perform a desired motion independently without manual or mechanical assistance being provided by a PT/PTA or a device, such as a wand or a cane, a finger-ladder device, or overhead pulleys.

## Strengthening Exercises

Strengthening exercises increase muscle strength, power, and endurance.

- Strength. The maximum tension that a muscle or muscle group can produce against resistance for one repetition. Engaging in progressive resistance exercises (PREs) that involve body weight or various equipment, such as weights, machines, or resistance bands, can improve strength. Compound exercises, such as squats, deadlifts, and bench presses, stress multiple muscle groups at once and are, therefore, more effective at building overall muscle strength (see **Box 21-1**).
- Power. The ability of a muscle or muscle group to generate force (work) within a specified time. Improving muscle power requires specific training exercises, such as plyometrics and ballistic movements.
- Endurance. A muscle or muscle group can perform repeated or sustained contractions over a specified period without fatigue. High-repetition, low-resistance exercises improve muscle endurance.

Different factors can affect muscle performance, including age, gender, genetics, and overall health. There are three main types of strengthening exercises. These include:

- Isometric exercises develop tension in the muscle without visible joint movement and changes in muscle length. When the patient cannot perform joint motion due to pain, inflammation, or surgical protocols, they can perform these exercises. An example of isometric exercises is quadriceps sets.
- Concentric/eccentric exercises develop tension in the muscle through dynamic concentric or eccentric muscular contractions (see **Figure 12-7**). A concentric muscular contraction causes the muscle to shorten, whereas an eccentric contraction causes the muscle to lengthen. Isotonic exercise is dynamic with a constant load (such as a cuff weight) but an uncontrolled movement speed. An example of an isotonic exercise is a biceps curl.

In the clinic, the PT/PTA can apply manual resistance to control the amount of resistance in the earlier stages of rehabilitation. However, quantifying the resistance for documentation is more difficult using this method.

- Isokinetic exercises are dynamic exercises having a predetermined velocity of muscle shortening or lengthening so that the force generated by the

### Box 12-1 Core Strengthening

Core strengthening refers to exercises that target the muscles of the abdomen, lumbar and cervical spine, and hips, which provide stability and support for the spine, and help with balance and posture. Examples of core exercises include:

- Plank: This exercise involves holding the body in a push-up position, but instead of doing push-ups, the patient maintains the position for a set amount of time.
- Russian Twist: This exercise involves sitting on the floor with the knees bent and feet flat, holding a weight in both hands and twisting the torso from side to side.
- Bicycle Crunch: This exercise involves lying supine with the hands behind the head, lifting one knee toward the chest while twisting to bring the opposite elbow toward the knee.
- Side Plank: This exercise involves holding the body in a side-lying push-up position instead of face down.

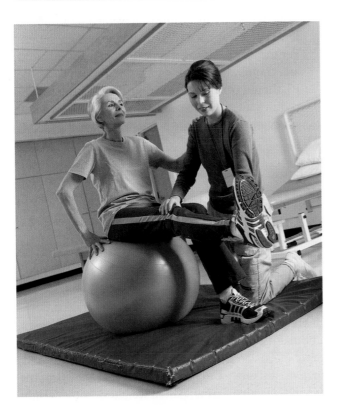

**Figure 12-7** Patient performing an isotonic exercise with her leg.

© Tyler Olson/Shutterstock

### What are flexibility exercises?

**Flexibility exercises** describe any therapeutic maneuver that increases soft-tissue mobility and improves ROM by elongating structures. Shortened and hypomobile structures need to be stretched.

muscle is maximal through the full ROM. Isokinetic exercises take place at a constant speed. Isokinetic exercises use specialized machines, such as Cybex, KinCom, or Biodex.

## Flexibility Exercises

There are several ways to increase flexibility, including:

- Manual passive static stretching is the manual application of an external force to move the involved body segment slightly beyond the point of tissue resistance and available ROM (see **Figure 12-8**). There is a lack of agreement on the ideal combination for the duration or the number of repetitions of a single stretch in a single session to achieve the best results. Applying heat to the muscle during the stretch and maintaining the stretch until muscle cooling occurs after removing the heat can enhance a stretch. Various neurophysiological techniques can reduce sensory-motor feedback and thereby increase muscle relaxation. Such techniques include proprioceptive neuromuscular facilitation (PNF) and muscle energy.
- Self-stretching is a stretching procedure that the patient can perform independently after receiving instruction from the PT or the PTA.
- Ballistic stretching is a forceful, rapid, intermittent stretch with high speed and intensity. When comparing the ballistic and static methods, most

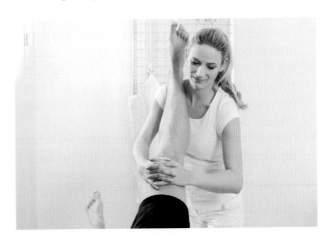

**Figure 12-8** A PT stretches a patient's hamstring muscles.

© Kzenon/Shutterstock

studies have found that both produce similar flexibility improvements, but the ballistic method appears to cause more residual muscle soreness.

Contraindications for stretching include sharp pain with joint movement, an incomplete bony union, a bony end feel, a recent fracture, acute inflammatory or infectious process, or where there is hypermobility.

## Balance and Coordination Exercises

Balance and coordination exercises help maintain and improve physical function, which can diminish with age. The findings from the examination may lead to the recommendation of some or all of the following.

- Double-leg stance exercises
- Single-leg stance exercises
- Heel-to-toe walk exercises
- Standing leg swing exercises
- Chair squat exercises

As the patient improves, they close their eyes or try standing on an unstable surface like a pillow or balance board.

Other activities that are often encouraged to help improve balance and coordination include:

- Tai Chi
- Yoga

## Functional Training

Functional training assists patients in returning to their prior level of function or the highest achievable function level. Functional exercises or activities incorporate balance and coordination with strength and flexibility. On a simplistic level, functional exercises use either an open or closed kinetic chain.

- Open kinetic chain. These are exercises where the limb or body part is free to move in space, usually not in contact with the ground or other surfaces, allowing for greater mobility and ROM. Examples include leg extensions, bicep curls, shoulder presses, and hamstring curls.
- Closed kinetic chain. These are exercises where the exercising limb or body part is fixed or stable, usually in contact with the ground or other surfaces. Since these exercises often require bearing weight and involve multiple joints working together, they are considered more functional than open kinetic chain exercises, especially for gait and balance. Examples include squats, lunges, push-ups, and the plank position.

## Soft-Tissue Techniques

- Massage. A systematic, mechanical stimulation of the body's soft tissue using rhythmically applied pressure and stretching for therapeutic purposes. Besides massage, other massage techniques are used, such as cross-fiber massage, connective tissue massage, soft-tissue mobilization, myofascial release, instrument-assisted soft-tissue mobilization, and acupressure.
- Dry needling. A relatively new technique, sometimes referred to as "intramuscular stimulation" or "trigger point dry needling," involves the insertion of fine, thin acupuncture needles into the skin to stimulate trigger points in the muscles to relieve pain, improve ROM, and reduce muscle tension by targeting areas of tightness or knots in the muscles. The effectiveness of dry needling is still being studied.
- Neural mobilization. Involves gentle, passive movements of the peripheral nerves in a specific direction and speed to stretch and mobilize the nerve tissue to relieve pain, numbness, tingling, and other symptoms associated with nerve damage or entrapment.
- Joint mobilizations. Involves the application of a gentle, passive force to a joint in a specific direction and speed to reduce pain, improve ROM, and enhance overall joint function. Joint manipulations are skilled passive, mechanical movements of high or low velocity applied to a specific joint or segment. Per the APTA, spinal and peripheral manipulations and mobilizations are among the interventions the PT should perform exclusively; however, these procedures are regulated differently by the individual states' physical therapy boards and regulations.

### KNOWLEDGE CHECK

What are the parameters of therapeutic exercise?
What are the three types of ROM?
What are the differences among isometric, isotonic, and isokinetic exercise?

## Gait Training

Because some patients with musculoskeletal pathologies may be unable to walk without assistive devices (or ambulatory aids), the PTA needs to teach these patients gait patterns and sequences that use assistive devices, such as walkers, crutches, or canes. The gait patterns are non–weight bearing, partial weight bearing, weight bearing as tolerated, and full weight bearing (FWB). Gait sequences or patterns are called three-point, two-point, four-point, swing-to, and swing-through.

## Orthotics and Prosthetics

Other physical therapy interventions for musculoskeletal disorders include orthotic and prosthetic devices. An **orthosis** (or brace) is an external device applied to body parts to provide support and stabilization, improve function, correct flexible deformities, prevent the progression of fixed deformities, and reduce pressure and pain by transferring the load from one area to another. A **prosthesis** is an artificial substitute for a missing body part. Prostheses are used for patients who have had amputations.

## Aquatic Therapy

Widespread interest has developed in aquatic therapy, a form of **hydrotherapy**, as a tool for rehabilitation. Among the psychological aspects, water motivates movement because painful joints and muscles can move more easily and painlessly in water. The indications for aquatic therapy include:

- Instances when partial weight-bearing ambulation is necessary
- To increase the ROM
- When standing balance needs to be improved
- When endurance/aerobic capacity needs to be improved
- When the goal is to increase muscle strength via active-assisted, gravity-assisted, active, or resisted exercise [6].

Contraindications to aquatic therapy include [6]:

- Incontinence
- Urinary tract infections
- Unprotected open wounds/menstruation
- Autonomic dysreflexia
- Heat intolerance
- Severe epilepsy/uncontrolled seizures
- Uncontrolled diabetes
- Unstable blood pressure
- Severe cardiac and/or pulmonary dysfunction

Once the clinician rules out any contraindications, they evaluate the patient's water safety skills, swimming ability, and general level of comfort in the water. The patient's needs and response determine the exact proportion and quantity of land and water activity. The following aquatic strategies/techniques can be used [7]:

- Position and direction of movement: A three-part progression moving from buoyancy-assisted exercises to buoyancy-supported and finally to buoyancy-resisted exercises. As with gravity, patient position and direction of movement can greatly alter the amount of assistance or resistance.

  - Buoyancy-assisted exercises involve movements toward the water's surface, similar to gravity-assisted exercises on land. For example, in the standing position, shoulder abduction and flexion, as well as the ascent phase of the squat, are considered buoyancy-assisted exercises. In the prone position, hip extension can be buoyancy assisted.
  - Buoyancy-supported exercises involve movements parallel to the bottom of the pool and similar to gravity-minimized positions on land. For example, in the standing position, horizontal shoulder abduction/adduction is an example of such activity, as is hip and shoulder abduction in the supine position.
  - Buoyancy-resisted exercises involve movements toward the bottom of the pool. For example, in the supine position, shoulder and hip extension and the squat's descent phase are considered buoyancy-resisted activities.

- Depth of water: Less support is provided by buoyancy in shallow water than in deeper water. In addition, modifications can be made by adding buoyant or resisted equipment.

- Lever arm length: As with land-based exercises, the lever arm length can be adjusted to change the amount of assistance or resistance. For example, performing buoyancy-assisted shoulder flexion in a standing position is easier with the elbow straight (i.e., long lever) than with the elbow flexed (i.e., short lever). Conversely, buoyancy-resisted shoulder abduction is more difficult with the elbow extended because of the long lever arm.

- Buoyant equipment: Buoyant equipment can be added to the lever arm to increase assistance (support for individuals in certain positions) or resistance. As the buoyancy of the equipment increases, the resistance also increases. Equipment designed to assist with patient positioning can be applied to the neck, extremities, or trunk.

- Viscosity: The water's viscous quality or density allows it to be used effectively as a resistive medium. When moving through the water, the body experiences a frontal resistance proportional to the presenting surface area. This resistance can be increased by enlarging the surface area or increasing the movement velocity.

- Water temperature: Variable temperature control for the water should be available, and the ambient air temperature should be 3°C higher than the water temperature for patient comfort. The body's ability to regulate temperature during an immersion exercise differs from that of a land exercise.

Water conducts temperature 25 times faster than air, and water retains heat 1,000 times more. With immersion, less skin is exposed to air, resulting in less opportunity to dissipate heat through normal sweating mechanisms. The following water temperatures are recommended based on activity:

- 26–33°C for aquatic exercises, including flexibility, strengthening, gait training, and relaxation. **Therapeutic exercise** in warm water (33°C) may benefit patients with painful musculoskeletal areas.
- 26–28°C should be used for cardiovascular training and aerobic exercise (active swimming).
- 22–26°C for intense and aerobic training.

The patient must enter the water slowly so that all systems can gradually accommodate to the new environment.

## Musculoskeletal Conditions

Several common traumatic injuries are as follows:

- Fracture. A bone fracture can be caused by high-force impacts, falls, and repetitive stress. Fractures may be classified according to direction, mechanism, whether or not the skin is broken, and location. The five most common fractures are the distal radius, proximal femur, ankle, proximal humerus, and metacarpal [8]. Two fracture types are specific to the skeletally immature patient: the greenstick (the bone cracks on one side but does not break completely) and the growth plate (an area in certain bones that allows the bone to grow). Symptoms of a fracture include pain, swelling, and difficulty moving the involved limb. Fracture diagnosis is best confirmed with radiographs. The type of fracture and its severity will determine the course of treatment, which may include immobilization, physical therapy, and, in severe cases, surgery.
- Sprain. An injury occurs when the ligaments, which connect bones, stretch or tear, because of a joint's sudden twisting, a fall, or overextension. The most common sprain areas are the ankle (lateral ligaments), knee (ACL), and wrist (radial). Symptoms include pain, swelling, and difficulty moving the involved joint. Treatment for a sprain typically involves rest, ice, compression, and elevation of the involved joint or area to reduce swelling and help with pain management. In severe cases, a brace or splint may be necessary to immobilize the joint or area and allow it to heal.
- Strain. Occurs when a muscle or tendon overstretches or tears from overuse, or a sudden, forceful movement. Symptoms of a muscle strain include pain, swelling, and muscle spasms. Treatment typically involves rest, ice, compression, and elevation of the involved structure to reduce swelling, and pain management, followed by strengthening and flexibility exercises. In severe cases, a brace or splint may be necessary to immobilize the area, or surgery may be required.

Several common overuse injuries are:

- Tendinopathy. A tendon is a strong and flexible fibrous connective tissue that attaches muscle to bone, allowing the muscles to generate force and movement. Tendinopathies are often the result of repetitive stress, overuse, or aging and commonly occur in the knee (patellar tendon) and elbow ("tennis elbow"). Symptoms include pain, weakness, and difficulty moving the involved joint. Treatment typically involves rest, ice, and exercises to help improve strength and flexibility in the tendon.
- Bursitis. Bursae are small fluid-filled sacs that cushion and lubricate joints and muscles throughout the body. Bursitis occurs when the bursae become inflamed by various factors, including overuse or repetitive motion, trauma or injury to the affected area, infection, or underlying medical conditions, such as gout or rheumatoid arthritis. Treatment typically involves a combination of protection, rest, ice, compression, and elevation (PRICE), nonsteroidal anti-inflammatory medications (NSAIDs), and exercises to help improve ROM, strengthen muscles, and prevent future episodes.

Musculoskeletal or orthopedic physical therapy occurs in various clinical settings, treating patients of different ages with various medical and physical problems. For example, young people may present with various orthopedic injuries, such as a knee ligament tear causing pain and difficulty walking. An older adult may require rehabilitation after total knee arthroplasty. The physical therapy treatment approaches are diverse depending on the patient's needs, the clinical setting, and the clinical experience of the PT and PTA. Goals in orthopedic physical therapy include maximizing the patient's function; alleviating pain; decreasing abnormal stress on joints; ensuring proper posture; and promoting tissue healing, ROM, and flexibility.

Various resources are available for students interested in the specialty area, including the Academy of Orthopaedic Physical Therapy (AOPT); the *Journal of Orthopaedic & Sports Physical Therapy* (JOSPT); and the Academy magazine, *Orthopaedic Physical Therapy Practice*. Within the AOPT, PTAs can also join the PTA Educational Interest Group.

# CASE STUDY

You are examining a 55-year-old female who has had neck and shoulder pain and numbness in her left arm and hand for about a month. Her primary care physician (PCP) recently prescribed rest, analgesics, and steroid injection into her shoulder that only temporarily relieved her symptoms, so her PCP referred her to physical therapy with a diagnosis of subacromial bursitis and tendinopathy of the left shoulder.

Your examination findings are:

- No red or yellow flags were present.
- Reports of neck and shoulder pain with numbness in the left arm and hand, described as deep, with an ache and occasional burning in the neck and shoulder, with an intensity that ranged from 0 to 9 on the visual analog scale (VAS). Aggravating factors include sleeping on the left side, punching forward with her left arm, and reaching behind her back.
- Poor overall posture with forward head and asymmetry between left and right upper body with atrophy in the left upper trapezius and the left scapula area.
- Cervical spine rotation was limited to 40° with ipsilateral-sided shoulder and arm pain and numbness pain reproduced with rotation to the left and a heavy sensation in the left arm. Left side flexion was also limited and painful on the ipsilateral side.
- MMT was normal except for the reproduction of immediate pain with left rotation and with left side flexion.
- The ROM assessment revealed an inability to actively lift the left arm above 30°. With active assistance using the right arm, the patient could achieve 145° flexion and maintain this position independently. Left upper extremity abduction measured 110°, but with anterior deviation and early activation of the scapula occurring from 40° and side flexion of the trunk. With scapula stabilization, the patient could only achieve 40° of abduction, but anterior deviation was still evident. On initial movement, the pain was experienced in the upper arm, but there was no change to the heavy feeling in her arm or hand. Horizontal adduction and hand behind the back were also limited.
- The upper limb tension tests (ULTTs) were all positive.
- Spurling's test was positive.

Based on the examination findings, discuss the following in your group:

- What conditions could be ruled out using the ULTT and Spurling tests?
- What would be your working hypothesis for a physical therapy diagnosis?
- If your hypothesis differs from the physician's, how would you approach this situation?
- What would be the main focus of your initial intervention?
- What would be your short- and long-term goals?

# CASE STUDY

You are observing a PT performing a lumbar spine examination. As part of the examination, the patient rides a stationary bicycle and, while riding it, the clinician asks the patient to sit up straight and then to bend forward.

1. What is the purpose of this test and how is the PT using it to help differentiate the causes of the patient's symptoms?
   The patient you are currently treating has a lumbar disc protrusion at the L4–5 level. Besides teaching the patient a home exercise program, you also want to educate the patient on positions to adopt and positions to avoid to help in the healing process.
2. Which positions will you advise the patient to avoid and which positions will you encourage the patient to adopt, and why?
   Any motion that produces a sacral nutation aggravates the patient's symptoms.
3. What lumbar spine and hip motions will you avoid so as not to provoke the patient's symptoms?
   You want to measure the ROM of the patient's lumbar spine as part of a reevaluation. Describe the different methods you could use to measure lumbar flexion and extension.

# Neurologic System

The neurologic examination uses a series of tests to evaluate the function of the PNS and CNS, and, to some degree, the autonomic nervous system (ANS). The length of the examination depends on the complexity of the patient's symptoms and medical history.

## Neurologic System Examination

A typical neurologic system examination consists of:

- Medical history, including questions about the patient's symptoms, medications, functional difficulties, and pertinent comorbidities
- Mental status assessment, including cognition (the ability to acquire, process, store, and use information during perception, attention, memory, language, problem-solving, and decision-making) and communication level
- Cranial nerve examination of the 12 cranial nerves
- Motor examination of the patient's muscle strength, ROM, muscle tone (e.g., rigidity, hypotonia, hypertonia), motor control (performance of smooth voluntary movements in a coordinated fashion), and gait (e.g., speed, ability to change directions on command), and perform other functions, including compensatory and preferred movement strategies
- Sensory examination of the patient's perception and ability to sense touch, pain, temperature, and vibration
- Reflex examination of normal (e.g., knee-jerk) and abnormal (e.g., Babinski) reflexes
- Coordination examination of the patient's ability to perform various coordination tests, such as finger-to-nose and heel-to-shin

The PTA works as a rehabilitation team member during the neurologic treatment (see **Figure 12-9**), considering both the therapeutic interventions and the psychosocial aspects of rehabilitation. In general, these aspects include the patient's psychological and social well-being. Specific psychosocial aspects of patient care in neurologic physical therapy may include:

- Patient's adaptation to disability
- Patient's and patient's family's stages of adjustment to the disease and disability
- Effects of impairments, functional limitations, and disability
- Effects of limitations on patient participation
- Patient's reintegration into the environment, family, work, and life

Neurologic physical therapy specializes in treating patients who have neurologic disorders affecting

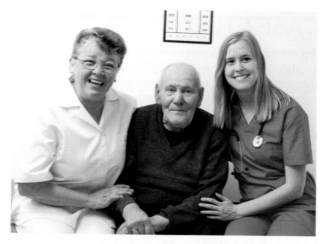

**Figure 12-9** Man with Parkinson's disease.
© Barabasa/Shutterstock

the structure and function of their nervous systems. The onset rate and course for neuromuscular conditions vary, with some being abrupt and devastating while others may be gradual, reversible, static, or progressive.

## Neurophysiologic Approaches

Numerous neurologic treatments to improve motor control exist, but as yet, research has not identified one neurophysiologic approach that is more effective than another and that most PTs use some or all of the following techniques to address specific patient problems.

### Constraint-Induced Movement Therapy

Constraint-induced movement therapy [9–14] has demonstrated significant and large improvements in upper extremity function using the concentrated and repetitive practice of the involved upper extremity with the restriction of movement in the uninvolved upper extremity through the use of mitts, sling, or brace so that the patient has to use their involved side to perform functional movements, thereby increasing the total number of movements that the involved side has to perform.

### Task-Oriented Approach

The task-oriented or systems approach is based on the current understanding of how normal movement emerges as an interaction among many systems, the environment, and the task, each contributing its aspect of control. Central to the functional/task-oriented approach to motor control is the idea that specific task-oriented training with extensive practice is essential to reacquiring skills and enhancing recovery [15]. Additionally, movement is organized around a behavioral goal (using behavioral-shaping techniques), constrained by the environment. Thus, the role of sensation in normal movement is not limited to a stimulus–response reflex mode but is also essential to the predictive and adaptive control of movement.

## Rood's Concept of Levels of Control

Rood's concept that sensory stimuli affect the motor response uses a series of positions and activities that go through the normal sequencing of motor development. Muscles are classified as either mobilizers or stabilizers. The development stages include:

- Mobility (reciprocal interaction)
- Stability (co-contraction)
- Controlled mobility (proximal muscles move while the distal muscles are fixed)
- Skill (proximal muscles are fixed while the distal muscles move)

## Impairment-Focused Interventions

Impairment-focused training includes developmental activity training, motor training, movement pattern training, and neuromuscular education or reeducation [15]. The central concept of this approach was using sensory input to modify the CNS and stimulate motor output. Two of the most popular approaches include neurodevelopmental treatment (NDT) and PNF.

- Neurodevelopmental treatment. The NDT approach evolved from the work of Karl and Berta Bobath, whose work focused on the hierarchical model of neurophysiologic function. The theoretical basis for this approach is that a maturational lag in integrating primitive postural reflexes is often found in learning-disabled children. Based on this finding, it was assumed that abnormal postural reflex activity and abnormal muscle tone were caused by the loss of *CNS* control at the brainstem and spinal cord levels. Thus the emphasis was on the inhibition/integration of primitive postural patterns, the promotion of the development of normal postural reactions, and the normalization of abnormal tone while avoiding abnormal and compensatory movement patterns. Current NDT theory recognizes that many factors can contribute to the loss of motor function in patients with neurological dysfunction, including the full spectrum of sensory and motor deficits. NDT therapy emphasizes the importance of postural control in skill learning.
- Proprioceptive neuromuscular facilitation. The concept of PNF (also termed complex motions) was developed by Dr. Hermann Kabat, then by Sherrington, and finally by Margaret Knott and Dorothy Voss.

## The Brunnstrom Approach

This approach was based on the hierarchical model using a combination of very precise observation of the sequential changes in motor function that typically occurred following stroke and an understanding of the reflex function of the nervous system. The Brunnstrom approach emphasized eliciting motor behavior in the sequence where it would occur using synergy patterns. Even though reinforcing synergy patterns is rarely used these days, except for stroke patients, Brunnstrom's detailed and accurate observations have enabled clinicians to document a patient's progress based on her seven stages of recovery.

## Ecological Systems Theory

The psychologist Urie Bronfenbrenner developed this theory to explain human development in the context of complex and interconnected social environments, with human development being shaped by various systems, ranging from the immediate family and community to broader cultural and societal contexts within four main systems:

Microsystem: This refers to the immediate environment in which an individual interacts, such as family, school, peers, and neighborhood, which can have a direct and significant impact on an individual's development.

Mesosystem: This refers to the connections between the different components of the microsystem. For example, the relationship between a child's school and family can influence their development, as can the relationship between a parent's work and family life.

Exosystem: This refers to the systems that indirectly impact an individual's development, such as government policies, mass media, and the workplace. These systems can affect the microsystem and mesosystem and shape an individual's experiences and opportunities.

Macrosystem: This refers to the broader cultural and societal contexts in which an individual lives, such as cultural values, beliefs, and norms. These systems can influence the other three systems and shape an individual's experiences and opportunities.

Bronfenbrenner's theory emphasizes the importance of understanding these connections and interactions to understand and promote healthy human development.

### Integrated Approach

Several factors must be considered when developing an effective treatment program for patients with developmental motor problems [16]:

- Variability in practice: Variable practice within a movement class will facilitate skill transfer to a novel condition of constant practice.
- Intratask and intertask organization: The practice order within a treatment session should be random or serial rather than involving the repetitive practice of one activity per treatment session, as the former creates regeneration of a motor plan, ultimately facilitating task recall.
- The specific motor learning tasks should involve functional and pre-gait activities (as appropriate). Functional activities include bed mobility, repositioning, and arising from the floor.

### Cognitive Rehabilitation

Cognitive rehabilitation is a systematic, goal-oriented treatment program designed to improve cognitive functions and functional abilities and increase self-management and independence following neurological damage to the CNS. Although the specific tasks are individualized to the patient's needs, treatment generally emphasizes restoring lost functions; teaching compensatory strategies to circumvent impaired cognitive functions; and improving competence in performing IADLs, such as managing medications, using the telephone, and handling finances. Cognitive rehabilitation has been postulated to maintain or improve language, memory, and other cognitive abilities in neurologically impaired individuals. There are several treatment approaches to cognitive rehabilitation, including retraining (also known as the transfer of training approach), restorative (repetitive exercise can restore lost functions and targets internal cognitive processes to generalize improvements in real-world environments), sensory integration (integration of basic sensorimotor functions), neurofunctional approach (retraining real-world skills rather than on retraining specific cognitive and perceptual processes), and compensatory (developing external prosthetic assistance for dysfunctions) [17].

## Neurologic Conditions

At the most fundamental level, all neurologic lesions are an upper motor neuron (UMN) lesion, a lower motor neuron (LMN) lesion, or a combination of both.

- UMN. A lesion of the neural pathway above the anterior horn cell or motor nuclei of the cranial nerves, characterized by spastic paralysis or paresis, little or no muscle atrophy, hyperreflexive stretch reflexes in a nonsegmental distribution, and pathological signs and reflexes. The PT/PTA must know the signs and symptoms of UMN lesions, which can constitute a medical emergency.
- LMN. A lesion affecting the nerve fibers traveling from the anterior horn of the spinal cord to the relevant muscle(s), characterized by muscle atrophy and hypotonus, a diminished or absent stretch reflex of the areas served by a spinal nerve root or a peripheral nerve and an absence of pathological signs or reflexes.

Neuromuscular disorders can affect many functions, such as movement, sensation, thinking, and communication. Most neuromuscular disorders are inherited or acquired:

- Inherited. These are genetic conditions that specific gene mutations can cause, which can be inherited from one or both parents and include:
    - Huntington's disease: A genetic disorder caused by a mutation in the Huntingtin (Htt) gene, resulting in progressive motor, cognitive, and psychiatric symptoms.
    - Spinocerebellar ataxia: A group of genetic disorders that affect coordination and balance, causing problems with movement, speech, and eye movements.
    - Friedreich's ataxia: A rare genetic disorder caused by a mutation in the frataxin (FXN) gene leading to coordination, muscle weakness, and speech problems.
    - Charcot-Marie-Tooth disease: A group of genetic disorders that affect the peripheral nerves, leading to muscle weakness, loss of sensation, and balance and coordination problems.
    - Neurofibromatosis: A genetic disorder that causes neural tumors, leading to neurological symptoms, such as loss of sensation, muscle weakness, and visual deficits.
    - Duchenne muscular dystrophy: A genetic disorder that affects muscle function, leading to progressive muscle weakness and atrophy.
    - Rett syndrome: A genetic disorder that affects brain development, causing problems with communication, movement, and coordination.

- Spinal muscular atrophy: A genetic disorder affecting the motor neurons in the spinal cord, leading to progressive muscle weakness and wasting.
- Acquired. These disorders can be caused by a range of factors, including:
  - Traumatic brain injury (TBI). A nondegenerative insult to the brain from an external mechanical force, possibly leading to permanent or temporary impairments of cognitive, physical, and psychosocial functions with an associated diminished or altered state of consciousness. TBI is the major cause of death related to injury among Americans younger than 45, with the highest risk for individuals aged 15–24. In individuals aged 75 and older, falls are the most common cause of TBI. Injuries are divided into several categories:
    - Focal injuries, which tend to be caused by contact forces.
    - Diffuse injuries, which are more likely to be caused by noncontact, acceleration–deceleration, or rotational forces.
    - Hypoxic-ischemic injury, which results from a lack of oxygenated blood flow to the brain tissue.
    - Increased intracranial pressure (ICP), which can lead to cerebral hypoxia, cerebral ischemia, cerebral edema, hydrocephalus, and brain herniation.

  Several clinical rating scales exist to evaluate change in the patient over time. Two of the more commonly used scales are the Glasgow Coma Scale (GCS), which defines the severity of TBI within 48 hours of injury (**Table 12-1**), and the Rancho Los Amigos Cognitive Functioning Scale, which can determine the severity of deficit in cognitive functioning.

  The initial physical therapy role typically involves an interdisciplinary team, including the patient and family, physician, speech-language pathologist, occupational therapist, rehabilitation nurse, case manager, medical social worker, and neuropsychologist to prevent indirect impairments (e.g., skin breakdown, increased ICP, and hypoxia), managing the effects of abnormal tone and spasticity, improving arousal through multisensory stimulation in a highly structured and consistent manner, and the early transition to sitting postures as soon as medically stable. During the later stages, physical therapy focuses on improving function and independence by improving mobility and strength, using assistive devices, and cognitive and behavioral therapies to help with memory, attention, and emotional regulation.
  - Spinal cord injury (SCI). The extent and seriousness of an SCI's consequences depend on the lesion's location and severity. SCIs are complete or incomplete. A complete loss of motor and sensory function below the level of the traumatic lesion characterizes a complete cord syndrome.
    - Tetraplegia refers to complete paralysis of all four extremities and the trunk, including the respiratory muscles, and results from cervical cord lesions.

**Table 12-1 Glasgow Coma Scale**

|  | Test | Patient response | Score |
|---|---|---|---|
| Eye-opening | Spontaneous<br>To speech<br>To pain<br>To pain | Opens eyes<br>Opens eyes<br>Opens eyes<br>Does not open | 4<br>3<br>2<br>1 |
| Best verbal response | Speech | A conversation carried out correctly<br>Confused, disoriented<br>Inappropriate words<br>Unintelligible sounds only<br>Mute | 5<br>4<br>3<br>2<br>1 |
| Best motor response | Commands<br>To pain<br>To pain<br>To pain<br>To pain<br>To pain | Follows simple commands<br>Pulls the examiner's hand away<br>Pulls part of the body away<br>Flexes body to pain<br>Decerebrates<br>No motor response | 6<br>5<br>4<br>3<br>2<br>1 |

○ Paraplegia refers to complete paralysis of all or part of the trunk and lower extremities resulting from lesions of the thoracic or lumbar spinal cord or cauda equina.

Incomplete cord syndromes have variable neurologic findings with partial loss of sensory and/or motor function below the level of injury. In the acute care setting, physical therapy addresses respiratory management (deep breathing exercises, assisted coughing, airway clearance, abdominal support) as appropriate, pain management, maintenance of joint ROM and prevention of contractures, selective strengthening, orientation to the vertical position and increased sitting tolerance, independence with bed mobility as appropriate, independence in body handling skills (coming to sit, sitting balance, rolling, ischial pressure relief) as appropriate. In the later stages, the focus shifts to emphasize independence in wheelchair transfers to a mat, bed, car, toilet, bathtub, and floor as appropriate; independence in wheelchair mobility and safety as appropriate; independence in preventative measures (self-skin inspection; self lower extremity ROM exercises) as appropriate; the identification of therapeutic equipment needs; and gait training as appropriate. In patients with complete SCI or incomplete SCI without functional ambulation skills, interventions may include bracing accompanied by instruction in alternative gait patterns. Upon discharge, the patient may require a home assessment and subsequent modifications (e.g., ramp, door widening).

• Vestibular disorders. Dizziness is one of the most common complaints adults report to physicians, and the prevalence increases with age [18]. Dizziness is not so much a disease but a symptom of a disease. The four main categories of dizziness that patients describe include:

○ Vertigo. An illusion of motion (an illusion is a misperception of a real stimulus) that represents a disorder of the vestibular-proprioceptive system.

○ Near-syncope. Due to reduced blood flow to the entire brain. Common causes include orthostatic hypotension (anemia, volume depletion, antihypertensive medications), cardiac disease (cardiomyopathy, dysrhythmias, aortic stenosis), vasovagal episodes (or neurocardiogenic syncope), and

hyperventilation (decreases $pCO_2$, which constricts blood vessels in the brain).

○ Dysequilibrium. Essentially a gait disorder, most often caused by cervical spondylosis. Other causes include extrapyramidal disease and cerebellar disease.

○ Psychophysiologic dizziness. The least understood; it is thought to be due to altered central integration of sensory signals arising from normal end organs. Some patients are overfocused on normal physiological sensations, while others (such as those with a panic syndrome) may have a neurochemical imbalance.

The etiology of peripheral and central vestibular deficits includes the following: age-related multisensory deficits, strokes and vascular insufficiencies, cerebellar degeneration, acoustic neuroma, chemical and drug toxicities, benign paroxysmal positional vertigo (BPPV), motion sickness, uncompensated Ménière disease, vestibular neuritis, labyrinthitis, and head trauma. Balance disorders are significant risk factors for falls in older individuals. Falls are the leading cause of serious injury and death in persons older than 65. The role of physical therapy includes implementing safety measures: sensory substitution, compensatory strategies, prescribing assistive and adaptive equipment as appropriate, repositioning maneuvers (in the case of BPPV), and vestibular rehabilitation exercises and activities, which can include:

• Habituation training—repetition of movement and positions that provoke dizziness and vertigo.
• Eye exercises progress from slow to fast, including up and down and side-to-side eye movements.
• Head motions in all directions, progressing from slow to fast movements.
• Functional mobility training, emphasizing turning, rapid changes of direction, and activities involving spatial and timing constraints.

• CVA (stroke). A CVA encompasses a heterogeneous group of pathophysiologic causes, including thrombosis, embolism, and hemorrhage that results in a sudden loss of circulation to an area of the brain, resulting in a corresponding loss of neurologic function. CVAs are either ischemic or hemorrhagic, although the two can coexist.

○ Ischemic. The most common type; results from a clot that blocks or impairs blood flow.

○ Hemorrhagic. Less common but is associated with higher mortality rates than

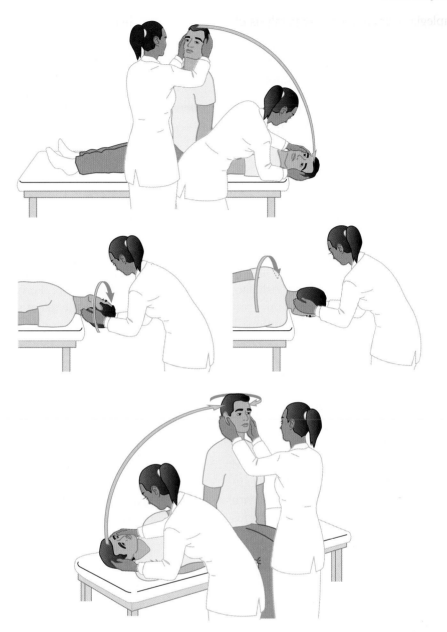

the ischemic variety [19]. Results from abnormal bleeding into the extravascular areas of the brain. Causes include but are not limited to intracranial aneurysms, hypertension, arteriovenous malformation (AVM), and anticoagulant therapy.

Common CVA symptoms include abrupt onset of hemiparesis, monoparesis, or quadriparesis; monocular or binocular visual loss; visual field deficits; diplopia; dysarthria; ataxia; vertigo; aphasia; or a sudden decrease in the level of consciousness. The treatment of CVA depends on the type of stroke and the time since the onset of symptoms.

○ Ischemic. Treatment may include thrombolytic therapy (administering tissue plasminogen activator [tPA] to dissolve the clot—most effective when given within 3–4.5 hours of the onset of symptoms), mechanical thrombectomy (using a catheter to remove the clot—most effective when given within 6 hours of the onset of symptoms), and antiplatelet and anticoagulant medications (to help prevent future blood clots from forming).

○ Hemorrhagic. Treatment may include controlling bleeding (e.g., medications and, sometimes, surgery) and monitoring and treatment for complications, such as seizures, swelling of the brain, and infections.

The recovery from a CVA depends on several factors, including the location and severity and the individual's age, sex, and number and type of comorbidities. Physical therapy aims to help individuals regain function and improve mobility, strength, and communication skills, including memory, attention, and problem-solving abilities. Assistive devices, such as wheelchairs, walkers, and canes, may be required to help with compensatory strategies with postural control and balance and address fall risks. The ability to perform sensorimotor, cognitive, or behavioral tasks involved with ADLs, such as gait, transfers, bed mobility, feeding, dressing, bathing, and toileting, can be improved through adaptation and training in the presence or absence of natural neurologic recovery. Strokes are largely preventable. Potentially modifiable risk factors include smoking, obesity, lack of exercise, diet, and excess alcohol consumption.

- Multiple sclerosis (MS): An inflammatory autoimmune demyelinating disease of the CNS—the PNS is rarely involved. MS patients commonly present with a mix of neuropsychological dysfunction depending on the location of the nerve demyelination, which tends to progress over years or decades. The diagnosis of MS is made by a neurologist based on the classic presentation of fatigue, weakness or numbness in the limbs, difficulty with coordination and balance, vision problems (blurred or double vision), muscle spasms and stiffness, bladder and bowel dysfunction, and cognitive impairment, including depression, memory, and attention problems. Medical management includes disease-modifying agents and management of relapses and symptoms. The physical therapy intervention is based on the impairments identified in the examination but typically includes regulation of activity level, relaxation, energy conservation techniques, normalization of muscle tone, adaptive/assistive device training, balance activities, gait training, exercises that emphasize core stabilization and trunk control, and patient and caregiver education.

- Parkinson's disease (PD): A progressive disorder that affects movement, causing tremors, stiffness, and difficulty with coordination and balance. Parkinsonism is a group of disorders that produce abnormalities of basal ganglia function. The three cardinal signs of PD are resting tremor, rigidity, and bradykinesia. Postural instability is another sign, but it emerges late in the disease. The medical management

for PD is largely pharmacologic and includes early neuroprotective and symptomatic therapy. Physical therapy aims to control signs and symptoms for as long as possible while attempting to prevent or minimize the secondary impairments associated with disuse and inactivity, including decreased ROM, weakness, and decreased aerobic capacity.

- Guillain–Barré syndrome (GBS): In its classic form, GBS is an acute inflammatory demyelinating polyneuropathy characterized by progressive symmetric ascending muscle weakness, paralysis, and hyporeflexia with or without sensory or autonomic symptoms. In severe cases, muscle weakness may lead to respiratory failure. Peripheral nerves and spinal roots are the major sites of demyelination, but cranial nerves also may be involved. GBS is believed to result from an autoimmune response—the typical GBS patient presents 2–4 weeks after a relatively benign respiratory or gastrointestinal illness complaining of dysesthesias of the fingers and lower extremity proximal muscle weakness. The weakness may progress over hours to days to involve the arms, truncal muscles, cranial nerves, and the muscles of respiration. The illness progresses over days to weeks. A plateau phase of persistent, unchanging symptoms ensues, followed days later by gradual symptom improvement. Up to one-third of patients require hospitalization for cardiac monitoring, plasma exchange, and mechanical ventilation during the disease. Pharmacological intervention often includes immunosuppressive and analgesic/narcotic medications. The role of physical therapy includes helping to maintain respiratory function, pulmonary (chest) physical therapy, prevention of indirect impairments (e.g., skin breakdown, contractures), splinting and positioning, muscle reeducation (through active assistance and active exercise progressing to resistive exercises), energy conservation techniques and activity pacing, and functional mobility and gait training progressions as appropriate.

- Amyotrophic lateral sclerosis (ALS): A slow, progressive degeneration of UMNs and LMNs characterizes ALS, commonly known as Lou Gehrig's disease. No single cause for ALS explains its entire pathology. UMN involvement of spinal cord tracts results in spastic weakness of the limbs (primary lateral sclerosis).

Later, the spread to other motor areas produces the classic combination of UMN and LMN dysfunction recognized as ALS. The medical intervention includes the use of disease-modifying agents for symptomatic management. The physical therapy role, which is restorative and geared toward remediating or improving impairments and functional limitations, includes maintenance of respiratory function (airway clearance techniques, cough facilitation, breathing exercises, chess stretching, suctioning, and incentive spirometry), prevention of indirect impairments (e.g., skin breakdown, contractures), splinting and positioning, aerobic exercises while carefully monitoring fatigue or overwork, functional training and progression, assistive devices, and adaptive equipment as appropriate, and patient, family, caregiver education.

- Encephalitis: An inflammatory infection of the brain parenchyma, usually caused by a viral infection, but it can also be caused by a bacterial, fungal, or parasitic infection or by an autoimmune reaction, producing a range of neurological symptoms, such as headache, fever, and seizures. As viral encephalitis is life-threatening, prompt identification and action by the PT/PTA are critical.
- Meningitis: An inflammation of the membranes covering the brain and spinal cord. Several factors influence the development of meningitis, including virulence of the strain, host defenses, and invader–host interactions. Swift identification by the PT/PTA can be life-saving. Classic symptoms (not evident in infants or seen often in older adults) include: headache; nuchal rigidity (discomfort on neck flexion); fever and chills; photophobia; vomiting; seizures; focal neurologic symptoms; altered sensorium (confusion may be the sole presenting complaint, especially in older adults).
- Brain neoplasm: Abnormal growths in the brain, which can be benign or cancerous but which cause a range of neurological symptoms, depending on the location, type, and size of the tumor.

Neurologic physical therapy occurs in acute care hospitals, skilled nursing facilities, rehabilitation hospitals, outpatient centers, or home care. Neurologic physical therapy approaches to treatments depend on the disease pathology and concentrate mostly on treating the patient's signs and symptoms. Impairments in neurologic physical therapy are pain, impaired balance and postural stability, impaired postural control, incoordination, delayed motor development, abnormal tone, and ineffective functional movement strategies.

The Academy of Neurologic Physical Therapy provides learning resources, such as the Journal of Neurologic Physical Therapy, special interest groups for specific neurologic diagnoses, information on current research initiatives, and opportunities for continuing education.

# A CASE STUDY

On your caseload today is a 27-year-old female patient diagnosed with relapsing-remitting multiple sclerosis (RRMS) that began 2 years ago. Three months within that year, the patient experienced her first relapse, which ultimately led to chronic fatigue, weakness, and impaired coordination of the lower extremities, impacting her ability to independently engage in ADLs. The patient has been prescribed physical therapy to help manage her weakness, incoordination, and fatigue and to learn techniques on how to self-manage her symptoms.

Your examination revealed:

- Subjective: reports of lower extremity weakness, gait difficulties, impaired balance and coordination, and fatigue.
- Current and Past Medical History: Unremarkable
- Social History: Patient lives with a partner in a bungalow with two steps to reach the entrance.
- Work History: Patient works as a fifth-grade teacher.
- Functional Status: Difficulty with simple housework due to fatigue and feelings of leg weakness prevents her from short walks outside the home.
- Self-Report Tests: Lower Extremity Function Questionnaire (LEFS): The patient scored 40/80.
- Fatigue Severity Scale (FSS): Patient scored a mean of 5.1.
- TUG: 10.8 seconds (just above the norm of ≤10 seconds).
- Berg Balance: 46/56 (an increased risk of falling)

- Neurologic:
  - Cranial nerve function tests: Normal except CN XII had decreased sensation and motor control over V1
  - Positive Babinski and clonus
  - LMN reflexes within normal limits (WNL) for upper extremity (UE)/lower extremity (LE)
  - Dermatomes: WNL
  - Myotomes: UE: WNL; LE: WNL
  - Resisted LE testing: WNL except knee flexors 4-/5, dorsiflexion (DF) and plantarflexion (PF) 4/5
  - Heel knee shin test: Minimal impairment
  - Finger-to-nose test: Minimal impairment with slightly less than normal control, speed, steadiness
  - Sensation testing: WNL for superficial and deep

Based on these findings, the physical therapy diagnosis is a 27-year-old female diagnosed with RRMS. In your groups, create:

A problem list for this patient and design both short-term (2-month) and long-term (6-month) goals.
Interventions to increase ROM, strength, balance, and aerobic conditioning.
A 12-week walking program.
A list of self-help strategies.

# Cardiopulmonary System

The heart is normally situated slightly to the left of the sternum in the human body. Unlike skeletal (striated) muscle, which has a neurogenic source for contraction (its motor nerve supply), cardiac muscle has a myogenic origin (an integral source of contraction). The heart has four chambers, two upper atria (singular: atrium) and two lower ventricles. Blood pumps through the heart chambers aided by four heart valves, which are flap-like structures that allow blood to flow in one direction. The left and right coronary arteries, which branch directly from the aorta near the aortic valve (sinus of Valsalva) supply the blood supply to the heart (coronary circulation). Every single beat of the heart involves a sequence of interrelated events known as the cardiac cycle (see **Box 12-2**). The cardiac cycle has three major stages: atrial systole, ventricular systole, and complete cardiac diastole.

- The atrial systole consists of the contraction of the atria. This contraction occurs during the last third of diastole and complete ventricular filling.
- The ventricular systole consists of the contraction of the ventricles and the flow of blood into the circulatory system.

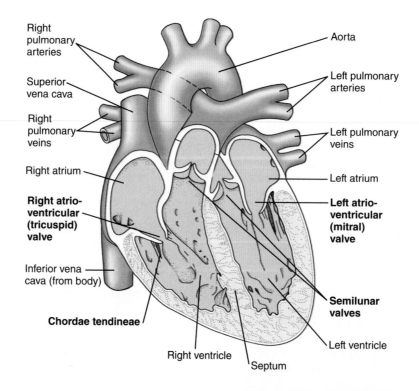

- The complete cardiac diastole involves the relaxation of the atria (atrial diastole) and ventricles (ventricular diastole) to prepare for refilling with circulating blood.

The magnitude at which the HR increases with increasing workloads depends on many factors, including age, fitness level, type of activity being performed, presence of disease, medications, blood volume, and environmental factors, such as temperature, humidity, and altitude. An inability of the heart to increase its rate with increasing workloads (chronotropic incompetence) should be of concern, even if the patient is taking beta-blockers [20]. Pulmonary arteries carry oxygen-deficient blood that has just returned from the body to the lungs.

The pulmonary system, also known as the respiratory system, which includes the lungs, airways, and respiratory muscles, exchanges oxygen and carbon dioxide between the body and the environment. The respiration process begins with inhaling air through the nose or mouth, which travels through the airways and into the lungs. The airways, which include the trachea, bronchi, and bronchioles, transport air to and from the lungs, while the respiratory muscles, including the diaphragm and intercostal muscles, help to control the volume and rate of breathing. The lungs exchange oxygen and carbon dioxide through tiny air sacs called alveoli, where oxygen is transferred into the bloodstream and carbon dioxide is removed. The respiratory system also plays a role in regulating acid–base balance and blood pressure.

## Cardiac Examination

The cardiovascular examination performed by the PT includes evaluation of the patient's medical status and history, physical examination, assessment of extremities, and the results of diagnostic tests. The patient's medical status and history assessment contain the patient's pain symptoms, including the differentiation among the types of pain (e.g., chest, angina, or myocardial infarction). Other patient symptoms can be **dyspnea** or shortness of breath, feelings of fatigue or generalized weakness, palpitations, such as heart rhythm abnormalities, dizziness, and edema. Physical examination of the patient with cardiac disorders assesses the patient's pulses, such as radial pulse, femoral pulse, popliteal pulse, and pedal pulse. It also includes listening to the patient's heart sounds, taking their blood pressure, and counting the respiratory rate (respiration).

---

### Box 12-2 Cardiac Terminology

- Pericardium: Fibrous, protective sac that encloses the heart.
- Epicardium: Inner layer of the pericardium.
- Myocardium: Heart muscle, the major portion of the heart.
- Endocardium: The smooth lining of the inner surface and cavities of the heart.
- Sinoatrial (SA) node: The main pacemaker of the heart, is located at the junction of the superior vena cava and right atrium. Under normal conditions, the SA node spontaneously generates an electrical impulse propagated to (and stimulates) the myocardium, causing a contraction.
- Stroke volume (SV): The amount of blood pumped out by the heart's left ventricle with each beat. The heart does not pump all the blood out of the ventricle—normally, only about two-thirds.
- Cardiac output (CO): The amount of blood discharged by each ventricle (not both ventricles combined) per minute, usually expressed as liters per minute. Factors influencing CO include venous pressure, HR, and left ventricular contractility [20]. CO is calculated by multiplying SV multiplied by HR. For example, if each ventricle has a rate of 72 beats per minute and ejects 70 mL with each beat, the CO = 72 beats/min × 0.07 L/beat = 5.0 L/min.
- Cardiac index: A valuable diagnostic and prognostic tool when treating patients with pulmonary hypertension (PH). Calculated as CO (liters) per unit time (minutes) divided by body surface area ($m^2$); normally calculated in liters per minute per square meter. The normal cardiac index ranges from 2.5 and 40.0 L/min/m.

---

## Cardiovascular signs and symptoms may include:

- Diaphoresis, which is excess sweating associated with decreased CO
- Decreased or absent pulses associated with peripheral vascular disease (PVD)
- Cyanotic skin, which is associated with decreased CO, or pallor, which is associated with PVD
- Skin temperature may indicate a lack of blood flow when it is cold
- Skin changes, such as pale, shiny, dry skin with loss of hair associated with PVD
- Bilateral edema can indicate congestive heart failure (CHF). Unilateral edema indicates thrombophlebitis or PVD.

The most accurate way to examine heart rhythm is to use an electrocardiogram (ECG). The other benefit of the ECG is that it is noninvasive. A typical ECG tracing of a normal heartbeat consists of a P wave, QRS complex, and T wave. The ST segment connects the QRS complex and the T wave.

P wave. The P wave is the electrical signature of the current that causes atrial contraction. Both the left and right atria contract simultaneously. Its relationship to QRS complexes determines a heart block [21].

The shape of the P waves may indicate atrial problems.

Irregular or absent P waves may indicate arrhythmia.

QRS complex. The QRS complex corresponds to the current that causes the contraction of the left and right ventricles. Abnormalities in the QRS complex may indicate bundle branch block (when wide), ventricular tachycardia, ventricular hypertrophy, or other ventricular abnormalities.

Very wide and deep Q waves indicate myocardial infarction that involves the full depth of the myocardium and has left a scar.

The R and S waves represent the contraction of the myocardium itself. The R wave is the first positive deflection in the ECG's QRS complex, representing the ventricles' depolarization. The S wave is the first negative deflection after the R wave in the QRS complex and represents the later stages of ventricular depolarization, as well as the early stages of ventricular repolarization. Changes in the R and S waves can be an indicator of heart problems, such as ventricular hypertrophy or myocardial infarction.

T wave. The T wave represents the repolarization (or relaxation) of the heart's ventricles, which occurs just before the heart muscle is ready to contract again. The T wave is usually a small, upward deflection on the ECG.

An abnormally tall or peaked T wave may be a sign of hyperkalemia (elevated levels of potassium in the blood).

A flattened or inverted T wave may be a sign of ischemia or other heart problems.

Interpreting ECG wave abnormalities occurs in conjunction with other clinical findings, such as symptoms and physical exam findings.

More invasive techniques can examine the cardiovascular system, including:

- Left heart catheterization/coronary angiogram [20]. This procedure involves inserting a catheter into a major artery (often the femoral or radial artery) and advancing retrograde through the aorta until it reaches the left ventricle. The catheter may then proceed into the left ventricle and is used to measure hemodynamic pressures during systole and diastole to examine left ventricular function (ejection fraction). The angiogram component involves injecting a radiopaque dye into the ostium of each coronary artery and observing blood flow through each artery to determine lesions or obstructions.
- Duplex ultrasonography. Duplex ultrasonography is the study of choice for evaluating venous insufficiency syndromes. Color-flow duplex imaging uses Doppler information to color code a two-dimensional sonogram. In the image, red indicates flow in one direction (relative to the transducer), and blue indicates flow in the other. With the latest-generation machines, the shade of the color may reflect the flow velocity (in the Doppler mode) or the flow volume (in the power Doppler mode).
- Magnetic resonance venography (MRV). MRV is the most sensitive and specific test for assessing deep and superficial venous disease in the lower legs and pelvis, areas not accessible with other modalities. MRV is particularly useful because it can help detect previously unsuspected nonvascular causes of leg pain and edema when the clinical presentation erroneously suggests venous insufficiency or obstruction.
- Direct contrast venography. Direct contrast venography is a labor-intensive and invasive imaging technique. In most centers, duplex sonography has replaced this direct contrast venography in the routine evaluation of venous disease.

The results of diagnostic tests can provide information about the HR, rhythm, conduction, areas of ischemia and infarction, increase in the heart size, and electrolyte imbalances. Electrolytes are mineral salts that conduct electricity in the body.

## Pulmonary Examination

The pulmonary examination (see **Figure 12-10**) performed by the PT provides a means of evaluating the patient through interviewing them about their chief complaints, such as a decreased ability to perform ADLs due to discomfort in breathing, such as dyspnea. The patient's history relative to their occupation needs to be assessed to evaluate, for example, for exposure to asbestos or silicon in their prior or present job. The PT must inquire about the patient's habits, such as smoking, alcohol consumption, or taking street drugs. The pulmonary physical therapy examination is like the cardiac examination, with the addition of inspection and palpation of the neck and thorax and listening to abnormal inspiration and expiration sounds. These sounds can be crackles (indicating a

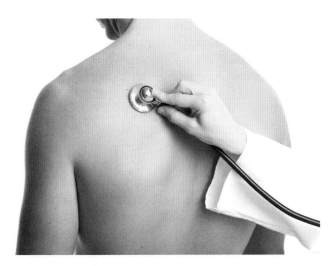

**Figure 12-10** PT performing auscultation of breath sounds.

© kurhan/Shutterstock

- Spirometry: This test measures how much air is inhaled and exhaled and at what speed. It is often used to diagnose and monitor COPD and asthma.
- Chest X-ray: This test produces images of the chest structures, including the lungs, heart, and blood vessels. It is commonly used to diagnose pneumonia, lung cancer, and other lung diseases.
- Computed tomography (CT) scan: This test uses X-rays to produce detailed images of the lungs and chest. It is often used to diagnose lung cancer, pulmonary embolism, and other lung diseases.
- Bronchoscopy: This test involves passing a thin, flexible tube with a camera down the throat and into the lungs to examine the airways and collect lung tissue or fluid samples. It is often used to diagnose lung infections, lung cancer, and other lung diseases.
- Pulse oximetry: This test uses a device that clips onto a finger to measure the oxygen saturation in the blood. It is often used to monitor the oxygen levels of people with respiratory conditions.
- Arterial blood gas test: This involves drawing blood from an artery to measure oxygen levels, carbon dioxide, and other gases in the blood. It is often used to diagnose and monitor respiratory failure and other lung diseases.

collapsed lung or pulmonary edema) or wheezes (indicating asthma or chronic obstructive pulmonary disease [COPD]). **Evaluation** of the patient's chest X-rays can detect abnormal material, such as blood, or a change in the lungs, such as collapse or fibrosis. The initial examination and evaluation must consider other test results. Several pulmonary diagnostic tests can help diagnose lung conditions and assess lung function. Some common tests include:

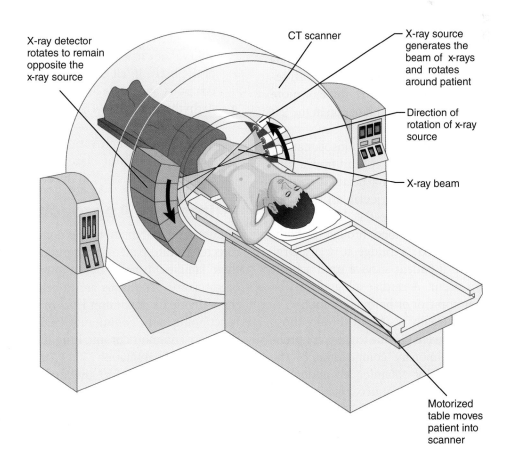

# Cardiopulmonary Surgery

There are several surgical procedures for the heart or blood vessels to treat a range of cardiac conditions, including:

- Heart valve repair. Surgery on defective heart valves is sometimes necessary in cases of mitral valve regurgitation. Surgical options include:
  - Mitral valve reconstruction with mitral annuloplasty, quadratic segmental resection, shortening of the elongated chordae, or posterior leaflet resection
  - Mitral valve replacement with either a mechanical valve (requiring lifelong anticoagulation) or a bioprosthetic porcine valve
- Percutaneous transluminal coronary angioplasty (PTCA). PTCA encompasses a variety of procedures used to treat patients with diseased arteries of the heart. Typically, PTCA involves threading a slender balloon-tipped catheter under fluoroscopy from an artery in the groin to a trouble spot in an artery of the heart. Once positioned correctly inside the lumen, the balloon is inflated, compressing the plaque and dilating the narrowed coronary artery, resulting in improved coronary blood flow, left ventricular function, and anginal relief.
- Coronary artery bypass graft (CABG). CABG surgery is a procedure that allows circumvention of an obstructed coronary artery using a healthy heart or vein taken from the patient's chest, leg, or arm (e.g., saphenous vein, internal mammary artery). CABG surgery often treats patients with severe coronary artery disease (CAD; three or more diseased arteries with impaired function in the left ventricle).
- Cardiac transplantation. Cardiac transplantation, the procedure by which another heart from a suitable donor replaces the failing heart, is used to treat end-stage CHF. A ventricular assist device (VAD) is a mechanical pump that helps a heart that is too weak to pump blood through the body. It is sometimes called "a bridge to transplant" since it can help a patient survive until a heart transplant can occur. A cardiac allograft can be sewn in a heterotopic or orthotopic position:
  - Heterotopic: usually restricted to only those patients with severe PH due to inherent problems (e.g., pulmonary compression of the recipient, difficulty obtaining an endomyocardial biopsy, need for anticoagulation).
  - Orthotopic: involves excision of the recipient's heart above the atrioventricular valves

and replacement with the donor's heart using either the classic Shumway-Lower technique or a bicaval anastomosis, which connects the superior and inferior vena cava (the two largest veins that return blood to the heart) of the donor's heart to the corresponding veins in the recipient. The graft includes the sinus node so that a sinus rhythm is possible after transplantation; however, some patients need lifelong pacing. Immunosuppression starts soon after surgery. Because the transplanted heart is denervated, it can respond to cardiovascular influences by humoral mechanisms but not by sympathetic or parasympathetic nerve stimulation.

- Transmyocardial revascularization (TMR). TMR is a laser surgery designed to improve myocardial oxygenation, eliminate or reduce angina, and improve the patient's cardiovascular function in those patients who are not candidates for bypass surgery or angioplasty. The surgeon makes an incision over the left breast to expose the heart. Using a laser, the surgeon interjects a strong energy pulse into the left ventricle, vaporizing the ventricular muscle and creating a transmural channel with a 1-mm diameter. Researchers do not thoroughly understand the precise physiologic mechanism for the efficacy of TMR.
- Aortic aneurysm repair. This involves replacing a weakened or bulging section of the aorta, the main artery that carries blood from the heart to the rest of the body. If left untreated, an aortic aneurysm can burst and cause life-threatening bleeding.
- Arrhythmia surgery. This procedure involves correcting abnormal heart rhythms, such as atrial fibrillation, through various procedures, such as catheter ablation or maze surgery (creating a series of small incisions in the atria).

## Pulmonary Approaches

Pulmonary rehabilitation is a continuum of services directed toward patients with pulmonary diseases and their families, usually by an interdisciplinary team of specialists. The goals are to achieve and maintain the individual's maximum level of independence and functioning in the community. COPDs and asthma are the most common chronic lung diseases that require pulmonary rehabilitation.

Pulmonary physical therapy interventions concentrate on secretion removal techniques. Secretion retention can interfere with ventilation and oxygen and carbon dioxide diffusion. Patients retaining secretions need an individualized program of secretion removal techniques directed to the areas of involvement.

Postural drainage techniques (also called chest physical therapy) are positional interventions. The patient is positioned so that the bronchus of the involved lung segment is perpendicular to the ground, and gravity assists in removing excessive secretions. Postural drainage drains and removes secretions from particular areas of the lungs. Besides the positioning, the PTA applies a percussion technique (using cupped hands) to a specific area of the patient's chest wall corresponding to an underlying lung segment to release pulmonary secretions.

# Cardiac and Pulmonary Conditions

Cardiac and pulmonary conditions can often coexist or influence each other.

- Cardiac conditions can include a wide range of conditions, such as CAD, heart failure, arrhythmias, and valve disorders.
- Pulmonary conditions can include a wide range of conditions that affect the lungs, such as asthma, COPD, pulmonary fibrosis, and lung cancer.

The following section describes some of the more common cardiopulmonary conditions.

### Congestive Heart Failure

**Congestive heart failure (CHF)** occurs when the heart fails to pump blood at a rate the metabolizing tissues require. CHF can be subdivided into systolic (left heart) and diastolic (right heart) dysfunction, both of which result in a decrease in SV.

- Systolic (impaired emptying of the heart) failure: A decrease in SV, which leads to activation of peripheral and central baroreflexes and chemoreflexes capable of eliciting marked increases in sympathetic nerve activity. Signs and symptoms of left-sided heart failure include progressive severity of (1) exertional dyspnea, (2) orthopnea (shortness of breath while lying flat), (3) paroxysmal nocturnal dyspnea, (4) dyspnea at rest, and (5) pulmonary edema.
- Diastolic (insufficient filling of the heart) failure: An altered relaxation of the ventricle (due to delayed calcium uptake and delayed calcium efflux) occurs in response to an increase in ventricular afterload (pressure overload). This impaired ventricle relaxation leads to impaired diastolic filling of the left ventricle and decreased SV. Signs and

symptoms of right-sided heart failure include ascites, congestive hepatomegaly, and anasarca (generalized edema).

### Coronary Artery Disease

CAD is a complex disease involving the lumen narrowing of one or more arteries that encircle and supply the heart, resulting in ischemia to the myocardium. Injury to the endothelial lining of arteries, an inflammatory reaction, thrombosis, calcification, and hemorrhage all contribute to arteriosclerosis or scarring of an artery wall. The clinical symptoms of CAD include any symptoms that may represent cardiac ischemia, such as an ache, pressure, pain, other discomforts, or possibly just decreased activity tolerance due to fatigue, shortness of breath, or palpitations.

### Angina Pectoris

Angina pectoris, commonly referred to as angina, results from myocardial ischemia caused by an imbalance between myocardial blood supply and oxygen demand, which causes myocardial cells to switch from aerobic to anaerobic metabolism, with a progressive impairment of metabolic, mechanical, and electrical functions. Angina can be stable (occurs during physical activity or stress and goes away with rest) or unstable (occurs at rest or with minimal activity and does not go away with rest). The symptoms of angina can include chest pain or discomfort, which may feel like pressure, squeezing, or fullness in the chest; pain or discomfort in the arms, neck, jaw, shoulder, or back; shortness of breath (dyspnea); fatigue; sweating; nausea or vomiting.

### Chronic Obstructive Pulmonary Disease

COPD is a generic term for lung diseases resulting in air trapping in the lungs, causing hyperinflation and a barrel chest deformity [22]. Airway narrowing, parenchymal destruction, and pulmonary vascular thickening characterize COPD. COPD can be subdivided into:

- Nonseptic obstructive pulmonary diseases include asthma, chronic bronchitis, emphysema, and $\alpha_1$-antitrypsin deficiency ($\alpha_1$ ATD).
- Septic obstructive pulmonary diseases include cystic fibrosis and bronchiectasis.

The medical management of chronic pulmonary disease includes smoking cessation, pharmacological agents, and supplemental oxygen.

## Restrictive Lung Disease

Restrictive lung disease is a grouping of diseases with differing etiologies. Unlike obstructive lung diseases, which cause airway obstruction and difficulty exhaling, restrictive lung diseases result in difficulty inhaling. Some examples of restrictive lung diseases include:

- Interstitial lung disease: A group of disorders that cause inflammation and scarring in the lung tissue, reducing the ability of the lungs to expand and fill with air.
- Sarcoidosis: A condition that causes the formation of granulomas, or small clusters of inflamed cells, in various parts of the body, including the lungs.
- Pulmonary fibrosis is when the lung tissue becomes scarred and stiff, reducing its ability to expand and fill with air.
- Obesity hypoventilation syndrome: A condition in which obesity causes the chest wall to become compressed, making it more difficult to breathe.

Symptoms of restrictive lung disease can include shortness of breath, cough, and chest pain.

Cardiovascular and pulmonary physical therapy treats patients with cardiac and pulmonary conditions that need physical therapy. In cardiovascular and pulmonary rehabilitation, the PTA must be able to reassess the patient as necessary, monitor the patient concerning treatment, monitor the patient's vital signs, and provide appropriate interventions. The clinical presentations of cardiovascular disease are diverse. CAD and CHF are the most common cardiac diagnoses referred for direct physical therapy interventions. Pulmonary rehabilitation is a continuum of services directed toward patients with pulmonary diseases and their families, usually by an interdisciplinary team of specialists. The goals of cardiovascular and pulmonary physical therapy are to achieve and maintain the individual's maximum level of independence and functioning in the community.

The Cardiovascular and Pulmonary section of the APTA publishes the Cardiopulmonary Physical Therapy Journal for information on current research. Another group, the American Association of Cardiovascular and Pulmonary Rehabilitation, provides educational opportunities for further study in this specialty area.

# Integumentary Physical Therapy

The integumentary system comprises the dermal and epidermal layers of the skin, hair follicles, nails, sebaceous glands, and sweat glands. The integument or skin is the body's largest organ system, constituting 15–20% of the body weight [23]. Key functions of the skin include:

- Protection against injury or invasion
- Secretion of oils that lubricate the skin
- Maintains homeostasis by fluid balance, regulation of body temperature
- Excretion of excess water, urea, and salt via sweat
- Maintenance of body shape
- Provides cosmetic appearance and identity
- Vitamin D synthesis
- Provides cutaneous sensation via receptors in the dermis

Anatomically, the skin has two distinct layers of tissue: the epidermis and the dermis. A third layer involved in the anatomical consideration of the skin is the subcutaneous fat cell layer directly under the dermis and above the muscle fascial layers [23]. The epidermis is the superficial, protective layer, while the dermis, considered the "true" skin because it contains sebaceous and sweat glands, blood vessels, lymphatics, nerves, collagen, and elastic fibers, is deeper and thicker than the epidermis [23]. Injury to the skin can occur in several ways:

- Abrasion: A wearing away of the upper layer of the skin due to applied friction force.
- Contusion: Caused when blood vessels are damaged or broken due to a direct blow to the skin.
- Ecchymosis: Skin discoloration caused by the escape of blood into the tissues from ruptured blood vessels.
- Hematoma: A localized collection of blood, usually clotted, in a tissue or organ.
- Excoriation: Lesion of traumatic nature with epidermal loss in a generally linear shape.
- Laceration: An injury involving skin penetration, in which the wound is deeper than the superficial skin level.
- Penetrating wound: A wound accompanied by disruption of the body surface that extends into the underlying tissue or a body cavity.
- Petechiae: Petechiae (tiny red spots in the skin that do not blanch when pressed upon) result from red blood leaking from capillaries into the skin (intradermal hemorrhages). Petechiae are less than 3 mm in diameter.
- Puncture: A wound made by a pointed object (like a nail).
- Ulcer: A lesion on the surface of the skin or the surface of the mucous membrane produced by the sloughing of inflammatory, necrotic tissue.

Wound healing involves four overlapping phases: hemostasis, inflammation, proliferation, and remodeling.

- Hemostasis: This phase begins immediately after injury and involves the formation of a blood clot to stop bleeding. Platelets in the blood form a temporary plug at the injury's site, which helps prevent further blood loss.
- Inflammation: This phase typically lasts several days and involves recruiting immune cells to the injury site. These cells remove dead tissue and pathogens and release growth factors that help promote the next healing phase.
- Proliferation: During this phase, new tissue forms to fill the wound. Fibroblasts, cells that produce collagen and other extracellular matrix proteins, form a scaffold for new tissue growth. Blood vessels also grow into the wound, providing oxygen and nutrients for healing.
- Remodeling: This final phase can last several months or even years and involves the remodeling and maturation of the new tissue. Collagen fibers are reorganized and cross-linked to form stronger, more resilient tissue. The blood vessels that infiltrated the wound are gradually removed.

Factors that can affect wound healing include the type and location of the wound, age, nutrition, comorbidities (e.g., diabetes or peripheral artery disease), and medications.

The PT and the PTA treating skin disorders have to be knowledgeable in the function and examination of the integumentary system and common skin disorders. During the skin examination and evaluation, the PT assesses the patient for pruritus (itching), rashes, excessive skin dryness, edema (swelling), unusual skin growths, changes in skin color and temperature, sensory integrity, pain, and soreness. The skin examination may indicate other system disorders, such as skin color changes showing cyanotic skin, characterized by bluish-gray discoloration; this could verify a lack of oxygen and excess carbon dioxide in the blood, which a respiratory disorder may cause. Circulatory, cardiac, or renal diseases can also cause edematous skin, and a positive examination for excessive skin dryness may indicate system dysfunction, such as diabetes or thyroid problems.

Besides treating skin disorders, a large part of integumentary physical therapy assesses wounds and burns (see **Figure 12-11**).

Some PTs specialize in wound management. Physical therapy wound examination and evaluation are complex processes resulting in information critical in determining the diagnosis and prognosis and developing the POC. The APTA's Guide to Physical

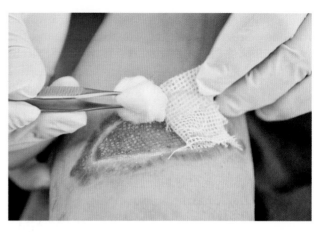

**Figure 12-11** PT assessing a wound.
© Anukool Manoton/Shutterstock

Therapist Practice provides a documentation template that delineates the necessary information to gather in the initial examination and evaluation of a wound regarding patient history, systems review, and tests and measures. Examples of tests and measures to establish wound characteristics include:

- Location of the wound
- Size, depth, and drainage of the wound
- Skin changes
- Involved tissue's color and temperature
- Involved extremity's girth, tissue, and sensation

The wound needs to be described using anatomical landmarks. For the wound size, the PT or the PTA can use a film grid or a clear plastic sheet to measure the length and width of the wound. Wound depth is assessed by inserting the tip of a sterile cotton swab into the deepest part of the base of the wound. Wound drainage indicates wound healing or infection.

- Serous: Presents as clear, light color with a thin, watery consistency. Serous exudate is considered normal in a healthy healing wound.
- Sanguinous: Present as red with a thin, watery consistency. Appears to be red due to the presence of blood or maybe brown if allowed to dehydrate. Typically indicative of new blood vessel growth or the disruption of blood vessels.
- Serosanguinous: Present as light red or pink, with a thin, watery consistency. This can be normal in a healthy healing wound.
- Seropurulent: Presents an opaque, yellow, or tan color with a thin, watery consistency. Seropurulent exudate may be an early warning sign of an impending infection.
- Purulent: Presents as a yellow or green with a thick, viscous consistency. This type of exudate is generally an indicator of wound infection.

Monitoring the healing process also involves tracking skin changes of the wound and around the wound during healing. The Red-Yellow-Black (RYB) system, or "color code" system, can describe the different stages of wound healing and provide a simple way to assess the progress of wound healing. In the RYB system for wounds, red, yellow, and black are used to describe the different tissues that can be present in a wound:

- Red: Healthy granulation tissue is typically bright red and indicates the proliferation phase of wound healing. Granulation tissue comprises new blood vessels and connective tissue, providing a scaffold for new tissue growth.
- Yellow: Yellow tissue in a wound can indicate slough, dead tissue that the body's natural processes have not yet removed. Slough is typically yellow or white and may be moist or dry.
- Black: Black tissue in a wound can indicate eschar, which is dead tissue that has dried and hardened. Eschar is typically black or brown and can be hard or soft.

Using the RYB system, the PT can quickly assess the progress of wound healing and determine whether additional interventions are needed to promote healing. For example, a wound with a large amount of yellow or black tissue may indicate the need for debridement.

The burn examination and evaluation performed by the PT is also complex because it considers the pathophysiology of the burn wound. For example, a burn wound has three zones: (1) the zone of coagulation, where the cells are dead; (2) the zone of stasis, where the cells are injured and can die without specialized treatment; and (3) the zone of hyperemia, where the injury is minimal, and the cells can recover. In addition, the severity of the damaged tissue classifies the burn degree as superficial, superficial partial thickness, deep partial thickness, and full thickness. For example, a common superficial burn is a sunburn. The damage in sunburn is limited to the outer layer of the skin, or epidermis, and is marked by tenderness, redness, and mild pain. The extent of the burned area

is ranked using the rule of nines for estimating the percentage of body surface areas.

Different percentages are used to classify children's burns. In addition, there are classifications regarding percentages of body area burned related to possible patient complications, such as respiratory involvement, smoke inhalation, and skin destruction.

The Vancouver Burn Scar Scale (VBSS), which assesses burn scar severity and functional impact, was developed to provide a standardized method for evaluating the physical, functional, and psychological impact of burn scars and to guide treatment planning and monitoring. The VBSS assesses burn scars based on the following parameters:

- Pigmentation: This refers to the color of the scar, which can range from normal skin color to hyperpigmented (darker than surrounding skin) or hypopigmented (lighter than surrounding skin).
- Vascularity: The amount and visibility of blood vessels in the scar, which can indicate the degree of inflammation and tissue remodeling.
- Pliability: The scar tissue's degree of flexibility and mobility, which can affect joint function and ROM.
- Height: The amount of elevation or depression of the scar compared to the surrounding skin.
- Symptoms: Any pain, itching, or other symptoms associated with the scar.

Each parameter scores on a scale of 0–3, with higher scores indicating greater severity or functional impact. The scores are then added up to provide an overall score for the scar, ranging from 0 to 15.

Various factors, including physical trauma, chemical exposure, radiation, infection, vascular insufficiency, and systemic diseases, can cause integumentary injuries. The following sections describe some of the more common integumentary conditions.

- Pressure ulcer. The terms "pressure ulcer" and "decubitus ulcer" are often used interchangeably, but because the common denominator of these ulcerations is pressure, a pressure ulcer is more accurate. Pressure ulcers result from sustained or prolonged pressure at levels greater than the capillary filling pressure on the tissue, which causes localized ischemia and/or tissue necrosis. Pressure against the skin over a bony prominence (**Table 12-2**) increases the risk of necrosis and ulceration.

Pressure ulcers can be graded using a four-stage system (**Table 12-3**).

Most pressure ulcers are avoidable. Prevention of pressure ulcers involves multiple members of the healthcare team. The groups of patients most

The rule of nines for an adult:
- The head represents 9%.
- Each upper extremity is 9%.
- The back of the trunk is 18%.
- The front of the trunk is 18%.
- Each LE is 18%.
- The perineum is the remaining 1%.

**Table 12-2** **Bony Prominences Associated With Pressure Ulcers**

| Supine | Prone | Side Lying | Seated |
|---|---|---|---|
| Occiput<br>Spine of scapula<br>The inferior angle of the scapula<br>Vertebral spinous processes<br>Medial epicondyle of humerus<br>Posterior iliac crest<br>Sacrum<br>Coccyx<br>Heel | Forehead<br>The anterior portion of the acromion process<br>Anterior head of the humerus<br>Sternum<br>Anterior superior iliac spine<br>Patella<br>Dorsum of foot | Ears<br>The lateral portion of the acromion process<br>The lateral head of the humerus<br>Lateral epicondyle of humerus<br>Greater trochanter<br>Head of the fibula<br>Lateral malleolus<br>Medial malleolus | Spine of scapula<br>Vertebral spinous processes<br>Ischial tuberosities |

**Table 12-3** **Pressure Ulcer Grading**

| Stage | Characteristics |
|---|---|
| Stage I | An observable pressure-related alteration of intact skin whose indicators, as compared to an adjacent or opposite area of the body, may include changes in skin color, skin temperature (warm or cool), tissue consistency (firm or boggy), and/or sensation (pain, itching). |
| Stage II | A partial thickness skin loss that involves the epidermis and/or dermis. The ulcer is superficial and presents clinically as an abrasion, a blister, or a shallow crater. |
| Stage III | A full-thickness skin loss involves damage or necrosis of subcutaneous tissue that may extend down to, but not through, underlying fascia. The ulcer presents clinically as a deep crater with or without undermining adjacent tissue. |
| Stage IV | A full-thickness skin loss with extensive destruction, tissue necrosis, or damage to muscle, bone, or supporting structures (e.g., tendon, joint capsule). Undermining or sinus tracts may be present. |

susceptible include older individuals, those with neurological impairment, and those who are acutely hospitalized. Other contributing factors to pressure ulcers include shear, friction, heat, maceration (softening associated with excessive moisture), medication, malnutrition, and muscle atrophy. Risk factors associated with ulcers include:

- Emaciation. Bony prominences should be protected and pressure distributed equally over large surface areas. The use of pressure distribution equipment, such as wheelchair cushions, custom mattresses, and alternating pressure mattress pads, is advocated. Patients should avoid movements that rub, drag, or scratch the skin.
- Immobilization. Patients should be turned every 2 hours when in bed, and weight shifting should occur every 15–20 minutes when seated.
- Decrease in activity level. Regular cardiovascular exercise are recommended with a gradual buildup of skin tolerance for new activities, equipment, and positions.
- Diabetes and other circulatory disorders. Regular skin inspections should occur.
- Incontinence. Good bowel and bladder care is paramount, with immediate cleansing after an episode of incontinence, and there should be current cleansing and drying of skin at least once daily. The skin should be inspected for areas of redness in the morning (a.m.) and evening (p.m.).
- Impaired mental status
- Arterial insufficiency ulcer. As the name suggests, these ulcers develop from a diminished blood supply. Arterial insufficiency ulcers are common in the diabetic population due to several metabolic abnormalities and occur most often on the distal aspects of the feet but may occur more proximally, depending on the location of the occluded artery. These ulcers have a punched-out appearance with a pale granulation base. Symptomatic patients may present with intermittent claudication, ischemic pain at rest, nonhealing ulceration, or frank

foot ischemia. Signs frequently associated with arterial ulcers include a loss of hair on the extremity, poor capillary refill in the toes, and brittle nails. The intervention focuses on cleansing the ulcer, resting, reducing risk factors, and limb protection. Patient education emphasizes:

- Washing and drying feet thoroughly
- Inspecting legs and feet daily
- Avoiding unnecessary leg elevation
- Wearing appropriately sized shoes with clean, seamless socks
- Using bandages as necessary and avoiding any unnecessary pressure
- Avoiding using heating pads or soaking feet in hot water

- Neuropathic ulcers. This type of ulcer is a secondary complication associated with neuropathy, such as that which occurs with diabetes. The pathophysiology of diabetic peripheral neuropathy is multifactorial but results in a loss of sensation in the foot. Unnoticed excessive heat or cold, pressure from a poorly fitting shoe, or damage from a blunt or sharp object inadvertently left in the shoe may cause blistering and ulceration. These factors, combined with poor arterial inflow, confer a high risk of limb loss. Neuropathic ulcers frequently occur in those areas that are most subjected to weight bearing, such as the heel, plantar metatarsal head areas, the tips of the most prominent toes (usually the first or second), and the tips of hammer toes. Ulcers also occur over the malleoli because these areas commonly are subjected to trauma.

- Venous insufficiency ulcers. Valvular incompetence in the high-pressure deep venous system, the low-pressure superficial venous system, or both causes venous insufficiency syndromes. The poor clearance of lactate, carbon dioxide, and other products of cellular respiration also contributes to the development of the syndrome. Untreated venous insufficiency in the deep or superficial system causes a progressive syndrome involving pain, swelling, skin changes, and eventual tissue breakdown. Most venous ulcers are caused by venous reflux that is purely or largely confined to the superficial venous system. Only a minority is caused by chronic DVT or valvular insufficiency in the deep veins. Venous ulcers typically are located over the medial malleolus area. They tend to be irregular in shape and possess a good granulation base. The most common subjective symptoms are leg aching, swelling, cramping, heaviness, and soreness, which are improved by walking or elevating the legs.

The intervention focuses on cleansing the ulcer and applying compression to control the edema. Patient education emphasizes:

- Elevating the ulcer above the heart when resting or sleeping
- Attempting active exercise, including frequent ROM exercises
- Inspecting legs and feet daily
- Wearing appropriately sized shoes with clean, seamless socks
- Using bandages as necessary and avoiding scratching or direct contact

The four primary principles of wound care are:

1. Wound cleansing: Removing loose cellular debris, devitalized tissue, metabolic wastes, bacteria, and topical agents that retard wound healing. The wound is cleansed initially and then at each dressing change.
2. Management of edema: Moisture levels in the wound should be balanced to optimize healing and prevent excessive fluid accumulation.
3. Reduction of necrosis: Targets harnessing endogenous systems (enzymes) to remove necrotic tissue in conjunction with dressings and debridement technologies. Harsh soaps, alcohol-based products, or harsh antiseptic agents should be avoided as they may erode the skin and create an imbalance in the hydration of the wound.
4. Control of microorganism level (bioburden management) aimed at reducing wound-bed microorganism levels through facilitating the body's normal immune response and using cleansing/debridement technologies and appropriate topical or systemic antimicrobials.

## Integumentary Interventions

Physical therapy's role in managing individuals with chronic wounds has extended to developing wound care centers within physical therapy departments. Wound interventions need treatments different from those for skin disorders (see **Figure 12-12**). Wound care interventions may consist of wound cleansing; wound debridement; wound dressing; and observing the patient's vital signs, nutritional considerations, and positioning (if necessary). Wound cleansing involves the removal of cellular debris, bacteria, or fungus utilizing different topical agents. Modalities such as electrotherapy, ultrasound, hydrotherapy, and negative-pressure therapy may assist in wound healing. Wound debridement removes necrotic tissue, bacteria, and fungus utilizing selective and nonselective

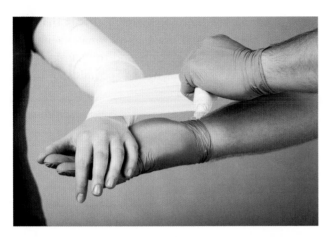

**Figure 12-12** Wound care bandaging.
© Photographee.eu/Shutterstock

debridement procedures. Physicians may prescribe topical agents to prevent and treat an infection or debride via enzymatic and autolytic debridement agents. Per the APTA [1], the PT is the only individual who can use sharp and surgical instruments, such as scalpels, forceps, and scissors to clean devitalized tissue in selective debridement procedures. Various wound dressings are available, and the PT and PTA must consider whether the wound is dry, moist, or infected when applying dressings. Patient education on wound care, preventative skin care practices, and lifestyle choices that promote good health may also be part of PT integumentary interventions.

Physical therapy for burn care consists of the following:

- Hydrotherapy using whirlpool or aquatic therapy
- Debridement
- Positioning of the affected body part
- ROM exercises
- Elastic or pressure garments to prevent scarring
- Edema control
- Strengthening exercises
- Breathing exercises
- Functional training

During wound and burn care, the PT and the PTA need to follow standards of safety and infection control, such as handwashing; wearing personal protective equipment, such as gloves, mask, eye protection, and gown; cleaning and discarding patient care equipment; environmental cleaning and disinfection of the work area; and occupational health and bloodborne pathogens standards.

Scar management involves various techniques to minimize the appearance and functional impact of scars. Several factors, including surgical incisions, wounds, burns, and skin conditions, such as acne, can cause scars. Some common scar management techniques include:

- Silicone therapy: Silicone sheets or gels can be applied to scars to help flatten and soften the tissue. Silicone hydrates and protects the skin and can be especially effective for hypertrophic scars and keloids.
- Compression therapy: Compression garments or bandages can help reduce swelling and improve blood flow to the scar tissue. Compression therapy can be especially effective for burn scars and hypertrophic scars.
- Massage: Gentle scar tissue massage can help improve circulation, reduce swelling, and promote tissue remodeling. Massage should be done with a moisturizer or oil to reduce friction and prevent further damage to the scar.
- Laser therapy: Laser treatment can reduce the redness and thickness of scars and improve their texture and appearance. Laser therapy can be effective for both hypertrophic scars and keloids.
- Surgery: In some cases, surgical intervention may be necessary to remove or revise a scar. Surgery may involve excision of the scar tissue, skin grafting, or flap surgery to reposition nearby tissue to cover the scar.

Patient education plays a critical role in the intervention and prevention of integumentary disorders. The clinician should determine those activities, positions, and postures that produce or reduce trauma to the skin and the level of safety awareness that the patient demonstrates during functional activities. In addition, the following should be addressed:

- The likelihood of future trauma to the skin
- Enhanced disease awareness and healthy behaviors
- Mechanisms of pressure ulcer development. These include assistive, adaptive, protective, orthotic, or prosthetic devices that produce or reduce skin trauma
- Avoidance of prolonged positions
- Safety awareness during self-care and use of devices and equipment
- Importance of ongoing activities/exercise program
- Daily, comprehensive skin inspection, paying particular attention to bony prominences
- Avoidance of harsh soaps, known irritants, temperature extremes, and exacerbating factors or triggers
- Avoidance of restrictive clothing and tight-fitting shoes and socks
- Incontinence management strategies
- Enhance ADLs, functional mobility, and safety
- Pressure relieving devices

- Enhance self-management of symptoms
- Edema management through leg/arm elevation, muscle pumping exercises, and compression therapy to facilitate the movement of excess fluid from the extremity
  - Compression wraps: Elastic or tubular bandages
  - Compression stockings, e.g., Jobst
  - Compression pump therapy
- Review of medications. The following medications can harm wound repair: NSAIDs, corticosteroids, immunosuppressives, anticoagulants, and prostaglandins.

PTs may specialize in caring for people with open wounds or burns. Specialized courses of study increase the knowledge of PTs and PTAs in this area. PTs and PTAs may become Certified Wound Care Specialists through several agencies, including the National Alliance of Wound Care and Ostomy and the American Board of Wound Management. Besides healing the wound or burn, goals include maintaining functional movements and strength and the prevention of further skin damage due to disease or pressure.

The APTA's Academy of Clinical Electrophysiology and Wound Care section provides a framework for PT entry-level skills. Research journals that can provide evidence-based practice information include *Advances in Skin & Wound Care* and the *Journal of the American College of Clinical Wound Specialists*.

## KNOWLEDGE CHECK

Why are physical agents used?

What assistive devices are used for gait?

What are the different types of neurologic interventions?

What is the purpose of cardiac rehabilitation?

What psychosocial care components are important to examine when working with a patient with a progressive neurologic disease?

What are the common symptoms of cardiopulmonary disease?

What diagnoses are being screened for with the Mini-Mental State Examination?

Why is it important for PTs to assess the skin of a patient?

Which practice areas overlap with all the other practice areas?

While each practice area differs, what is the common patient goal they share?

# References

1. American Physical Therapy Association: Guide to Physical Therapist Practice 3.0. Alexandria, VA, American Physical Therapy Association, 2014

2. Morris C, Chaitow L, Janda V: Functional Examination for Low Back Syndromes, in Morris C (ed): Low Back Syndromes: Integrated Clinical Management. New York, McGraw-Hill, 2006, pp 333–416

3. Resnick DN, Morris C: History and Physical Examination for Low Back Syndromes, in Morris C (ed): Low Back Syndromes: Integrated Clinical Management. New York, McGraw-Hill, 2006, pp 305–331

4. Downs MB, Laporte C: Conflicting dermatome maps: educational and clinical implications. J Orthop Sports Phys Ther 41(6):427–434, 2011

5. O'Sullivan SB, Schmitz TJ, Fulk G: Examination of Sensory Function, in O'Sullivan SB, Schmitz TJ, Fulk G (ed): Physical Rehabilitation, 7th ed. Philadelphia, PA, F.A. Davis, 2019

6. Martin G: Aquatic Therapy in Rehabilitation, in Prentice WE, Voight ML (eds): Techniques in Musculoskeletal Rehabilitation. New York, McGraw-Hill, 2001, pp 279–287

7. Thein-Brody L: Aquatic Physical Therapy, in Hall C, Thein-Brody L (eds): Therapeutic Exercise: Moving Toward Function. Baltimore, MD, Lippincott Williams & Wilkins, 2005, pp 330–347

8. Bergh C, Wennergren D, Möller M, et al: Fracture incidence in adults in relation to age and gender: a study of 27,169 fractures in the Swedish Fracture Register in a well-defined catchment area. PLoS One 15(12):e0244291, 2020

9. Hoare B, Wasiak J, Imms C, et al: Constraint-induced movement therapy in the treatment of the upper limb in children with hemiplegic cerebral palsy. Cochrane Database Syst Rev (2):CD004149, 2007

10. Wu CY, Chen CL, Tsai WC, et al: A randomized controlled trial of modified constraint-induced movement therapy for elderly stroke survivors: changes in motor impairment, daily functioning, and quality of life. Arch Phys Med Rehabil 88(3):273–278, 2007

11. Boake C, Noser EA, Ro T, et al: Constraint-induced movement therapy during early stroke rehabilitation. Neurorehabil Neural Repair 21(1):14–24, 2007

12. Mark VW, Taub E, Morris DM: Neuroplasticity and constraint-induced movement therapy. Eura Medicophys 42(3):269–284, 2006

13. Morris DM, Taub E, Mark VW: Constraint-induced movement therapy: characterizing the intervention protocol. Eura Medicophys 42(3):257–268, 2006

14. Smania N: Constraint-induced movement therapy: an original concept in rehabilitation. Eura Medicophys 42(3):239–240, 2006

15. O'Sullivan SB: Strategies to Improve Motor Function, in O'Sullivan SB, Schmitz TJ (eds): Physical Rehabilitation. Philadelphia, PA, F.A. Davis, 2007, pp 471–522

16. Winstein CJ: Motor Learning Considerations in Stroke Rehabilitation, in Duncan PW, Badke MB (eds): Stroke Rehabilitation: The Recovery of Motor Control. Chicago, Yearbook Medical Publishers, Inc., 1987, pp 109–134

17. Unsworth CA: Cognitive and Perceptual Dysfunction, in O'Sullivan SB, Schmitz TJ (eds): Physical Rehabilitation. Philadelphia, PA, F.A. Davis, 2007, pp 1149–1188

18. Sloane PD, Coeytaux RR, Beck RS, et al: Dizziness: state of the science. Ann Intern Med 134(9 Pt 2):823–832, 2001

19. Locksley HB: Hemorrhagic strokes. Principal causes, natural history, and treatment. Med Clin North Am 52(5): 1193–1212, 1968

20. Grimes K: Heart Disease, in O'Sullivan SB, Schmitz TJ (eds): Physical Rehabilitation. Philadelphia, PA, F.A. Davis, 2007, pp 589–641

21. Cahalin LP: Cardiovascular Evaluation, in DeTurk WE, Cahalin LP (eds): Cardiovascular and Pulmonary Physical Therapy: An Evidence-Based Approach. New York, McGraw-Hill, 2004, pp 273–324

22. Wells C: Pulmonary Pathology, in DeTurk WE, Cahalin LP (eds): Cardiovascular and Pulmonary Physical Therapy: An Evidence-Based Approach. New York, McGraw-Hill, 2004, pp 151–188

23. Richard RL, Ward RS: Burns, in O'Sullivan SB, Schmitz TJ (eds): Physical Rehabilitation. Philadelphia, PA, F.A. Davis, 2007, pp 1091–1115

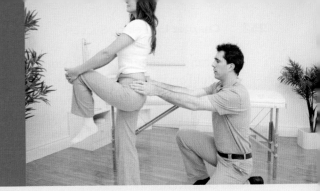

# CHAPTER 13

# Lifelong Success

## OBJECTIVES

- Identify attributes that lead to successful careers.
- Describe strategies for developing a satisfying career.
- Develop strategies to gain employment.
- Create a career plan.

## KEY TERMS

competence                    initiative                    networking

As students enter a new professional program, it may be difficult to imagine career success and project future happiness. If one stops to consider their life's journey, it may be very helpful to consider developing skills and a mindset that can lead to those goals. Developing skills and enhancing personality traits may be the difference between a satisfying job and one that just pays the bills.

## Attributes of Successful People

Success is a subjective concept, and what constitutes success can vary greatly from person to person. However, there are certain attributes and qualities that are commonly associated with successful people. Some of the most important attributes of successful people include:

- A positive can-do attitude: Successful people have a positive outlook on life and see challenges as opportunities for growth and improvement. They

maintain a can-do attitude and remain optimistic, even in the face of adversity.

- Hard work: Successful people will put in the time and effort required to achieve their goals. They are persistent, determined, and unafraid to work hard to reach their full potential.

- Self-discipline: Successful people possess strong self-discipline, which allows them to focus on their goals and avoid distractions. They can prioritize their tasks, set boundaries, and avoid procrastination.

- Strong work ethic: Successful people have a strong work ethic and take pride in their work. They are committed to excellence and will put in the extra effort required to achieve their goals.

- Adaptability: Successful people are adaptable and able to adjust to changing circumstances. They can pivot and change direction when necessary and are not afraid to take calculated risks.

- Good communication skills: Successful people have strong communication skills, which allows them to articulate their ideas and goals effectively.

They can communicate with people at all levels and build and maintain strong relationships.

- Emotional intelligence: Successful people possess high levels of emotional intelligence, which allows them to understand and manage their own emotions and the emotions of others. They can build strong relationships, resolve conflicts, and lead effectively.
- Continuous learning: Successful people are life-long learners who seek new opportunities to grow and improve. They are open to new ideas and will invest in self-development.

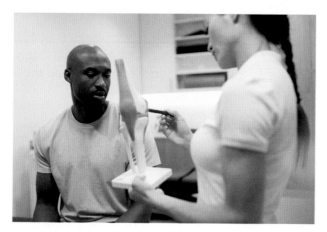

© Hero Images/Getty Images

**KNOWLEDGE CHECK**

What are the attributes of successful people?

# Developing a Career

## Mentors

As a student, it may be helpful to identify working members of the profession who might act as mentors. Mentors can assist students in navigating the transition from the classroom to the clinic to their first job. Mentors may be found through joining the national, state, and college physical therapy organizations, via alumni of the college the student is attending, or through hometown physical therapy community members. Creating a relationship with a mentor can help a student understand the expectations and behaviors that will lead them to job opportunities and career success. The American Physical Therapy Association (APTA) offers a mentoring program for new graduates that connects them to seasoned professionals who can answer questions and help guide their early career decisions.

The APTA has many opportunities for students to network, starting with the student assembly. The student assembly was created to help students understand the APTA, connect with the current leadership and members, and connect with other students across the United States and the world. Leaders communicate with students via Twitter, Facebook, and Skype. Student leaders have created a blog called The Pulse, the Pulse Podcast, and a monthly Facebook live chat and have also developed a network of core ambassadors to help communicate opportunities and information to all students. Students can attend the National Student Conclave, the Next Conference, Combined Sections, and the House of Delegates and National Assembly meeting of physical therapist (PT)/physical therapist assistant (PTA) leaders. Special interest groups exist at the state chapter level to help connect students from area colleges and universities and allow networking with the state chapter. These opportunities allow networking and learning within the physical therapy community to help students find their niche.

## Career Development

Before beginning a job search, students should identify their career goals to help them identify if a potential employer meets their career values and how they will best fit within the company and assist them in

According to the APTA, some questions graduates should ask themselves include:

**Financial Considerations**

- How is the management of the facility set up?
- What opportunities are available for advancement?
- What are the wages and benefits?

**Professional Development Considerations**

- Does the facility provide opportunities for continuing education?
- Does the facility have a mentoring program?
- Does the facility have a plan for growth and sustainability?

**Ethical and Legal Considerations**

- How does the business handle its financial operations?
- Do PTs control patient care decisions?
- What is the role of PTAs and physical therapy aides?

**Quality of Care Considerations**

- What is the job description of the PT and PTA?
- What input do the employees have in physical therapy, policies and procedures, and quality improvement practices?
- What are the policies for providing quality care and concern for patient outcomes?

identifying the attributes that will benefit the company. Skill surveys are available online to assist graduates in identifying career goals and creating a list of skills that can highlight their interests and strengths; personality assessments can identify values and personality traits. Graduates can use these assessments to create resumes and evaluate job opportunities. Career-Intelligence.com and https://careerwise.minnstate.edu/ are two websites that feature these assessments.

The APTA has created a document, Considerations for Practice Opportunities and Professional Development, to assist graduates in assessing whether certain job openings meet their professional goals.

# Physical Therapy Employment

After completing PT/PTA programs and passing the licensure examination, PTs/PTAs are ready to enter the physical therapy workforce. Students should begin their academic preparation with this end goal in mind. Several strategies will assist the student in gaining employment.

## Networking

Students may underestimate the value of making relationships to their ability to find employment. Creating relationships with PTs and PTAs not only provides the graduate with a possible reference when applying for a job but may ultimately be a way for one to get an interview. Students can begin making these connections during clinical experiences. Getting to know their clinical instructor and other organization employees will help make those valuable contacts. Another avenue to explore is participation in volunteer activities within the components and sections of the APTA. Students will meet national and local leaders within the profession and may find job prospects through these relationships. If students form relationships during their academic preparation, it is much more likely that, as graduates, they will have opportunities to interview with the employers of their choice.

### KNOWLEDGE CHECK

What is the value of mentor and networking?

## Cover Letter

A cover letter is an opportunity to introduce you to a potential employer. Before creating a cover letter,

a graduate should do their homework. A cover letter should be specific to each job or each employer to which the graduate sends it [3]. The cover letter requires research to determine to whom to direct the letter: human resource manager, physical therapy department supervisor, clinic owner, etc. If possible, the letter should be directed to a specific person. In addition, the graduate should learn about the philosophy and mission of the employer. This information will help identify how the graduate can contribute to the employer's success. Graduates should also identify any connections that they have to the company. An example might be that the graduate was encouraged to contact them by a clinical instructor or that the graduate read an article about the company's great work in a trade magazine. Creating a good cover letter can be the difference between getting an interview and not.

## Resume

The resume contains a summary of personal information, educational information, professional qualifications and experience, and references [3]. Candidates can provide resumes before an interview if a cover letter is not used. It is also acceptable to send a resume with a cover letter, or an applicant may provide it at an interview; it is best to inquire which the employer would prefer [4]. As a statement, the resume must be perfect, computer-typed, and printed on high-quality paper (such as a 20-pound white bond). It should not be sloppy with spelling mistakes, be handwritten, or typewritten [4].

### Why do you need a resume

- To show a desire to work and a work ethic by describing that you could work and hold a job while in high school or during the PTA program
- To show flexibility by describing that you could work various shifts or weekends or attended evening or weekend classes
- To express ambition by describing previous work experience or advancement in school or a local chapter of the physical therapy professional organization
- To express dedication by describing membership in the APTA or the state professional organization or long-term employment

There are two types of resumes: chronological and functional [5]. A chronological resume lists experiences in reverse order, with the most recent one first. It is the more common type of resume. A functional resume lists the skills a prospective employee possesses. Healthcare professionals do not typically utilize it.

A chronological resume is divided into the following sections:

- Identification: Includes the name and address of the PT/PTA.
- Career objective: The desire to grow or work with a special patient population such as geriatric, pediatric, or orthopedic. This section is important for a new graduate with no professional experience but who wants to work with a certain patient population.
- Work experience: Includes all full-time and relevant part-time positions, education, activities, and honors.
- Education: Includes names and addresses of the educational institution, dates of attendance, degree earned (or anticipated to be earned), the date the degree was earned, honors obtained, licensure number, special course work, and seminars. Grades and grade point averages are not typically included in the resume. Prospective employers should ask for the prospective employee's consent to obtain academic records, educational program information, and references.
- Activities: Include professional, civic, and/ or volunteer activities demonstrating positive work habits, leadership, and acceptance of responsibility. The honors section may be omitted for a new graduate if all honors are academic.

## References

References can describe the applicant's clinical and professional experience (and achievements) and character. Faculty members, clinical instructors, clinical supervisors, and/or former employers can provide references describing clinical and professional experience. Family, friends, or clergy can provide references describing the applicant's character.

## Interview

Although interviewing as a selection tool is generally considered an unsuccessful method for picking the best worker (the literature indicates that the best way of selecting someone for a position is based on a person's credentials and not the interview [5]), interviews remain the main selection tool in the healthcare industry. The strengths and weaknesses displayed during an interview are the strengths and weaknesses that the person will display as an employee [4].

The requirements that some healthcare managers look for in a job applicant include:

- Neat and clean appearance
- Showing a pleasant personality
- Exhibiting a desire to work and a work ethic
- Describing himself or herself as flexible, ambitious, and dedicated
- Having the best presentation [5]
- Understanding the company and what the applicant might contribute as an employee [4]

Like health care in general, in physical therapy, during an interview, employers look for decision-making style, communication skills, poise, tact, ability to work with others, leadership skills, achievement record, and a sense of personal direction. In physical therapy, a physical therapy director (or supervisor or manager) or a member of the personnel department can conduct interviews. The interview aims to meet with the prospective employee, exchange questions and answers, and obtain enough information about the prospective employee to make an informed decision.

### How should you prepare for the interview?

- Professional preparation: education, experience, and professional activities
- Physical preparation: resume, references, attire, and communication skills
- Mental preparation: knowing the information in the resume and the cover letter and being able to ask and answer questions

### Professional Preparation for the Interview

Professional preparation for the interview involves the PT's/PTA's education, experience, and activities. For a PT/PTA, professional preparation starts in the program by conscientiously studying the material, applying learned information at school and clinical settings, and joining the national professional organization (APTA) and the state physical therapy professional organization. In addition, participating as a student and as a licensed graduate in seminars and meetings at the local chapter or national level increases the professional network, ultimately helping with the interview process.

## Physical Preparation for the Interview

Physical preparation for the interview involves the resume, cover letter, portfolio of work, follow-up correspondence, and physical appearance.

**Attire and Communication Skills.** Physical preparation for the interview also involves dressing professionally and using appropriate verbal and non-verbal communication. Clothing must be clean, neat, and conservative. A business suit or sports jacket is typically appropriate for men or women. Trendy hairstyles, makeup, jewelry, and scents should be kept at a minimum. Be particularly sensitive to breath odor; avoid the smell of smoke or alcohol. Tattoos should be covered, if possible, and piercings removed if distracting.

Verbal communication should show interpersonal skills such as poise and tact. Be courteous to everyone in the business, including administrative assistants, professional personnel, custodial staff, etc. Nonverbal communication should show confidence and consistency in verbal and nonverbal cues. Some appropriate nonverbal communication signs include sitting upright (with both feet on the floor) and slightly forward in the chair, looking straight at the interviewer, using a firm handshake, and maintaining focus and interest in the interview. Signs of nervousness, such as fidgeting, restlessness, or chewing gum, can be detrimental to the interviewee.

**Mental Preparation for the Interview.** Mental preparation means being prepared for the interview, knowing the information in the resume and the cover letter, and being able to answer questions. It also includes knowing personal information, answers to typical interview questions, and information about the prospective employer. Questions are typically informational, encouraging discussions. Answers such as yes or no are not appropriate. Answer the interviewer's questions clearly and directly. Do not interrupt the interviewer. When possible, prepare specific examples of your strengths so the interviewer clearly understands when the graduate has displayed a particular trait [4]. An example of this might include a specific time when the graduate faced a difficult clinical decision and how they handled the situation. A prospective employer should not ask questions about a person's age, religion, race, marital status, political interests, social interests, national origin, whether renting or owning a home,

training not related to the job, birthplace, height and weight, native language, spouse's occupation, sexual preferences, and the number of dependents. When such questions are asked, the interviewee should use tactful answers.

---

Questions to ask a prospective employer during the interview include:

- Advantages and disadvantages of working for the organization
- Available benefits
- Work hours
- Vacation, sick, and personal leave time
- Salary range and description of job requirements
- Provision of professional liability insurance by the employer

---

After hiring a person, the employer can ask questions related to insurance to obtain the following information.

- Whether the person can work legally in the United States
- Person's age
- Spouse's information
- Dependent information
- Citizenship information
- Membership in professional organizations (although this information should be in the resume)
- Minority status for affirmative action plans
- Religious holidays to make work accommodations

## Follow-Up Activities

Regardless of whether being hired, the graduate should send a thank you note the same day as the interview or as soon as possible. A personal phone call thanking the interviewers for the opportunity to meet with them and expressing continued interest in the position a few days after the interview can also be a powerful tool. The graduate should not leave the potential of standing out from the other applicants for a position to chance, but instead show appreciation for the opportunity to interview. [4].

### KNOWLEDGE CHECK

What strategies are necessary to land your dream job?

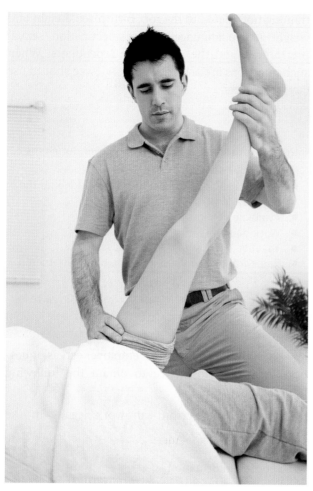

© wavebreakmedia/Shutterstock

**Box 13-1** PTA Advanced Proficiency Pathways

The PTA Advanced Proficiency Pathways are a set of guidelines and competencies that outline the knowledge and skills that PTAs should possess to provide high-quality patient care and help PTAs develop expertise and increase their value as members of the rehabilitation team. The Advanced Proficiency Pathways focus on six core areas of competency:

1. Clinical decision-making: PTAs should be able to use their knowledge of anatomy, physiology, and kinesiology to make informed decisions about patient care.
2. Interventions: PTAs should be able to implement various interventions to help patients achieve their goals, including manual therapy, exercise, and modalities.
3. Patient education: PTAs should be able to educate patients about their conditions, treatments, and how to participate in their own care.
4. Documentation: PTAs should be able to accurately document patient information and progress and communicate effectively with other healthcare team members.
5. Evidence-based practice: PTAs should be knowledgeable about the latest research and be able to apply it to their practice.
6. Professionalism: PTAs should demonstrate professional behavior and adhere to ethical standards in every aspect of their practice.

## Continuing Competence

While identifying career goals, new graduates should consider what areas or topics of physical therapy they found most interesting in school. Because PTA education prepares graduates to work with entry-level skills, students can utilize their interest areas to develop a continuing education plan. This plan will help graduates develop skills that may set them apart from others in the workforce. It can be a valuable tool when applying for jobs or creating opportunities for specialization. Some students find that returning to college for degrees in athletic training, massage therapy, or certification in lymphedema care, for example, can open doors that might not otherwise be possible.

For the PTA, an avenue for developing skills and leadership is the Physical Therapist Assistant Advanced Proficiency Pathways program through the APTA (see **Box 13-1**). PTAs who want to develop specific skills within a specified area of work can utilize these programs to move from entry-level knowledge to an advanced skill level.

Advanced proficiency can be in several specialized areas: acute care, cardiovascular/pulmonary, geriatrics, oncology, orthopedics, pediatrics, and wound care.

As students advance through their educational program, they are immersed in reading research and identifying evidence-based practice. This practice should continue after graduation and can lead graduates to identify areas of practice that interest them. Creating journal reading groups with other professionals can help to facilitate learning and collegiality between practitioners. Learning through journal readings and continuing education courses will help to develop a deeper understanding of physical therapy questions and may even lead graduates to their own research.

An additional component of continuing competency is that many states require continuing education for licensure renewal. This requirement aims to increase knowledge, clinical competence, enthusiasm, and contentment in professional work and improve benefits to the business. The number of hours varies by state, but research shows that clinicians in states that require continuing education hours complete more than those in states that do not require continuing education [6].

## Leadership Development

John Maxwell, in his book *The 21 Indispensable Qualities of a Leader* [1], outlines the attributes of leaders and how to develop them. According to Maxwell, the attributes that lead to success include optimism, commitment, passion, **competence**, **initiative**, flexibility, generosity, and relationships [1]. Leadership development is an ongoing process that refers to the process of improving and refining the skills, knowledge, and abilities of individuals in leadership positions. Leadership development aims to help leaders become more effective and successful in their roles and support the growth and success of the organizations they lead. Leadership development can take many forms, including:

- Formal education: Formal education in leadership and management can provide individuals with a strong foundation in leadership theory and practice. This can include degrees in business administration, management, or leadership, as well as professional certifications.
- On-the-job training: On-the-job training can help leaders develop practical skills and experience in leading and managing teams. This can include shadowing experienced leaders, participating in leadership development programs, and attending workshops and training sessions.
- Coaching and mentoring: Coaching and mentoring can help leaders develop their skills and abilities in specific areas, such as communication, conflict resolution, or decision-making. Coaches and mentors can provide personalized guidance and support to help leaders grow and develop in their roles.
- Self-reflection and self-awareness: Self-reflection and self-awareness are important components of leadership development. Leaders who take the time to reflect on their strengths and weaknesses, and to understand their own values, beliefs, and motivations, can become more effective and confident in their leadership roles.
- Networking: **Networking** with other leaders and professionals can provide opportunities to learn from others, share experiences and insights, and build professional relationships.

There are key differences between being a leader and being a manager:

- Leaders inspire trust and inspire others to do better. They focus on why things occur and have a long-range perspective. Honest, inspiring, competent, and credible leaders can influence other people's behaviors.
- Managers focus more on day-to-day activities and functions and work to control the functions of their employees.

Both roles are important and have a place in business and success, and PTs/PTAs may have opportunities for both leadership and management roles in their careers. PTs/PTAs can find opportunities for leadership development through the APTA, continuing education workshops, and the many books that have been written on the subject. The RM Barney Poole Leadership Academy, developed by the Georgia chapter of the APTA, is a seminar that teaches skills for visionary change. The APTA's Health Policy and Administration Section has developed a leadership certificate called LAMP (Leadership, Administration, Management, and Professionalism). This program requires a series of courses, projects, and mentoring to help the person develop these skills. These activities may lead to APTA, work, and community leadership roles.

Opportunities within the APTA can occur at the state chapter, the section level, or the national level. The Commission on Education in Physical Therapy Education and the Federation of State Boards of Physical Therapy also rely on volunteers and leaders to assist in their missions. Reviewing PTA educational programs for quality and assisting in writing the National Physical Therapy Examination requires leaders from every part of the United States and those with various expertise.

Leadership within the workplace can also be a gratifying endeavor. PTs/PTAs can become team leaders, be employed in supervisory positions such as minimum data set coordinators or rehabilitation team leaders in skilled nursing facilities, or become clinical instructors for PT/PTA programs. Some PTs/PTAs may also choose to continue their careers as instructors within PT/PTA programs. In addition, success within the workplace may also take the form of ownership in physical therapy clinics.

Leadership within the community requires only two things: a cause and passion. Looking at the needs of the community and developing strategies of hope and change can be related to the profession, such as developing a support group for patients who have multiple sclerosis and their families, leading exercise classes for people who have arthritis at the community pool, or leading the local efforts for Special Olympics. Or, it may relate to things outside of health care, such as working with the local child protection group; food bank; or a civic club such as Kiwanis, Rotary, or the Optimist Club.

## Discussion Questions

1. Describe a person you feel is successful and list the attributes that make you feel this way.
2. Brainstorm at least three questions that an employer might ask during an interview.
3. Brainstorm three questions that a PT/PTA might ask a potential employer.
4. Discuss your career goals in 5 years, 10 years, 15 years, and so on.

## Learning Opportunities

1. Write a resume.
2. Interview a classmate or be interviewed by a classmate.
3. Create a plan to develop the attributes of successful people.
4. Develop a timeline of career goals and connect them to activities to assist you in achieving them.

## References

1. Maxwell JC: The 21 Indispensable Qualities of a Leader. Nashville, TN, Thomas Nelson, 1999
2. Yate M: Knock'em Dead Cover Letters, 9th ed. Avon, MA, Adams Media, 2010
3. Bolles RN: What Color Is Your Parachute? A Practical Manual for Job-Hunters and Career-Changers. New York, NY, Ten Speed Press, 2010
4. Drafke MW: Working in Health Care: What You Need to Know to Succeed. Philadelphia, PA, F.A. Davis Company, 2002
5. Landers MR, McWhorter JW, Krum LL, et al: Mandatory continuing education in physical therapy: survey of physical therapists in states with and states without a mandate. Phys Ther 85(9):861–871, 2005

# Appendix A

# APTA Strategic Plan 2022-2025

| | |
|---|---|
| **Mission** | Building a community that advances the profession of physical therapy to improve the health of society. |
| **Vision for the Physical Therapy Profession** | Transforming society by optimizing movement to improve the human experience. |
| **Commitment to Diversity, Equity, and Inclusion** | APTA is committed to increasing diversity, equity, and inclusion in the association, profession, and society. |

| Member Value | Sustainable Profession | Quality of Care | Demand and Access |
|---|---|---|---|
| **GOALS** | | | |
| Increase member value by ensuring that APTA's community delivers unmatched opportunities to belong, engage, and contribute. | Improve the long-term sustainability of the profession by leading efforts to increase payment, reduce the cost of education, and strengthen provider health and well-being. | Elevate the quality of care provided by PTs and PTAs to improve health outcomes for populations, communities, and individuals. | Drive demand for and access to physical therapy as a proven pathway to improve the human experience. |
| **OUTCOMES** | | | |
| APTA will grow membership market share to extend the reach and impact of the APTA community. | APTA resources on financial literacy and published program comparisons will drive decision making to lower individual education costs. | A portfolio of new APTA evidence-based resources will drive quality of care evolutions to impact health at all levels. | Use of and demand for physical therapist services as a primary entry point of care for consumers will increase. |
| The profession will realize improvement in diversity and representation. | Physical therapists and physical therapist assistants will be paid fairly and will spend more time with patients than with paperwork. | A record number of members will seek career advancement through specialization, residency, fellowship, continuing education, and/or certifications. | The APTA community will collaborate to reach more consumers, drive demand for physical therapy, and expand the markets and venues that promote the profession. |
| **APTA CONNECTED OPERATIONAL PLANS** | | | |
| Diversity, Equity, and Inclusion Action Plan (Publication: 2022) | APTA Public Policy Priorities A Vision for Excellence in Physical Therapy Education | APTA Scientific Research Priorities for the Physical Therapy Profession | Physical Therapy Value Project (Publication: 2022) |

| | |
|---|---|
| **Better Together** | To maximize its effectiveness, reach, and impact, APTA collaborates with stakeholders, including components, external organizations, public sector entities, and consumers. To improve the health of society, we believe every stakeholder in the APTA community has a role to play. |

# Appendix B

## Problem-Solving Algorithm Utilized by PTAs in Patient/Client Intervention

This algorithm, developed by the American Physical Therapy Association's Departments of Education, Accreditation, and Practice, is intended to reflect current policies and positions on the problem-solving processes utilized by physical therapist assistants (PTAs) in the provision of selected interventions. The controlling assumptions are essential to understanding and applying this algorithm (see **Figure B-1**). (This document can be found in A Normative Model of Physical Therapist Assistant Education: Version 2007.)

- The physical therapist (PT) integrates the five elements of patient/client management— examination, evaluation, diagnosis, prognosis, and intervention—in a manner designed to optimize outcomes. The PT bears responsibility for completing the examination, evaluation, diagnosis, and prognosis. The PT's plan of care (POC) may involve the PTA to assist with selected interventions. This algorithm represents the decision-making of the PTA within the intervention element.

- The PT will direct and supervise the PTA consistent with the APTA House of Delegates (HOD) positions, including Direction and Supervision of the Physical Therapist Assistant (HOD P06-05-18-26); APTA core documents, including Standards of Ethical Conduct for the PTA; federal and state legal practice standards; and institutional regulations.

- All selected interventions are directed and supervised by the PT. Additionally, the PT remains responsible for the physical therapy services provided when the PT's POC involves the PTA to assist with selected interventions.

- Selected intervention(s) includes the procedural intervention, associated data collection, and communication, including written documentation associated with the safe, effective, and efficient completion of the task.

- The algorithm may represent the thought processes involved in a patient/client interaction or episode of care. Entry into the algorithm will depend on the point at which the PT directs the PTA to provide selected interventions.

- Communication between the PT and PTA regarding patient/client care is ongoing. The algorithm does not intend to imply a limitation or restriction on communication between the PT and PTA (see **Figure B-2**).

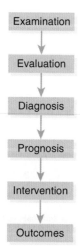

**Figure B-1** Controlling assumptions.

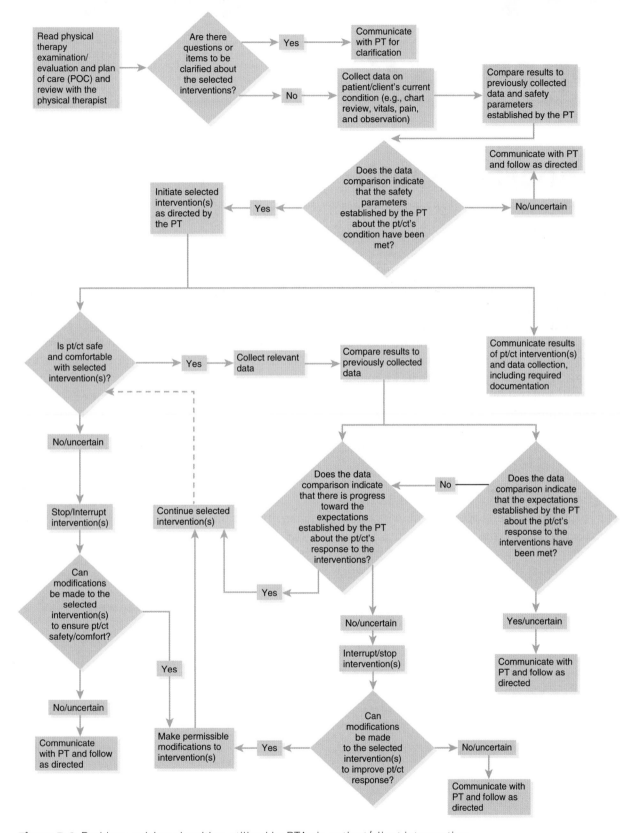

**Figure B-2** Problem-solving algorithm utilized by PTAs in patient/client intervention.

# Appendix C

## Hippocratic Oath

I swear by Apollo the physician, and Aesculapius, and Health, and All-heal, and all the gods and goddesses, that, according to my ability and judgment, I will keep this Oath and this stipulation: to reckon him who taught me this Art equally dear to me as my parents, to share my substance with him, and relieve his necessities if required; to look upon his offspring in the same footing as my own brothers, and to teach them this art, if they shall wish to learn it, without fee or stipulation; and that by precept, lecture, and every other mode of instruction, I will impart a knowledge of the Art to my own sons, and those of my teachers, and to disciples bound by a stipulation and oath according to the law of medicine, but to none others.

I will follow that system of regimen which, according to my ability and judgment, I consider for the benefit of my patients, and abstain from whatever is deleterious and mischievous.

I will give no deadly medicine to any one if asked, nor suggest any such counsel; and in like manner I will not give to a woman a pessary to produce abortion. With purity and with holiness I will pass my life and practice my Art. I will not cut persons laboring under the stone, but will leave this to be done by men who are practitioners of this work.

Into whatever houses I enter, I will go into them for the benefit of the sick, and will abstain from every voluntary act of mischief and corruption; and, further from the seduction of females or males, of free men and slaves.

Whatever, in connection with my professional practice or not, in connection with it, I see or hear, in the life of men, which ought not to be spoken of abroad, I will not divulge, as reckoning that all such should be kept secret.

While I continue to keep this Oath unviolated, may it be granted to me to enjoy life and the practice of the art, respected by all men, in all times! But should I trespass and violate this Oath, may the reverse be my lot!

# Appendix D

# Patient's Bill of Rights

1. The patient has the right to considerate and respectful care.
2. The patient has the right to obtain, from their certified provider, complete current information regarding their diagnosis, treatment, and prognosis in terms the patient can reasonably be expected to understand. When it is not advisable to give such information to the patient, the information should be made available to an appropriate person on their behalf.
3. The patient has the right to receive from their certified provider information to make informed consent prior to the start of any procedure or treatment. This shall include such information as the medically significant risks involved with any procedure and probable duration of incapacitation. Where medically appropriate, alternatives for care or treatment should be explained to the patient.
4. The patient has the right to refuse any and all treatment to the extent permitted by law and to be informed of any of the medical consequences of their action.
5. The patient has the right to every consideration of privacy concerning their own medical care program limited only by state statutes, rules, regulations, or imminent danger to the individual or others.
6. The patient has the right to be advised if the clinician, hospital, clinic, or others propose to engage in or perform human experimentation affecting their care or treatment. The patient has the right to refuse to participate in such research projects.
7. The patient has the privilege to examine and receive an explanation of the bill.
8. Insurance companies may not discriminate against children who have preexisting conditions.
9. Insurance companies may not cancel coverage based upon prior illness or errors in application for insurance. Additionally, coverage may not be limited based upon total lifetime coverage limits.
10. Insurance companies may not limit the consumer's choice of healthcare providers including which emergency room location a patient may access.
11. Patients may appeal denied services to an independent third party.
12. Young adults may remain on their parent's insurance until age 26.
13. Patients will receive preventative care without cost, such as mammograms, immunizations, and prenatal and new baby care.

# Appendix E

# American Physical Therapy Association's Code of Ethics for Physical Therapists

HOD S06-09-07-12 [Amended HOD S06-00-12-23; HOD 06-91-05-05; HOD 06-87-11-17; HOD 06-81-06-18; HOD 06-78-06-08; HOD 06-78-06-07; HOD 06-77-18-30; HOD 06-77-17-27; Initial HOD 06-73-13-24] [Standard].

## Preamble

The Code of Ethics for the Physical Therapist (Code of Ethics) delineates the ethical obligations of all physical therapists as determined by the House of Delegates of the American Physical Therapy Association (APTA). The purposes of this Code of Ethics are to:

1. Define the ethical principles that form the foundation of physical therapist practice in patient/client management, consultation, education, research, and administration.
2. Provide standards of behavior and performance that form the basis of professional accountability to the public.
3. Provide guidance for physical therapists facing ethical challenges, regardless of their professional roles and responsibilities.
4. Educate physical therapists, students, other healthcare professionals, regulators, and the public regarding the core values, ethical principles, and standards that guide the professional conduct of the physical therapist.
5. Establish the standards by which the APTA can determine if a physical therapist has engaged in unethical conduct.

No code of ethics is exhaustive nor can it address every situation. Physical therapists are encouraged to seek additional advice or consultation in instances where the guidance of the Code of Ethics may not be definitive.

This Code of Ethics is built upon the five roles of the physical therapist (management of patients/clients, consultation, education, research, and administration), the core values of the profession, and the multiple realms of ethical action (individual, organizational, and societal). Physical therapist practice is guided by a set of seven core values: accountability, altruism, compassion/caring, excellence, integrity, professional duty, and social responsibility. Throughout the document the primary core values that support specific principles are indicated in parentheses. Unless a specific role is indicated in the principle, the duties and obligations being delineated pertain to the five roles of the physical therapist. Fundamental to the Code of Ethics is the special obligation of physical therapists to empower, educate, and enable those with impairments, activity limitations, participation restrictions, and disabilities to facilitate greater independence, health, wellness, and enhanced quality of life.

## Principle #1

Physical therapists shall respect the inherent dignity and rights of all individuals.

(Core Values: Compassion/Caring, Integrity)

- 1A.
  Physical therapists shall act in a respectful manner toward each person regardless of age, gender, race, nationality, religion, ethnicity, social or economic status, sexual orientation, health condition, or disability.

- 1B.
Physical therapists shall recognize their personal biases and shall not discriminate against others in physical therapist practice, consultation, education, research, and administration.

# Principle #2

Physical therapists shall be trustworthy and compassionate in addressing the rights and needs of patients/clients.

(Core Values: Altruism, Compassion/Caring, Professional Duty)

- 2A.
Physical therapists shall adhere to the core values of the profession and shall act in the best interests of patients/clients over the interests of the physical therapist.
- 2B.
Physical therapists shall provide physical therapy services with compassionate and caring behaviors that incorporate the individual and cultural differences of patients/clients.
- 2C.
Physical therapists shall provide the information necessary to allow patients or their surrogates to make informed decisions about physical therapy care or participation in clinical research.
- 2D.
Physical therapists shall collaborate with patients/clients to empower them in decisions about their health care.
- 2E.
Physical therapists shall protect confidential patient/client information and may disclose confidential information to appropriate authorities only when allowed or as required by law.

# Principle #3

Physical therapists shall be accountable for making sound professional judgments.

(Core Values: Excellence, Integrity)

- 3A.
Physical therapists shall demonstrate independent and objective professional judgment in the patient's/client's best interest in all practice settings.
- 3B.
Physical therapists shall demonstrate professional judgment informed by professional standards,

evidence (including current literature and established best practice), practitioner experience, and patient/client values.
- 3C.
Physical therapists shall make judgments within their scope of practice and level of expertise and shall communicate with, collaborate with, or refer to peers or other healthcare professionals when necessary.
- 3D.
Physical therapists shall not engage in conflicts of interest that interfere with professional judgment.
- 3E.
Physical therapists shall provide appropriate direction of and communication with physical therapist assistants and support personnel.

# Principle #4

Physical therapists shall demonstrate integrity in their relationships with patients/clients, families, colleagues, students, research participants, other healthcare providers, employers, payers, and the public.

(Core Value: Integrity)

- 4A.
Physical therapists shall provide truthful, accurate, and relevant information and shall not make misleading representations.
- 4B.
Physical therapists shall not exploit persons over whom they have supervisory, evaluative, or other authority (e.g., patients/clients, students, supervisees, research participants, or employees).
- 4C.
Physical therapists shall discourage misconduct by healthcare professionals and report illegal or unethical acts to the relevant authority, when appropriate.
- 4D.
Physical therapists shall report suspected cases of abuse involving children or vulnerable adults to the appropriate authority, subject to law.
- 4E.
Physical therapists shall not engage in any sexual relationship with any of their patients/clients, supervisees, or students.
- 4F.
Physical therapists shall not harass anyone verbally, physically, emotionally, or sexually.

# Principle #5

Physical therapists shall fulfill their legal and professional obligations.

(Core Values: Professional Duty, Accountability)

- 5A.
  Physical therapists shall comply with applicable local, state, and federal laws and regulations.
- 5B.
  Physical therapists shall have primary responsibility for supervision of physical therapist assistants and support personnel.
- 5C.
  Physical therapists involved in research shall abide by accepted standards governing protection of research participants.
- 5D.
  Physical therapists shall encourage colleagues with physical, psychological, or substance-related impairments that may adversely impact their professional responsibilities to seek assistance or counsel.
- 5E.
  Physical therapists who have knowledge that a colleague is unable to perform their professional responsibilities with reasonable skill and safety shall report this information to the appropriate authority.
- 5F.
  Physical therapists shall provide notice and information about alternatives for obtaining care in the event the physical therapist terminates the provider relationship while the patient/client continues to need physical therapy services.

# Principle #6

Physical therapists shall enhance their expertise through the lifelong acquisition and refinement of knowledge, skills, abilities, and professional behaviors.

(Core Value: Excellence)

- 6A.
  Physical therapists shall achieve and maintain professional competence.
- 6B.
  Physical therapists shall take responsibility for their professional development based on critical self-assessment and reflection on changes in physical therapist practice, education, healthcare delivery, and technology.

- 6C.
  Physical therapists shall evaluate the strength of evidence and applicability of content presented during professional development activities before integrating the content or techniques into practice.
- 6D.
  Physical therapists shall cultivate practice environments that support professional development, lifelong learning, and excellence.

# Principle #7

Physical therapists shall promote organizational behaviors and business practices that benefit patients/clients and society.

(Core Values: Integrity, Accountability)

- 7A.
  Physical therapists shall promote practice environments that support autonomous and accountable professional judgments.
- 7B.
  Physical therapists shall seek remuneration as is deserved and reasonable for physical therapist services.
- 7C.
  Physical therapists shall not accept gifts or other considerations that influence or give an appearance of influencing their professional judgment.
- 7D.
  Physical therapists shall fully disclose any financial interest they have in products or services that they recommend to patients/clients.
- 7E.
  Physical therapists shall be aware of charges and shall ensure that documentation and coding for physical therapy services accurately reflect the nature and extent of the services provided.
- 7F.
  Physical therapists shall refrain from employment arrangements, or other arrangements, that prevent physical therapists from fulfilling professional obligations to patients/clients.

# Principle #8

Physical therapists shall participate in efforts to meet the health needs of people locally, nationally, or globally.

(Core Value: Social Responsibility)

- 8A.
  Physical therapists shall provide pro bono physical therapy services or support organizations

that meet the health needs of people who are economically disadvantaged, uninsured, and underinsured.

- 8B.
  Physical therapists shall advocate to reduce health disparities and healthcare inequities, improve access to healthcare services, and address the health, wellness, and preventive healthcare needs of people.

- 8C.
  Physical therapists shall be responsible stewards of healthcare resources and shall avoid overutilization or underutilization of physical therapy services.

- 8D.
  Physical therapists shall educate members of the public about the benefits of physical therapy and the unique role of the physical therapist.

# Appendix F

# APTA Guide for Conduct of the Physical Therapist Assistant

## Purpose

The APTA Guide for Conduct of the Physical Therapist Assistant (Guide) is intended to serve physical therapist assistants in interpreting the Standards of Ethical Conduct for the Physical Therapist Assistant (Standards of Ethical Conduct) of the American Physical Therapy Association (APTA). The APTA House of Delegates in June of 2009 adopted the revised Standards of Ethical Conduct, which became effective July 1, 2010.

The Guide provides a framework by which physical therapist assistants may determine the propriety of their conduct. It also is intended to guide the development of physical therapist assistant students. The Standards of Ethical Conduct and the Guide apply to all physical therapist assistants. These guidelines are subject to change as the dynamics of the profession change and as new patterns of health care delivery are developed and accepted by the professional community and the public.

## Interpreting the Standards of Ethical Conduct

The interpretations expressed in this Guide reflect the opinions, decisions, and advice of the Ethics and Judicial Committee (EJC). The interpretations are set forth according to topic. These interpretations are intended to assist a physical therapist assistant in applying general ethical standards to specific situations. They address some but not all topics addressed in the Standards of Ethical Conduct and should not be considered inclusive of all situations that could evolve.

This Guide is subject to change, and the Ethics and Judicial Committee will monitor and revise the Guide to address additional topics and standards when and as needed.

## Preamble to the Standards of Ethical Conduct

### The Preamble states as follows:

The Standards of Ethical Conduct for the Physical Therapist Assistant (Standards of Ethical Conduct) delineate the ethical obligations of all physical therapist assistants as determined by the House of Delegates of the American Physical Therapy Association (APTA). The Standards of Ethical Conduct provide a foundation for conduct to which all physical therapist assistants shall adhere. Fundamental to the Standards of Ethical Conduct is the special obligation of physical therapist assistants to enable patients/clients to achieve greater independence, health and wellness, and enhanced quality of life. No document that delineates ethical standards can address every situation. Physical therapist assistants are encouraged to seek advice or consultation in instances where the guidance of the Standards of Ethical Conduct may not be definitive.

**Interpretation:** Upon the Standards of Ethical Conduct for the Physical Therapist Assistant being amended effective July 1, 2010, all the lettered standards contain the word "shall" and are mandatory ethical obligations. The language contained in the Standards of Ethical Conduct is intended to better explain and further clarify existing ethical obligations. These ethical obligations predate the revised Standards of Ethical Conduct.

Although various words have changed, many of the obligations are the same. Consequently, the addition of the word "shall" serves to reinforce and clarify existing ethical obligations. A significant reason that the Standards of Ethical Conduct were revised was to provide physical therapist assistants with a document that was clear enough to be read on its own without the need to seek extensive additional interpretation.

The Preamble states that "[n]o document that delineates ethical standards can address every situation." The Preamble also states that physical therapist assistants "are encouraged to seek additional advice or consultation in instances where the guidance of the Standards of Ethical Conduct may not be definitive."

Potential sources for advice or counsel include third parties and the myriad resources available on the APTA website. Inherent in a physical therapist assistant's ethical decision-making process is the examination of his or her unique set of facts relative to the Standards of Ethical Conduct.

# Topics

## Respect

### Standard 1A states as follows:

1A. Physical therapist assistants shall act in a respectful manner toward each person regardless of age, gender, race, nationality, religion, ethnicity, social or economic status, sexual orientation, health condition, or disability.

**Interpretation:** Standard 1A addresses the display of respect toward others. Unfortunately, there is no universal consensus about what respect looks like in every situation. For example, direct eye contact is viewed as respectful and courteous in some cultures and inappropriate in others. It is up to the individual to assess the appropriateness of behavior in various situations.

## Altruism

### Standard 2A states as follows:

2A. Physical therapist assistants shall act in the best interests of patients/clients over the interests of the physical therapist assistant.

**Interpretation:** Standard 2A addresses acting in the best interest of patients and clients over the interests of the physical therapist assistant. Often this is done without thought, but, sometimes, especially at the end of the day when the clinician is fatigued and ready to go home, it is a conscious decision. For example, the physical therapist assistant may need to make a decision between leaving on time and staying at work longer to see a patient who was 15 minutes late for an appointment.

## Sound Decisions

### Standard 3C states as follows:

3C. Physical therapist assistants shall make decisions based upon their level of competence and consistent with patient/client values.

**Interpretation:** To fulfill 3C, the physical therapist assistant must be knowledgeable about his or her legal scope of work as well as level of competence. As a physical therapist assistant gains experience and additional knowledge, there may be areas of physical therapy interventions in which he or she displays advanced skills. At the same time, other previously gained knowledge and skill may be lost due to lack of use. To make sound decisions, the physical therapist assistant must be able to self-reflect on his or her current level of competence.

## Supervision

### Standard 3E states as follows:

3E. Physical therapist assistants shall provide physical therapy services under the direction and supervision of a physical therapist and shall communicate with the physical therapist when patient/client status requires modifications to the established plan of care.

**Interpretation:** Standard 3E goes beyond simply stating that the physical therapist assistant operates under the supervision of the physical therapist. Although a physical therapist retains responsibility for the patient or client throughout the episode of care, this standard requires the physical therapist assistant to take action by communicating with the supervising physical therapist when changes in the individual's status indicate that modifications to the plan of care may be needed. Further information on supervision via APTA policies and resources is available on the APTA website.

## Integrity in Relationships

### Standard 4 states as follows:

4. Physical therapist assistants shall demonstrate integrity in their relationships with patients/clients, families, colleagues, students, other health care providers, employers, payers, and the public.

**Interpretation:** Standard 4 addresses the need for integrity in relationships. This is not limited to relationships with patients and clients but includes everyone physical therapist assistants come into contact with in the normal provision of physical therapist services. For example, demonstrating integrity could encompass working collaboratively with the health care team and taking responsibility for one's role as a member of that team.

## Reporting

### Standard 4C states as follows:

> 4C. Physical therapist assistants shall discourage misconduct by health care professionals and report illegal or unethical acts to the relevant authority, when appropriate.

**Interpretation:** Physical therapist assistants shall seek to discourage misconduct by health care professionals. Discouraging misconduct can be accomplished through a number of mechanisms. The following is not an exhaustive list:

- Do not engage in misconduct; instead, set a good example for health care professionals and others working in their immediate environment.
- Encourage or recommend to the appropriate individuals that health care and other professionals, such as legal counsel, conduct regular (such as annual) training that addresses federal and state law requirements, such as billing, best practices, harassment, and security and privacy; as such training can educate health care professionals on what to do and not to do.
- Encourage or recommend to the appropriate individuals other types of training that are not law based, such as bystander training.
- Assist in creating a culture that is positive and civil to all.
- If in a management position, consider how promotion and hiring decisions can impact the organization.
- Access professional association resources when considering best practices.
- Revisit policies and procedures each year to remain current.

Many other mechanisms may exist to discourage misconduct. The physical therapist assistant should be creative, open-minded, fair, and impartial in considering how to best meet this ethical obligation. Doing so can actively foster an environment in which misconduct does not occur. The main focus when thinking about misconduct is creating an action plan on prevention. Consider that reporting may never make the alleged victim whole or undo the misconduct.

If misconduct has not been prevented, then reporting issues must be considered. This ethical obligation states that the physical therapist assistant reports to the "relevant authority, when appropriate." Before examining the meaning of these words it is important to note that reporting intersects with corporate policies and legal obligations. It is beyond the scope of this interpretation to provide legal advice regarding laws and policies; however, an analysis of reporting cannot end with understanding one's ethical obligations. One may need to seek advice of legal counsel who will take into consideration laws and policies and seek to discover the facts and circumstances.

With respect to ethical obligations, the term "when appropriate" is a fact-based decision and will be impacted by requirements of the law. If a law requires the physical therapist assistant to take an action, then, of course, it is appropriate to do so. If there is no legal requirement and no corporate policy, then the physical therapist assistant must consider what is appropriate given the facts and situation. It may not be appropriate if the physical therapist does not know what occurred, or because there is no legal requirement to act and the physical therapist assistant does not want to assume legal responsibility, or because the matter is being resolved internally. There are many different reasons that something may or may not be appropriate.

If the physical therapist assistant has determined that it is appropriate to report, the ethical obligation requires him or her to consider what entity or person is the "relevant authority." Relevant authority can be a supervisor, human resources, an attorney, the Equal Employment Opportunities Commission, the licensing board, the Better Business Bureau, Office of the Insurance Commissioner, the Medicare hotline, the Office of the Inspector General hotline, the US Department of Health and Human Services, an institution using their internal grievance procedures, the Office of Civil Rights, or another federal, state, city, or local agency, or a state or federal court, among others.

Once the physical therapist assistant has decided to report, he or she must be mindful that reporting does not end his or her involvement, which can include office, regulatory, and/or legal proceedings. In this context, the physical therapist assistant may be asked to be a witness, to testify, or to provide written information.

## Sexual Harassment

### Standard 4F states as follows:

4F. Physical therapist assistants shall not harass anyone verbally, physically, emotionally, or sexually.

**Interpretation:** As noted in the House of Delegates policy titled "Sexual Harassment," "[m]embers of the association have an obligation to comply with applicable legal prohibitions against sexual harassment...." This statement is in line with Standard 4F that prohibits physical therapist assistants from harassing anyone verbally, physically, emotionally, or sexually. While the standard is clear, it is important for APTA to restate this point, namely that physical therapist assistants shall not harass anyone, period. The association has zero tolerance for any form of harassment, specifically including sexual harassment.

## Exploitation

### Standard 4E states as follows:

4E. Physical therapist assistants shall not engage in any sexual relationship with any of their patients/clients, supervisees, or students.

**Interpretation:** The statement is clear—sexual relationships with their patients or clients, supervisees, or students are prohibited. This component of Standard 4 is consistent with Standard 4B, which states:

4B. Physical therapist assistants shall not exploit persons over whom they have supervisory, evaluative, or other authority (eg, patients and clients, students, supervisees, research participants, or employees).

Consider this excerpt from the EJC Opinion titled Topic: Sexual Relationships With Patients or Former Patients (modified for physical therapist assistants):

A physical therapist [assistant] stands in a relationship of trust to each patient and has an ethical obligation to act in the patient's best interest and to avoid any exploitation or abuse of the patient. Thus, if a physical therapist [assistant] has natural feelings of attraction toward a patient, he or she must sublimate those feelings in order to avoid sexual exploitation of the patient.

One's ethical decision making process should focus on whether the patient or client, supervisee, or student is being exploited. In this context, questions have been asked about whether one can have a sexual relationship once the patient or client relationship ends. To this question, the EJC has opined as follows:

The Committee does not believe it feasible to establish any bright-line rule for when, if ever, initiation of a romantic/sexual relationship with a former patient would be ethically permissible.

The Committee imagines that in some cases a romantic/sexual relationship would not offend ... if initiated with a former patient soon after the termination of treatment, while in others such a relationship might never be appropriate.

## Colleague Impairment

### Standard 5D and 5E state as follows:

5D. Physical therapist assistants shall encourage colleagues with physical, psychological, or substance-related impairments that may adversely impact their professional responsibilities to seek assistance or counsel.

5E. Physical therapist assistants who have knowledge that a colleague is unable to perform their professional responsibilities with reasonable skill and safety shall report this information to the appropriate authority.

**Interpretation:** The central tenet of Standard 5D and 5E is that inaction is not an option for a physical therapist assistant when faced with the circumstances described. Standard 5D states that a physical therapist assistant shall encourage colleagues to seek assistance or counsel while Standard 5E addresses reporting information to the appropriate authority.

5D and 5E both require a factual determination on the physical therapist assistant's part. This may be challenging in the sense that the physical therapist assistant might not know or easily be able to determine whether someone in fact has a physical, psychological, or substance-related impairment. In addition, it might be difficult to determine whether such impairment may be adversely affecting someone's work responsibilities.

Moreover, once the physical therapist assistant does make these determinations, the obligation under 5D centers not on reporting, but on encouraging the colleague to seek assistance, while the obligation under 5E does focus on reporting. But note that 5E discusses reporting when a colleague is unable to perform; whereas, 5D discusses encouraging colleagues to seek assistance when the impairment may adversely affect their professional responsibilities. So, 5D discusses something that may be affecting performance, whereas 5E addresses a situation in which someone clearly is unable to perform. The 2 situations are distinct. In addition, it is important to note that 5E does not mandate to whom the physical therapist assistant reports; it provides discretion to determine the appropriate authority.

The EJC Opinion titled Topic: Topic: Preserving Confidences; Physical Therapist's Reporting Obligation With Respect to Unethical, Incompetent, or Illegal Acts provides further information on the complexities of reporting.

## Clinical Competence

**Standard 6A states as follows:**

6A. Physical therapist assistants shall achieve and maintain clinical competence.

**Interpretation:** 6A should cause physical therapist assistants to reflect on their current level of clinical competence, to identify and address gaps in clinical competence, and to commit to the maintenance of clinical competence throughout their career. The supervising physical therapist can be a valuable partner in identifying areas of knowledge and skill that the physical therapist assistant needs for clinical competence and to meet the needs of the individual physical therapist, which may vary according to areas of interest and expertise.

Further, the physical therapist assistant may request that the physical therapist serve as a mentor to assist him or her in acquiring the needed knowledge and skills. Additional resources on Continuing Competence are available on the APTA website.

## Lifelong Learning

**Standard 6C states as follows:**

6C. Physical therapist assistants shall support practice environments that support career development and lifelong learning.

**Interpretation:** 6C points out the physical therapist assistant's obligation to support an environment conducive to career development and learning. The essential idea here is that the physical therapist assistant encourages and contributes to his or her career development and lifelong learning, whether or not the employer provides support.

## Organizational and Business Practices

**Standard 7 states as follows:**

7. Physical therapist assistants shall support organizational behaviors and business practices that benefit patients/clients and society.

**Interpretation:** Standard 7 reflects a shift in the Standards of Ethical Conduct. One criticism of the former version was that it addressed primarily face-to-face clinical practice settings. Accordingly, Standard 7 addresses ethical obligations in organizational and business practices on both patient and client and societal levels.

## Documenting Interventions

**Standard 7D states as follows:**

7D. Physical therapist assistants shall ensure that documentation for their interventions accurately reflects the nature and extent of the services provided.

**Interpretation:** 7D addresses the need for physical therapist assistants to make sure that they thoroughly and accurately document the interventions they provide to patients and clients and document related data collected from the patient or client. The focus of this Standard is on ensuring documentation of the services rendered, including the nature and extent of such services.

## Support—Health Needs

**Standard 8A states as follows:**

8A. Physical therapist assistants shall support organizations that meet the health needs of people who are economically disadvantaged, uninsured, and underinsured.

**Interpretation:** 8A addresses the issue of support for those least likely to be able to afford physical therapist services. The standard does not specify the type of support that is required. Physical therapist assistants may express support through volunteerism, financial contributions, advocacy, education, or simply promoting their work in conversations with colleagues.

When providing such services, including pro bono services, physical therapist assistants must comply with applicable laws, and as such work under the direction and supervision of a physical therapist. Additional resources on pro bono services are available on the APTA website.

Issued by the Ethics and Judicial Committee American Physical Therapy Association October 1981

**Last Amended:** March 2019
**Contact:** ejc@apta.org

# Appendix G

# Answers to Knowledge Check Questions

## Chapter 1

**Which positive learning traits do you employ?**
Student-specific answers

**Which negative learning traits do you have?**
Student-specific answers

**What are the five learning styles?**
Visual, Auditory, Kinesthetic, Analytic (Linear), Spatial

**Which learning style is most comfortable for you?**
Student-specific answers

**What does SQ3R stand for?**
*Survey* the reading, consider *questions* that will be answered, *read* with purpose, stop periodically to *recite* what has been read, and *review* notes taken while completing the reading.

**What college resources should a student look for when studying?**
The library and librarians, Student Services—tutors, study and test-taking skill instruction—and instructor office hours for questions.

**Why should a student review and organize their classroom notes?**
Understanding material requires students to manipulate the information to make connections between what they currently know and the new material being learned. Using the information to solve problems creates memory of the material that is more long-lasting.

**What is the value in reviewing the mistakes made on an exam?**
It creates an attitude of self-assessment that allows students to correct misunderstanding and develop an awareness of areas of the information that require more study.

**What strategies help students learn deeply?**
When studying, the student should compare and contrast the concepts to be learned, relate the information to what the student already understands, and connect the information to future clinical practice to give it context in practice.

## Chapter 2

**What two historical events developed the profession?**
World War I and the poliomyelitis epidemic

**Who were the first physical therapists (PTs)?**
Marguerite Sanderson and Mary McMillan

**What major accomplishments in the development of the profession can be attributed to Mary McMillan?**
Mary McMillan was in charge of the training of reconstruction aides and went on to develop the curriculum for the first physical therapy program.

**What was the purpose of the American Physiotherapy Association?**
The purpose was to establish and maintain professional and scientific standards for individuals who were involved with the profession of physical therapeutics.

**What events changed the PT from a technician to a professional?**
The American Physiotherapy Association wanted to create a standardized education, encourage regulation of practice, and provide a central registry for physiotherapists. The name "physical therapist" was adopted to prevent society from mistaking physiotherapists with physicians.

**What caused the development of physical therapist assistant (PTA) education?**
Due to an ever-increasing number of elderly and a society that was becoming more health conscious, the demand for physical therapy services expanded, allowing for the expansion of physical therapy education to include PTAs.

**What is direct access and how did it change physical therapy practice?**
Direct access allows patients and clients to seek physical therapy services without first seeing a physician.

**What was the impact of the Balanced Budget Act on physical therapy services?**
The Balanced Budget Act applied an annual cap per beneficiary for outpatient rehabilitation services. This caused a reduction of services for Medicare patients and resulted in decreased job opportunities for new graduates and decreased income for PTs and PTAs.

**How did the APTA's Vision 2020 change physical therapy education and practice?**
The American Physical Therapy Association (APTA) Vision 2020 successfully moved the entry-level degree to the doctorate level, advocated for all states to allow for direct access, created a vision for future professionals to use evidence to make clinical decisions, and promoted professionalism in practice.

**What do the following terms mean: autonomous practice, direct access, practitioner of choice, evidence-based practice, and professionalism?**
Autonomous practice recognizes that PTs have the skills and knowledge to evaluate patients, create musculoskeletal diagnoses, and not require supervision by other professionals.

Direct access allows patients and clients to access physical therapy services without first seeing a physician.

Practitioner of choice recognizes that PTs have the appropriate skills and knowledge to treat patients and that physical therapy should be a covered service in healthcare insurance programs for problems related to movement, function, and health.

Evidence-based practice promotes the use of research when making patient care decisions.

Professionalism includes the skills, knowledge, attitudes, and behaviors that allow respectful interaction with patients and clients.

**What are the seven guiding principles of the current APTA vision?**
Identity, quality, collaboration, innovation, consumer-centered care, access/equity, advocacy

**What are the benefits of belonging to the professional organization of physical therapy?**
The APTA offers the following membership benefits: resources for learning, student debt management tools, advocacy for practice initiatives, public awareness campaigns, career development, networking and career advancement opportunities, evidence-based practice tools, physical therapy news, resources to understand and apply payment policies, and discount and value programs.

# Chapter 3

**What portions of the patient and client management model can the PTA perform?**
The PTA will use examination skills, such as tests and measures, to assess the patient's progress during the episode of care. PTAs will also participate in interventions that are part of the plan of care (POC).

**What are the differences among an impairment, an activity limitation, a participation restriction, and a disability?**
Impairments are problems that relate to a body part or its function. Activity limitations are problems people have with performing functional activities. Participation restriction describes the patient's inability to be involved within their environment. Disability is the inability to perform or participate in activities or tasks that change their social roles.

**How are a medical diagnosis and a physical therapy diagnosis different?**
A medical diagnosis is made by a physician who labels the patient's illness or disorder. A physical therapy diagnosis is made by a PT to label the patient's impairments, functional limitations, and participation restrictions.

**What are some examples of interventions within a POC?**

1. Patient or client instruction
2. Airway clearance techniques (assistive technology)
3. Biophysical agents, including electrotherapeutic modalities
4. Functional training in self-care and domestic, work, community, social, and civic life
5. Integumentary repair and protection techniques
6. Manual therapy techniques
7. Motor function training
8. Therapeutic exercise

**What conditions indicate that a patient should be discharged from physical therapy?**

Patients are discharged from physical therapy episodes of care when they have achieved their anticipated goals and expected outcomes, have plateaued in progression toward their goals, or no longer desire to participate in physical therapy interventions.

**What are clinical practice guidelines?**

Clinical practice guidelines are documented practice patterns, based on research evidence, that help PTs develop effective and efficient plans of care for specific diagnoses and impairments.

**Where would a patient receive physical therapy services if they are too ill to be cared for at home, but do not need hospitalization?**

Patients in this situation are placed in subacute care facilities, which may be available within a subacute hospital or a skilled nursing facility.

**Which settings utilize healthcare teams to treat patients/clients?**

Healthcare teams are found in acute care hospitals, subacute care facilities, skilled nursing facilities, outpatient facilities, rehabilitation hospitals, chronic care facilities, hospice care facilities, home health care, and school systems. Teams are found anywhere a PT and a PTA work together, as well as where other professionals are working with shared patients/clients.

**What condition needs to exist in order for a patient to be eligible for home health services?**

To be eligible, the patient has to be homebound, meaning that he or she requires physical assistance to leave home.

**Which practice areas overlap with all the other practice areas?**

Because orthopedic, neurologic, cardiovascular, and integumentary are body system–based practice areas, they will overlap into the practice areas that are based on other attributes (pediatrics, geriatrics, oncology, women's health).

**While each of the practice areas is different, what is the common patient goal that they all share?**

Regardless of practice, all patient goals are focused on the patient achieving the highest function possible.

**What kinds of topics are part of a policy and procedure manual?**

Policy and procedure manuals include things such as leave policies, dress codes, salary and wage practices, training expectations, safety standards and practices, disciplinary practices, etc.

**What are the purposes of departmental meetings in a physical therapy department?**

Departmental meetings are used to disseminate information important to the business of the department as a whole. Staff meetings provide time to discuss strategies to improve practices or solve problems. Team meetings allow for the coordination of patient care. Supervisory meetings between PTs and PTAs are used specifically to discuss individual patient care. Strategic planning meetings are used to plan for future departmental goals.

**What is the role of all department members in fiscal responsibility?**

Every department member should utilize the resources of the business in a responsible manner, as it affects the overall success of the business. Members should recognize that in addition to their interaction with patients/clients, thoughtful use of electricity, water, and supplies makes a difference in the fiscal outcome for the department or business.

**Which of the quality assurance activities is the evaluation of the necessity, quality, effectiveness, or efficiency of physical therapy services?**

Utilization review

**What is an example of risk management?**

Risk management includes the following:

- Identification of healthcare delivery problems in an institution (as evidenced by previous lawsuits and patient or staff complaints)
- Development of standards and guidelines to enhance the quality of care
- Anticipation of problems that may arise in the future

**What are some topics that would address the goal of physical therapy in promoting wellness and disease prevention?**

Examples of health promotion could be the PT's assessments of a patient's/client's:

- Behavioral health risks (such as smoking or drug abuse)
- Level of physical fitness
- Psychological function (such as memory, reasoning ability, depression, anxiety, or memory)
- Social activities
- Other clinical findings (such as nutrition or hydration)

# Chapter 4

## What are the levels of PTA supervision?

General supervision requires that the PT be available to supervise the PTA at a minimum by telecommunications. Direct supervision requires that the PT be physically present to supervise the PTA. During direct personal supervision, the PT is continuously directing and supervising all of the care provided to the patient.

## What are some of the tasks that a PTA may perform?

POC review; provision of procedural interventions; patient instruction; patient progression; data collection; documentation; safety; cardiopulmonary resuscitation (CPR) and emergency procedures; resource management; communication; and promotion of health, wellness, and prevention

## What components of care can only be performed by the PT?

The PTA cannot perform an evaluation, develop or change the POC, or write a discharge plan.

## What are the supervision requirements of the PT working with the PTA?

Each state will have laws regarding supervision of PTAs, including the number of assistive personnel each PT can supervise, the specific level of supervision, and the timing of supervision.

## What are the differences among the three types of healthcare teams?

Intradisciplinary team members work together within the same discipline. In a multidisciplinary team, members work separately and independently in their different disciplines. They do not meet or try to collaborate with each other. The interprofessional team members work together within all disciplines to set goals relevant to a patient's/client's individual case. All the members collaborate in decision-making; however, the evaluations and interventions are done independently.

## What are the roles of occupational therapists and certified occupational therapy assistants?

Occupational therapists (OTs) and certified occupational therapy assistants (COTAs) help people improve their ability to perform tasks in their daily living and working environments. They work with individuals who have conditions that are mentally, physically, developmentally, or emotionally disabling. They also help these individuals to develop, recover, or maintain daily living and work skills. OTs help patients and clients not only to improve their basic motor functions and reasoning abilities but also to compensate for permanent loss of function.

## How might the PT and PTA interact with the speech-language pathologist on the healthcare team?

Speech-language pathologists can provide information to the healthcare team that will assist them in communicating effectively with the patient/client. They also can help the team understand cognitive impairments that can help the members interact with the patient/client successfully.

# Chapter 5

## Where does the PT obtain information for the examination?

The PT obtains information for the examination from data collected from the patient's medical chart, review of intake paperwork, and interviewing and examining the patient.

## What is the difference between an examination and an evaluation?

An examination is the process of obtaining a history, performing relevant systems reviews, and selecting and administering specific tests and measures. An evaluation is a dynamic process in which the PT makes clinical judgments based on data gathered during the examination.

## When working with a patient who has a progressive neurologic disease, what psychosocial care components are important to exam?

Specific psychosocial aspects of patient care in neurologic physical therapy may include the following:

- Patient's adaptation to disability
- Patient's and patient's family's stages of adjustment to the disease and disability
- Effects of impairments, functional limitations, and disability
- Effects of limitations in patient's participation
- Patient's reintegration into environment, family, work, and life

## What are the common symptoms of cardiopulmonary disease?

Cardiovascular signs and symptoms may include the following:

- Diaphoresis, which is excess sweating associated with decreased cardiac output
- Decreased or absent pulses associated with peripheral vascular disease (PVD)
- Cyanotic skin, which is associated with decreased cardiac output; or pallor, which is associated with PVD

- Skin temperature may indicate a lack of blood flow when it is cold.
- Skin changes, such as pale, shiny, or dry skin, with loss of hair are associated with PVD.
- Bilateral edema can be an indication of congestive heart failure. Unilateral edema indicates thrombophlebitis or PVD.

## What pediatric screening tool is common in elementary-aged children?

A variety of standardized tests are available to compare the older child's functional abilities, such as the Peabody Developmental Motor Scales or the Bruininks–Oseretsky Test of Motor Proficiency.

## What diagnoses are being screened for with the Mini-Mental State Examination?

The Mini-Mental State Examination is an assessment of the patient's cognitive changes in orientation, attention, math, recall, and language.

## Why are environmental examinations important?

Environmental examinations check for an obstacle in a patient's/client's home that may present with safety concerns. Things that may be assessed are adequate lighting, flooring, and stairs that may present with tripping hazards, clutter, or unsafe furniture that pose a fall risk, etc.

## Why is it important for PTs to assess the skin of a patient?

The skin is an important barrier to infectious agents, the first line of the immune system defense. Loss of skin integrity can lead to pain, inflammation, or systemic infection. Skin can also be an indicator of internal health concerns, such as liver or blood and circulatory conditions.

## What will a POC include?

The POC will identify the patient's impairments, functional long-term goals and expected outcomes, and the interventions that will be utilized to meet the goals. The intensity, frequency, and duration of the episode of care will also be identified.

## How will a POC be used by a PTA?

The PTA will utilize the POC and their clinical judgment to determine what activities they will perform with the patient during every visit to physical therapy.

## What are the parameters of therapeutic exercise?

Therapeutic exercise parameters include the frequency, duration, repetitions, sets, intensity, and mode of the exercise.

## What are the three types of range of motion?

The three types of range of motion (ROM) include passive, active assistive, and active.

## What are the differences among isometric, isotonic, and isokinetic exercise?

- Isometric exercises develop tension in the muscle without visible joint movement and changes in muscle length.
- Isotonic exercises develop tension in the muscle through dynamic concentric or eccentric muscular contractions. Concentric muscular contraction causes the muscle to shorten, whereas eccentric muscular contraction causes the muscle to lengthen. Isotonic exercise is a dynamic exercise with a constant load (such as a weight) but uncontrolled speed of movement.
- Isokinetic exercises are dynamic exercises having a predetermined velocity of muscle shortening or lengthening, so that the force generated by the muscle is maximal through the full ROM. Isokinetic exercises take place at a constant speed.

## Why are physical agents used?

- To reduce or eliminate soft-tissue inflammation
- To speed the healing time of a soft-tissue injury
- To decrease pain
- To modify muscular tone
- To remodel scar tissue
- To increase connective tissue extensibility and length

## Why are assistive devices used for gait?

Assistive devices are used during gait to allow patients to walk safely and more effectively.

## What are the different types of neurologic interventions?

Some examples of neurologic interventions include neurodevelopmental treatment, proprioceptive neuromuscular facilitation, sensory stimulation, and movement therapy.

## What is the purpose of cardiac rehabilitation?

Cardiac rehabilitation assists patients with cardiac dysfunctions to develop safe exercise habits; improve cardiovascular and pulmonary endurance; and learn about healthy living topics, such as diet, smoking cessation, and the use of medication.

# Chapter 6

## What is the difference between medical ethics and medical law?

Medical ethics is a system of principles governing medical conduct. Ethics is a system of moral principles or standards governing a person's conduct.

Morals are the basis for ethical conduct. They are an individual's beliefs, principles, and values about what is right and wrong. Medical law is the establishment of social rules for conduct. A violation of medical law may create criminal and civil liability. Lawmakers frequently turn to policy statements, including medical ethics statements of professional organizations, when creating laws affecting that profession.

### How are beneficence and nonmaleficence alike and how are they different?

Beneficence is the ethical principle that emphasizes doing the best for the patient. Beneficence requires actions to benefit the patient. Nonmaleficence is the ethical principle that exhorts practitioners to "do no harm." Nonmaleficence is an obligation to not do harmful actions.

### What do the terms "justice" and "veracity" mean?

Justice is an ethical principle that mandates that a healthcare provider distribute fair and equal treatment to every patient. Veracity is an ethical principle that binds the healthcare provider and the patient in a relationship to tell the truth.

### What does confidentiality mean?

Confidentiality is an ethical principle that requires a healthcare provider to maintain privacy by not sharing or divulging to a third party privileged or entrusted patient information.

### What protections are contained in HIPAA?

The Health Insurance Portability and Accountability Act (HIPAA) includes protections for any health information that is individually identifiable and dictates under what conditions and with whom information can be shared, and it gives patients rights over their health information. It requires covered users to have appropriate policies and procedures in place to ensure that information is protected.

### What information is considered personal health information?

Information that is included as personal health information includes things such as names, addresses, birth dates, social security numbers, etc., that can provide enough information to be linked to an individual person.

### What are good practices to prevent breaking confidentiality and HIPAA?

Examples of reasonable safeguards that a covered entity needs to implement may include the following:

- Avoiding the use of the patient's name in public hallways

- Speaking quietly when discussing a patient's condition in the waiting room with the patient/patient's family
- When making private phone calls, verifying the identity of the person you are speaking to
- Leaving limited voice mail information
- Locking file cabinets or records rooms
- Requiring additional passwords on computers used by all employees working in the facility

### What is the first step to identifying cultural competence?

Cultural competence requires a person's openness and willingness to learn about cultural issues and the ability to understand a person's own biases, values, attitudes, beliefs, and behaviors.

### What patient/client characteristics make up cultural diversity?

Cultural diversity can be addressed through awareness/acceptance of the following patient/client characteristics:

- Racial characteristics and national origin
- Religious affiliations
- Physical size
- Spoken language
- Sexual orientation
- Physical and mental disability
- Age
- Gender
- Socioeconomic status
- Political orientation
- Geographic location
- Occupational status

### What are the strategies to develop cultural competence?

1. Identify personal cultural biases.
2. Understand general cultural differences.
3. Accept and respect cultural differences.
4. Apply cultural understanding.

### What is ethnocentrism?

Ethnocentrism is the act of judging another culture based upon one's own cultural customs and standards.

### What things should be included when asking a patient for informed consent?

Elements of informed consent to be discussed with the patient/client include the following:

- The nature of the decision or the procedure (such as a clear description of the proposed intervention)

- Reasonable alternatives to the proposed intervention
- The relevant risks, benefits, and uncertainties related to each alternative
- Assessment of patient understanding
- The patient's acceptance of the intervention

## What standards should a PTA adhere to in order to act ethically and professionally?

- Provide respectful and compassionate care for the patient, including sensitivity to individual and cultural differences.
- Act on behalf of the patient/client while being sensitive to the patient's/client's vulnerability.
- Work under the direction and supervision of the PT.
- Comply with laws and regulations governing physical therapy.
- Maintain competence in the provision of selected physical therapy interventions.
- Make judgments commensurate with one's educational and legal qualifications.
- Protect the public and the profession from unethical, incompetent, and illegal acts.

## What are the eight value-based behaviors of the PTA?

1. Altruism
2. Caring and compassion
3. Continuing competence
4. Duty
5. Integrity
6. PT/PTA collaboration
7. Responsibility
8. Social responsibility

## Which of the core values of a PTA is described as the devotion to the interest of a patient/client?
Altruism

# Chapter 7

## What type of laws are utilized by the Centers for Medicare and Medicaid Services to apply rules and regulations?
Federal statutes are utilized to create Medicare and Medicaid rules and regulations.

## What is included in Title I of the Americans with Disabilities Act (ADA)?
Title I of the ADA protects people with disabilities against employment discrimination. Discrimination applies to an employee's recruitment, selection, training, benefits, promotion, discipline, and retention.

## What does the Individuals with Disabilities Education Act of 1997 require for compliance?

- To ensure that all children with disabilities have available to them a free, appropriate public education that emphasizes special education and related services designed to meet their unique needs and prepare them for employment and independent living
- To ensure that the rights of children with disabilities and parents of such children are protected
- To assist states, localities, educational service agencies, and federal agencies to provide for the education of all children with disabilities
- To assist states in the implementation of a statewide, comprehensive, coordinated, multidisciplinary, interagency system of early intervention services for infants and toddlers with disabilities and their families
- To ensure that educators and parents have the necessary tools to improve educational results for children with disabilities by supporting systemic change; coordinated research and personnel preparation; coordinated technical assistance, dissemination, and support; and technology development and media services
- To assess and ensure the effectiveness of efforts to educate children with disabilities

## What are the requirements for practice included in regulatory practice acts?
Requirements of regulatory practice acts include the following:

- Requirements for licensure of professionals educated in the United States
- Requirements for licensure of foreign-educated or foreign-trained professionals
- Requirements for continuing professional education
- Requirements for practice within the state pursuant to temporary licensure
- Requirements for periodic relicensure
- Requirements for mandatory reporting of perceived unethical conduct within the scope of permissible practice
- Restrictions, if any, on independent or autonomous practice called practice without referral
- Provisions establishing licensure boards to administer professional licensure
- Provisions defining grounds and procedures for disciplinary action

## What are the APTA policies regarding licensure?

The APTA requires that the PTs should be licensed and PTAs should be licensed or certified. They should be graduates of a Commission on Accreditation in Physical Therapy Education (CAPTE)-accredited program (or meet the regulations if foreign trained) and pass a competency-based exam. State regulations should provide title protection, allow for disciplinary action, and define the scope of practice. State regulations should also direct the supervision of PTAs by PTs.

## What does OSHA regulate?

The Occupational Safety and Health Administration (OSHA) is a federal government regulatory agency concerned with the health and safety of workers.

## What is bloodborne pathogen training?

Bloodborne pathogen training is part of OSHA regulations that require employers to train at-risk workers in procedures to decrease the possible exposure to bloodborne pathogens during their work tasks.

## What are the recommendations of universal precautions?

Universal precautions represent OSHA's recommendations to control and protect employees from exposure to all human blood and other potentially infectious materials. The Bloodborne Pathogens standard (BPS) requires all blood and other potentially infectious materials to be considered infectious regardless of the perceived risk of an individual patient or patient population. Healthcare workers should utilize precautions, such as the utilization of personal protective equipment, when appropriate.

## What is a sign of domestic abuse?

Domestic violence, also called domestic abuse or battering, occurs between people in intimate relationships and takes many forms, including coercion; threats; intimidation; isolation; and emotional, sexual, and physical abuse. Some signs that PTs or PTAs may notice include physical symptoms related to stress, hypervigilance and very guarded behaviors, suicide attempts, eating disorders, self-mutilation, self-harm, and overuse of pain medications and other drugs.

## Explain the types of abuse.

- Physical violence, such as hitting, kicking, or in general hurting the victim using physical force
- Sexual violence, such as forcing the victim to have sexual intercourse or to engage in other sexual activities against the intimate partner's will
- Using children as pawns, such as accusing the intimate partner of bad parenting, threatening to take the children away, or using the children to relay messages to the partner
- Denial and blame, such as denying that the abuse occurred or shifting responsibility for the abusive behavior onto the partner
- Coercion and threats, such as threatening to hurt other family members, pets, children, or self
- Economic abuse, such as controlling finances, refusing to share money, sabotaging the partner's work performance, making the partner account for money spent, or not allowing the partner to work outside the home
- Intimidation, such as using certain actions, looks, or gestures to instill fear, and breaking things, abusing pets, or destroying property
- Emotional abuse, such as insults, criticism, or name calling
- Isolation, such as limiting the partner's contact with family and friends, requiring permission to leave the house, not allowing the partner to attend work or school, or controlling the partner's activities and social events
- Privilege, such as making all major decisions, defining the roles in the relationship, being in charge of the home and social life, or treating the partner as a servant or possession

## What behaviors might an abuser use to control the healthcare provider?

An abuser's tactics to control the healthcare providers may include the following:

- Intimidating healthcare professionals with a variety of threats or acts
- Portraying himself or herself as a good provider and caregiver and/or consistently praising healthcare professionals
- Harassing healthcare professionals by repeated phone calls, threats of legal action, and/or false reports to superiors about supposed breaches of confidentiality, inappropriate treatment, or rude behavior
- Splitting healthcare teams by creating divisiveness among professionals

## How can a healthcare provider help a person who is abused?

Healthcare providers can assist the person by screening for domestic violence, creating emergency protocols, and having a list of appropriate referrals for community agencies.

## What is negligence?

It is the failure to give reasonable care or the giving of unreasonable care. A healthcare practitioner is negligent only when harm occurred to the patient/client.

### What are examples of malpractice?

Some examples of malpractice would be burns due to defective equipment, utilization of broken equipment, a patient fall during gait training, exercise injuries, and actions/inaction that are inconsistent with ethical principles and standards of practice.

# Chapter 8

### What is the ability to imagine oneself in another person's place and to understand their feelings, ideas, desires, and actions?

Empathy

### What is the difference between empathy and sympathy?

Empathy is genuinely feeling our patients'/clients' feelings, ideas, desires, and emotions. Sympathy is understanding the patients'/clients' feelings, ideas, desires, and emotions, but not really feeling them.

### What are the three stages of empathy?

The first stage, the cognitive stage, involves getting into the position of the other person. This stage involves listening to the patient/client and trying to imagine what it must be like for the patient/client to experience what he or she is describing. The second stage, the crossing over stage, is the most significant because for a moment or so the PT/PTA can feel himself or herself as the patient/client, living in the patient's/client's world. Then, in the third stage (coming back to own feelings stage), the PT/PTA comes back to his or her own person and feels a special alliance with the patient.

### What attributes assist in creating a healthy therapeutic relationship with patients/clients?

The attributes that help to create a therapeutic relationship with the patient include punctuality, friendliness, cultural sensitivity, communication that is understandable to the patient, behaviors that are patient-focused, knowledgeable interactions, trustworthiness, helpfulness, and a comforting manner.

### What strategies can a PTA use when working with people who do not assist in creating a healthy therapeutic relationship?

When working with difficult people, PTAs can employ the following strategies: stay calm, act respectfully, ignore rudeness, redirect the patient to the present, focus on the problem to be solved by listening to the patient, and understand that you may not be able to change the situation.

### What personal and professional characteristics should be explored when creating an effective PT/PTA team?

In order to create a good working relationship with the PT, the team should discuss their backgrounds and beliefs. Understanding each other's education, the state laws, professional and ethical standards, and personal standards can assist the team in creating an effective PT–PTA team.

### What are the purposes of verbal communication?

- To establish a rapport with the patient/client and/or the patient's/client's family/caregiver
- To enhance the relationship among the patient/client, his or her family/caregiver, and the PT/PTA
- To obtain information concerning the patient's/client's condition and progress
- To transmit pertinent information to other healthcare professionals and providers and supportive personnel
- To provide education and instructions to the patient/client and patient's/client's family/caregiver
- To increase the patient's/client's adherence to education and the continuum of care at home
- To decrease the patient's/client's health risks

### What challenges occur when communicating with people from different cultural backgrounds?

When working with people with different cultural backgrounds, the PTA may encounter challenges, such as different worldviews, languages, and backgrounds. Inappropriate judgments, ethnocentrism, and decreased cultural competence can cause inadequate interactions with patients/clients.

### What are some possible negative effects of using family members as interpreters?

Patients may not feel comfortable being forthright when using family members as interpreters. Additionally, inaccurate language interpretation may occur if the family member changes the language transmission to prevent embarrassment or uncomfortable feelings. Finally, issues of confidentiality and informed consent are difficult when professional interpreters are not employed in language barrier situations.

### What is the difference between open and closed questions?

An open question requires responses that require some length, rather than "yes" or "no" answers that closed questions require.

### What type of listening is used to gather specific information that will help assess a patient's symptoms?

Directed listening

## What are the methods of effective listening?

- The PT/PTA focuses his or her attention on the patient.
- The PT/PTA helps the patient to feel free to talk by smiling and looking at the patient.
- The PT/PTA pays attention to the patient's non-verbal communication, such as gestures, facial expressions, tone of voice, and body posture.
- The PT/PTA asks the patient to clarify the meaning of words and the feelings involved or to enlarge the statement.
- The PT/PTA repeats the patient's message to understand completely the meaning and the content of the message. Reflective listening allows the PTA to clarify what the patient has stated and the patient can then correct any misperceptions.
- The PT/PTA takes notes as necessary to help remember or document what was said.
- The PT/PTA uses body language, such as nonverbal gestures (leaning forward, nodding the head, keeping eye contact, or keeping hands at his or her side), to show involvement in the patient's message.
- The PT/PTA does not abruptly interrupt the patient and thus gives adequate time to present the full message.
- The PT/PTA empathizes with the patient.

## What are the barriers to effective listening?

Ineffective listeners typically listen on and off and typically listen to words, ideas, or opinions. Ineffective listeners consider the patient boring and are absorbed in their own thoughts. This type of listener often daydreams when another person is speaking. Ineffective listeners have favorite ideas, prejudices, and points of view and can become defensive when challenged.

## What postures are most useful when creating a therapeutic relationship?

Open postures assist in creating a therapeutic relationship. Some examples of open postures include standing or sitting with arms at the sides and legs uncrossed, standing or sitting straight, standing or sitting positioned at the same eye level with the receiver, and facing the other person.

## How might cultural differences change the way you verbally and nonverbally interact with a patient/client?

Some examples of changes that may be necessary include not looking the patient in the eyes, changing the distance between PTA and patient, avoiding certain gestures, or changing therapeutic touch practices.

## What is the value of giving a patient information in writing?

Written information helps to reinforce the activities that occurred and assist the patient in remembering details that may often be forgotten.

## What are some good practices to employ when providing a home exercise program?

When creating a home exercise program, utilize the patient's primary language, avoid technical or complex words, utilize pictures, and use font of 12 or larger. Use high contrast to assist people with visual impairments. Include all pertinent information and make the information concise to promote compliance with the home exercise program.

# Chapter 9

## What are the instructional formats utilized to teach patients/clients?

Clinical instruction modes for patients/clients can take the following formats:

- Discussions
- Demonstrations
- Presentations
- Lectures
- Audiovisual materials or web-based learning methods
- Return demonstrations
- Illustrations of written information

## What instructional activities will improve learning?

The following activities will improve learning:

- Respect for the patient's values, preferences, and expressed needs
- An overview of the objectives and purpose of the learning activity
- A description of how the learning activity fits with the patient's personal goals
- An environment that is quiet and appropriate for learning
- Reduction of conditions that have a negative impact on learning, such as pain or discomfort, anxiety, fear, frustration, feelings of failure, humiliation, embarrassment, boredom, or time pressures
- A teaching plan that is logical and sequential, using patient-friendly language, and being understandable for the patient given his or her own personal traits (e.g., culture, age, intellect, and educational levels)
- Ample time for practice and answering questions

- Specific instructions to ensure that the clinician and patient have the same perceptions
- Appropriate assessment of learning immediately following the teaching and in subsequent treatment sessions
- Involvement of family members or friends to provide a support system for the patient

## What should the PTA do in order to effectively communicate during patient education?

The therapist should communicate clearly and simply by using everyday words, rephrasing as necessary, and explaining new words. To ensure the message gets to the patient, besides speaking and writing, the therapist can use other materials, such as audiotapes, videotapes/DVDs, support groups, hotlines, and websites, for online information. In addition, the patient's understanding of information can be verified by asking open-ended questions and asking the patient to demonstrate how he or she will accomplish the instructions.

## What are the obstacles to learning that may be present when teaching a patient?

Some barriers to learning include learning impairments, visual and auditory impairments, lack of concentration, or lack of motivation.

## What strategies should a PTA employ to decrease obstacles to learning?

Some strategies to decrease obstacles to learning include the following:

- Adjust the teaching method to the patient's learning style or needs
- Focus on the patient's concerns
- Include family or a friend who is supportive of the patient
- Teach information in smaller chunks
- Create opportunities for practice
- Write in plain language
- Use multisensory instruction
- Create a learning environment
- Adjust methods for those who have visual or auditory impairment
- Use language interpreters
- Adjust communication styles with cultural sensitivity

# Chapter 10

## What are the purposes for documentation?

Documentation is used for reimbursement, assurance of quality care, assurance of continuity of care, legal reasons, research and education, and marketing.

## What are the recommendations for effective documentation?

The APTA makes the following documentation recommendations:

- The documentation must be consistent with the APTA's Standards of Practice and all jurisdictional and regulatory requirements.
- Every visit/encounter requires documentation.
- All documentation must be legible and use medically approved abbreviations or symbols.
- All documentation must be written in black or blue ink, and the mistakes must be crossed out with a single line through the error, initialed, and dated by the PTA.
- When utilizing electronic health records, security measures to ensure patient confidentiality must be utilized.
- Each intervention session must be documented; the patient's name and identification number must be on each page of the documentation record.
- Informed consent for the interventions must be signed by a competent adult. If the adult is not competent, the consent must be signed by the patient's/client's legal guardian. If the patient is a minor, the consent must be signed by the parent or an appointed guardian.
- Each document must be dated and signed by the PT/PTA using their first and last names and their professional designation. Professional license number may be included, but it is optional.
- All communications with other healthcare providers or healthcare professionals must be recorded.
- PT students' notes should be cosigned by the PTs.
- PTA students' notes should be cosigned by the PTs and/or PTAs.
- Nonlicensed personnel notes should be cosigned by the PT.
- Documentation of referral sources or self-referral should occur within the initial documentation.
- Cancellations and no-shows should be documented.

## What is the difference between problem-oriented medical records and source-oriented medical records?

Problem-oriented medical records list the patient's problems in order of importance and then connect them to the intervention. Source-oriented medical records are organized by the medical department that is providing the service.

## What do the four sections of the SOAP format represent?

Subjective, Objective, Assessment, Plan

**What information is found in the initial evaluation?**

The initial evaluation identifies the reason for the referral, the functional limitations, the PT assessment, goals and outcomes, and the intervention plan.

**What are the differences among a treatment note, a progress report, and a discharge report?**

A treatment note provides information about the patient's current status, the intervention provided, assessment of the progress or lack of progress of the patient's condition, and the plan for the following intervention. A progress report is a documentation of the care from the time of evaluation to the writing of the progress note. The PT will outline the patient's current status and progress toward meeting the goals and outcomes outlined in the initial evaluation. A discharge report represents a final outline of the patient's episode of care, including meeting of goals and outcomes and reason for discharge from PT services.

**What information is found in the subjective section of the SOAP format?**

Information located in the subjective section includes things that the patient or patient's family have communicated to the PTA, such as symptoms, functional losses, or aggravating factors.

**What information is found in the objective section of the SOAP format?**

Information located in the objective section includes signs of disease or dysfunction that are noted by the PTA, interventions performed by the PTA, descriptions of patient functions, tests and measures performed, and patient education provided.

**How is the assessment section of the SOAP format different than the subjective and objective?**

The assessment section discusses the patient's response to intervention and the effectiveness of the intervention, and also comments about the patient's progress/lack of progress toward the goals established by the PT in the initial examination and evaluation.

**What components should be present in the Plan section of the SOAP format?**

The plan data of the progress SOAP note contains information that the PTA may need to apply regarding the patient's interventions before and during the treatment session(s) or between the sessions. They also indicate when the next session will take place or how many sessions are to be scheduled.

**What is the regulatory designation of a physical therapist assistant?**

The regulatory designation for the physical therapist assistant is PTA.

**What types of information should be included in documentation to provide verification of professional judgment?**

PTAs should include evidence-based practice using researched clinical guidelines and approved PT protocols to demonstrate professional judgment.

**What are the advantages and disadvantages of electronic medical records?**

The benefits of computerized documentation include the following:

- Submitting information to insurance companies electronically
- Monitoring the clinician's productivity
- Tracking patients' visits
- Easing patient scheduling
- Minimizing documentation paperwork
- Integrating billing
- Maximizing efficiency
- Increasing reimbursement
- Improved communication among healthcare teams

The negative consequences of using electronic records include the following:

- Distraction of documentation while working with the patient
- Concerns for safeguarding the information from malicious entities
- Cost of upgrading hardware and software to maintain an operational system
- Need for a backup system of documentation if the electronic system fails

# Chapter 11

**What is the money paid by the patient to the healthcare professional each time a service is provided called?**

Co-pay

**What is the difference between eligibility and prior authorization?**

Eligibility is the process of determining whether a patient qualifies for benefits. Prior authorization is a process that requires the patient or provider to contact the insurance company to determine if a service can be provided.

**What are CPT codes and ICD-10 codes?**

International Classification of Diseases, Tenth Revision (ICD-10) codes are standardized classification of diagnoses for all healthcare providers. Current Procedural

Terminology (CPT) codes are numbers that identify specific procedures and are used for billing.

## What benefits are paid for by Medicare Part A and Medicare Part B?

Medicare Part A will pay for inpatient care in hospitals, skilled nursing facilities, and hospice care. Medicare Part B pays for doctors' services and outpatient care.

## What is the prospective payment system?

The prospective payment system (PPS) is a fixed payment that is matched to diagnosis classifications, known as diagnosis-related groups (DRGs), in the acute care setting.

## What are the new payment models being implemented in skilled nursing facilities, outpatient facilities, and home health agencies?

Skilled nursing facilities will begin implementing the Patient-Driven Payment Model became effective in October 2019. The Home Health Patient-Driven Groupings Model began in January 2020 and be a similar program for home health agencies. Outpatient services began the Quality Payment Program in 2019. This program is divided into the Merit-Based Incentive Payment System and the Advanced Alternative Payment Model.

## Who is eligible for Medicaid services?

Medicaid services are designed for children, nonelderly low-income parents, other caretaker relatives, pregnant women, nonelderly individuals with disabilities, and low-income elderly people.

## What is the difference between private insurance and health maintenance organizations?

Private insurance companies provide insurance to individuals and employees through employer-provided plans. A health maintenance organization (HMO) is a form of managed care. Managed care provides healthcare services by a limited number of healthcare professionals for a fixed prepaid fee.

## What are the three reasons for reading research?

The three reasons to read research include to determine quality improvement practices, to answer specific practice questions, and to learn about current research and current practice topics.

## What are the steps to a successful search strategy?

Step one is to be clear about the purpose of the information the learner is reading. Step two is to create an understanding of foundational concepts and terminology. Step three is to choose the most appropriate search database and to use it in the most effective way possible.

## What are the levels of evidence?

Levels of evidence refers to the amount of confidence the reader can place in the research based on the study design.

## Why is it important to assess the levels of evidence?

Each level of evidence provides a different type of usefulness that should be linked to the question being researched.

## What is found in each part of a research article?

The *title and abstract* create interest in the article and summarize its contents.

The *introduction* describes the reason that authors chose to perform the research and state the hypothesis.

The *methods* section describes what process was undertaken during the research including the validity and study design.

The *results* section highlights the research findings in an objective way.

The *discussion and conclusions* section allows the authors to describe what they think the results mean and what conclusions can be drawn from the research. The authors also point out flaws that they found in doing the research.

## What is validity?

Validity refers to how effective the tool used is at measuring what it intended to measure.

## What is reliability?

Reliability in research refers to the ability of the research activity to show the same results when repeated by another researcher.

# Chapter 12

## What are the attributes of successful people?

The attributes of successful people are optimism, commitment, passion, competence, initiative, flexibility, generosity, and developing good relationships.

## What is the value of a mentor and networking?

Mentors can assist students in navigating the transition from the classroom to clinic to the first job. Networking with other professionals can lead to occasions to learn and share information, and may lead to jobs and other professional opportunities.

## What strategies are necessary to land your dream job?

Graduates should start their job search by identifying their career goals and researching job opportunities, looking for those that match their goals. Career skill surveys and personality assessments can help to identify attributes that graduates can highlight in their resume and job interviews. Graduates should take time to prepare their resume and should practice for the interview.

**What lifelong activities will provide the PTA with job satisfaction?**
Graduates will find opportunities to continue learning after graduation and should consider leadership opportunities within the place of employment; components and sections of the APTA; and their community.

# Appendix H

# American Physical Therapy Association's Standards of Ethical Conduct for Physical Therapist Assistants

Standards of Ethical Conduct for the Physical Therapist Assistant HOD S06-09-20-18 [Amended HOD S06-00-13-24; HOD 06-91-06-07; Initial HOD 06-82-04-08] [Standard]

## Preamble

The Standards of Ethical Conduct for the Physical Therapist Assistant (Standards of Ethical Conduct) delineate the ethical obligations of all physical therapist assistants as determined by the House of Delegates of the American Physical Therapy Association (APTA). The Standards of Ethical Conduct provide a foundation for conduct to which all physical therapist assistants shall adhere. Fundamental to the Standards of Ethical Conduct is the special obligation of physical therapist assistants to enable patients/clients to achieve greater independence, health and wellness, and enhanced quality of life.

No document that delineates ethical standards can address every situation. Physical therapist assistants are encouraged to seek additional advice or consultation in instances where the guidance of the Standards of Ethical Conduct may not be definitive.

## Standards

Standard #1: Physical therapist assistants shall respect the inherent dignity, and rights, of all individuals.

- 1A.
  Physical therapist assistants shall act in a respectful manner toward each person regardless of age,

gender, race, nationality, religion, ethnicity, social or economic status, sexual orientation, health condition, or disability.
- 1B.
  Physical therapist assistants shall recognize their personal biases and shall not discriminate against others in the provision of physical therapy services.

Standard #2: Physical therapist assistants shall be trustworthy and compassionate in addressing the rights and needs of patients/clients.

- 2A.
  Physical therapist assistants shall act in the best interests of patients/clients over the interests of the physical therapist assistant.
- 2B.
  Physical therapist assistants shall provide physical therapy interventions with compassionate and caring behaviors that incorporate the individual and cultural differences of patients/clients.
- 2C.
  Physical therapist assistants shall provide patients/clients with information regarding the interventions they provide.
- 2D.
  Physical therapist assistants shall protect confidential patient/client information and, in collaboration with the physical therapist, may disclose confidential information to appropriate authorities only when allowed or as required by law.

Standard #3: Physical therapist assistants shall make sound decisions in collaboration with the physical therapist and within the boundaries established by laws and regulations.

- 3A.
  Physical therapist assistants shall make objective decisions in the patient's/client's best interest in all practice settings.
- 3B.
  Physical therapist assistants shall be guided by information about best practice regarding physical therapy interventions.
- 3C.
  Physical therapist assistants shall make decisions based upon their level of competence and consistent with patient/client values.
- 3D.
  Physical therapist assistants shall not engage in conflicts of interest that interfere with making sound decisions.
- 3E.
  Physical therapist assistants shall provide physical therapy services under the direction and supervision of a physical therapist and shall communicate with the physical therapist when patient/client status requires modifications to the established plan of care.

Standard #4: Physical therapist assistants shall demonstrate integrity in their relationships with patients/clients, families, colleagues, students, other healthcare providers, employers, payers, and the public.

- 4A.
  Physical therapist assistants shall provide truthful, accurate, and relevant information and shall not make misleading representations.
- 4B.
  Physical therapist assistants shall not exploit persons over whom they have supervisory, evaluative, or other authority (e.g., patients/clients, students, supervisees, research participants, or employees).
- 4C.
  Physical therapist assistants shall discourage misconduct by healthcare professionals and report illegal or unethical acts to the relevant authority, when appropriate.
- 4D.
  Physical therapist assistants shall report suspected cases of abuse involving children or vulnerable adults to the supervising physical therapist and the appropriate authority, subject to law.

- 4E.
  Physical therapist assistants shall not engage in any sexual relationship with any of their patients/clients, supervisees, or students.
- 4F.
  Physical therapist assistants shall not harass anyone verbally, physically, emotionally, or sexually.

Standard #5: Physical therapist assistants shall fulfill their legal and ethical obligations.

- 5A.
  Physical therapist assistants shall comply with applicable local, state, and federal laws and regulations.
- 5B.
  Physical therapist assistants shall support the supervisory role of the physical therapist to ensure quality care and promote patient/client safety.
- 5C.
  Physical therapist assistants involved in research shall abide by accepted standards governing protection of research participants.
- 5D.
  Physical therapist assistants shall encourage colleagues with physical, psychological, or substance-related impairments that may adversely impact their professional responsibilities to seek assistance of counsel.
- 5E.
  Physical therapist assistants who have knowledge that a colleague is unable to perform their professional responsibilities with reasonable skill and safety shall report this information to the appropriate authority.

Standard #6: Physical therapist assistants shall enhance their competence through the lifelong acquisition and refinement of knowledge, skills, and abilities.

- 6A.
  Physical therapist assistants shall achieve and maintain clinical competence.
- 6B.
  Physical therapist assistants shall engage in lifelong learning consistent with changes in their roles and responsibilities and advances in the practice of physical therapy.
- 6C.
  Physical therapist assistants shall support practice environments that support career development and lifelong learning.

Standard #7: Physical therapist assistants shall support organizational behaviors and business practices that benefit patients/clients and society.

- 7A.
  Physical therapist assistants shall promote work environments that support ethical and accountable decision-making.
- 7B.
  Physical therapist assistants shall not accept gifts or other considerations that influence or give an appearance of influencing their decisions.
- 7C.
  Physical therapist assistants shall fully disclose any financial interest they have in products or services that they recommend to patients/clients.
- 7D.
  Physical therapist assistants shall ensure that documentation for their interventions accurately reflects the nature and extent of the services provided.
- 7E.
  Physical therapist assistants shall refrain from employment arrangements, or other arrangements, that prevent physical therapist assistants from fulfilling ethical obligations to patients/clients.

Standard #8: Physical therapist assistants shall participate in efforts to meet the health needs of people locally, nationally, or globally.

- 8A.
  Physical therapist assistants shall support organizations that meet the health needs of people who are economically disadvantaged, uninsured, and underinsured.
- 8B.
  Physical therapist assistants shall advocate for people with impairments, activity limitations, participation restrictions, and disabilities in order to promote their participation in community and society.
- 8C.
  Physical therapist assistants shall be responsible stewards of healthcare resources by collaborating with physical therapists in order to avoid overutilization of physical therapy services.
- 8D.
  Physical therapist assistants shall educate members of the public about the benefits of physical therapy.

# Glossary

## A

**abuse** Actions that are improper, inappropriate, outside acceptable standards of professional conduct, or medically unnecessary. For example, a provider performs and bills for an unnecessary treatment.

**American Physical Therapy Association (APTA)** An individual membership professional organization representing member physical therapists (PTs), physical therapist assistants (PTAs), and students of physical therapy.

**Americans with Disabilities Act (ADA)** Federal law that prohibits discrimination and ensures equal opportunity for persons with disabilities in employment, state and local government services, public accommodations, commercial facilities, and transportation.

**APGAR screening** A system of evaluating an infant's physical condition at birth; the infant's heart rate, respiration, muscle tone, response to stimuli, and color are rated at 1 minute, and again at 5 minutes after birth.

**assembly** A group of members from the same category and who provide means for members to communicate and contribute at the national level to their future governance.

**assessment data** Data that include an appraisal or evaluation of a patient's condition based on clinical and laboratory data, medical history, and the patient's accounts of symptoms; data included in the "A" section of the SOAP note; in the SOAP note, they provide the rationale for the necessity of the skilled physical therapy services, interpret the data, and give meaning to the data.

**autonomous practice** Physical therapy settings PTs are responsible for practicing autonomously and collaboratively to provide best practice to the patient/client. Independent, self-determined, professional judgments and actions characterize such PT practice.

**autonomy** The ability to act independently of others.

## B

**bloodborne pathogens standards (BPS)** A group of rules that provide information for preventing occupational infections in employees who have a reasonable risk of coming in contact with bloodborne infections, such as HIV or hepatitis.

**board of directors (BOD)** A governing body to carry out the mandates and policies established by the house of delegates (HOD) and to communicate issues to internal and external personnel, committees, and agencies.

## C

**capitation** A reimbursement method that pays the provider a monthly fee based on the number of patients enrolled in the insurance plan.

**case mix** A PT comes across a variety of patient cases with different complexities.

**case studies** A type of research that is a description and an analysis of a single person with a particular diagnosis.

**Centers for Medicare and Medicaid Services (CMS)** A federal agency that administers the major healthcare programs in the United States. The programs include Medicare, Medicaid, and the Children's Health Insurance Program (CHIP).

**Children's Health Insurance Program (CHIP)** Provides health coverage to children in families who earn too much to qualify for Medicaid but cannot afford private insurance.

**Children's Health Insurance Program Reauthorization Act (CHIPRA)** A federal law enacted in 2009 to reauthorize CHIP. The law provided funding for CHIP and made changes to the program to improve access to health care for low-income children and pregnant women.

**claims** Payment request submitted to the insurance provider or payer for patient services rendered. This is usually raised by a PT or their healthcare facility.

**client** An individual who seeks physical therapy services to maintain health or a business that hires a PT for consultation.

**clinical practice guidelines** A recommendation that outlines appropriate examination and evaluation of patients with a particular diagnosis. The outline also includes evidence-based interventions. The recommendations are made based on research studies and are intended to improve patient care decisions.

**closed question** A question that requires a "yes" or "no" answer.

**coinsurance** A cost-sharing arrangement typically used with a deductible in which the policyholder and the insurance company each pay a certain percentage of the covered medical expenses.

**combined sections meeting (CSM)** APTA's most popular national education meeting, usually occurs in early February, to provide educational and business sessions for all sections and product demonstrations.

**Commission on Accreditation in Physical Therapy Education (CAPTE)** An accrediting agency that grants accreditation to qualified entry-level education programs for PTs and PTAs.

**communication** The use of words, sounds, signs, or behaviors to impart information to someone else.

**competence** The ability to complete a task well and to a certain professional standard.

**congestive heart failure (CHF)** The inability of the heart to pump enough blood to maintain adequate circulation of the blood to meet the body's metabolic needs.

**consumer-driven healthcare plans** A type of healthcare insurance plan that places more responsibility on the patient to manage their healthcare expenses, which is designed to encourage patients to become more involved in their health care.

**copayment** A monetary amount the patient pays to healthcare professionals each time a service is provided.

**cryotherapy** Therapeutic application of cold such as an ice or cold pack.

**cultural competence** A group of skills, behaviors, and attitudes that individuals acquire that allow them to provide effective clinical care to patients from a variety of cultural differences, such as ethnicity, race, age, or gender.

**Current Procedural Terminology (CPT)** A list of descriptive terms that contain five-character numeric codes assigned to nearly every healthcare service.

# D

**deductible** A portion of the healthcare costs the patient must pay before getting benefits from the insurance company.

**dementia** A progressive, irreversible decline in mental function.

**diagnosis** A step that involves identifying the patient's health problem and determining the underlying cause or causes

**diagnosis-related groups (DRGs)** A classification system that categorizes patients into groups based on their diagnosis, procedures performed, age, and other relevant factors. Understanding their influence on physical therapy practice is important for ensuring continuity of care and optimizing patient outcomes.

**direct access** The legal right of patients to seek evaluation and treatment from a PT without the need for a referral or prescription from a physician or other healthcare provider. This model allows for more immediate and potentially more cost-effective care, as it bypasses the initial step of consulting a primary care doctor for a referral.

**direct personal supervision** The PT is physically present and immediately available to direct and supervise tasks performed by the PTA.

**direct supervision** The PT will need to be physically present and immediately available to supervise the PTA.

**disability** The inability to engage in age-specific, gender-related, and sex-specific roles in a particular social context and physical environment; it is also any restriction or lack of ability (resulting from an injury) to perform an activity in a manner or within the range considered normal for a human being.

**domestic violence** A pattern of abusive behavior that keeps one partner in a position of power over the other partner through the use of fear, intimidation, and control.

**durable medical equipment (DME)** Devices or medical equipment used at home that help in the treatment or management of a medical condition. It includes assistive devices, orthotics and prosthetics, mobility aids, therapeutic equipment, pain management devices, etc.

**duration** A part of an exercise prescription that indicates the length of time the exercise is necessary.

**dyspnea** Inability to breathe or difficulty breathing (shortness of breath).

**dystonia** Impaired tone due to prolonged muscular contractions causing twisting of body parts.

# E

**economic abuse** Attempting to or making a person financially dependent, such as maintaining total control over financial resources, withholding access to money, or forbidding attendance at school or employment.

**edema** Accumulation of large amounts of fluid in the tissues of the body; swelling.

**electronic medical/health record (EMR/EHR)** Digital versions of medical records that allow healthcare providers to store, manage, and access patient health information electronically.

**emotional abuse** Undermining a person's sense of self-worth by doing things such as criticizing constantly, calling names, belittling one's abilities, or damaging a partner's relationship with the children.

**empathy** The feeling that you understand and share another person's experiences and emotions.

**ethics** Rules of behavior based on ideas about what is morally good or bad.

**ethnocentrism** The universal tendency of human beings to think that their ways of thinking, acting, and believing are the only right, proper, and natural ways; universal phenomenon in that most people tend to believe that their ways of living, believing, and acting are right, proper, and morally correct.

**evaluation** The use of information to make a judgment about a patient's condition.

**evidence-based practice** A practice that accesses, applies, and integrates evidence to guide clinical decision-making to provide best practice for the patient/client. It includes integrating the best available research, clinical expertise, patient/client values and circumstances related to patient/client management, practice management, and healthcare policy decision-making.

**examination** The use of tests and measures to gather information about a patient's condition.

# F

**fee-for-service (FFS)** A payment for specific healthcare services provided to a patient. The payment can be made by the patient or by an insurance carrier.

**flaccidity** A state of tone in the muscle that produces weak and floppy limbs.

**flexibility exercises** Activities that cause lengthening of soft tissues.

**fraud** The intentional deception or misrepresentation of fact that can cause unauthorized benefit or payment, for example, a provider that bills Medicare for services or supplies they did not perform.

**frequency** The number of times that an exercise is repeated daily, weekly, or monthly.

**functional limitations** Restrictions of the ability to perform a physical action, activity, or task in an efficient, typically expected, or competent manner.

**functional outcome report (FOR)** A measurement of a patient's function at examination and evaluation that is required by Medicare for payment; will also include a goal outcome and will periodically be updated to provide Medicare with information about a patient's progress toward the discharge functional outcome goal.

# G

**gatekeeper** The one who refers patients to specialists or subspecialists for care.

**general supervision** The PT is available to direct care provided by the PTA by a minimum of telecommunication.

**goals** Functional activities that are the intended response to the physical therapy intervention and that are set by the PT, the patient, and the patient's family/caregivers.

**Guide to Physical Therapist Practice 4.0** The guide written to provide a comprehensive description of accepted PT practice, to reduce unwarranted variation in physical therapy treatments, improve the quality of physical therapy practice, enhance consumer satisfaction by maintaining and improving function and movement, promote appropriate utilization of healthcare services, and reduce the cost of treatment. The guide introduces the patient and client management model, which comprises the elements involved in patient/client management: examination, evaluation, diagnosis, prognosis, intervention, and outcomes.

# H

**Health Insurance Portability and Accountability Act (HIPAA)** Federal law that, among other things, provides rules that govern to whom, in what format, and when information about a patient can be released to others.

**health maintenance organization (HMO)** An organization that provides health care to people who make payments to it and who agree to use the doctors, hospitals, etc., that belong to the organization.

**history** Gathering information about the individual's past and current status. The patient/client history accounts for the patient's/client's past and current health status.

**House of Delegates (HOD)** A highest policymaking body of the APTA comprising chapter voting delegates; section, assembly, PTA Caucus nonvoting delegates; and consultants.

**hydrotherapy** Physical therapy intervention using water.

**hypertonia** Increased muscular tension above normal resting level.

**hypotonia** Decreased muscular tension below normal resting level.

# I

**informed consent** An agreement by a patient that grants permission for an intervention after having been provided information about the risks, benefits, etc.

**initiative** A personal characteristic that demonstrates the willingness and awareness to perform tasks without being directed to do so by someone else.

**interprofessional team** A group of healthcare individuals of different specialties that work together for a specific goal or purpose.

**intervention** Skilled techniques and activities that make up the treatment plan. This step involves implementing a plan of care (POC) that includes physical therapy interventions designed to improve the patient's functional status, reduce impairments, and increase participation.

**intradisciplinary team** A group of healthcare professionals from the same specialty that work together for a specific goal or purpose.

# K

**kinesthesia** A sensation that provides information about position and movement.

# L

**learning** The process of assimilating, understanding, and utilizing information that is being taught.

**levels of evidence** A grading that is assigned to research that is based on its quality, validity, reliability, and applicability and gives readers information that helps to inform their decision-making.

# M

**Medicaid** A government program that provides money for healthcare services when patients cannot pay for themselves.

**medical diagnosis** Physician's identification of the cause of the patient's illness or discomfort.

**Medicare Advantage** An optional health plan that replaced Medicare + Choice that includes health plans offered by private companies but approved by Medicare.

**Medicare Part A–hospital insurance** Pays for inpatient care in hospitals, including critical access hospitals and skilled nursing facilities, hospice care, and some home health care.

**Medicare Part B–supplementary medical insurance** Pays for doctors' services and outpatient care.

**Medicare Part D–Prescription Drug Coverage** An optional benefit available to individuals enrolled in Medicare Part A and/or Medicare Part B. The plan covers a wide range of prescription drugs and offers different levels of coverage and cost-sharing, such as deductibles, copays, and coinsurance.

**Medicare** A medical program that provides money for medical care of older adults.

**Merit-Based Incentive Payment System (MIPS)** Aims for a healthcare system that is more value-based than volume-based. It scores providers into four categories based on their performance: quality, cost, improvement activities, and promoting interoperability.

**morals** Concerning what is right and wrong in human behavior.

**multidisciplinary team** Composed of different healthcare professionals who make treatment recommendations that facilitate quality patient care but do not necessarily have common goals.

# N

**networking** A cultivation of relationships with professionals within a field of study.

# O

**objective data** Data included in the "O" section of the SOAP note; they include information gathered by the healthcare provider through examination or assessment (or reassessment) of the patient; in the SOAP note, information that can be observed, measured, or reproduced by another healthcare provider with the same training as the initial provider.

**observational studies** A research method in which the scientist watches the effect without trying to change who is exposed to the test or treatment and draws conclusions from the observations.

**Occupational Safety and Health Administration (OSHA)** A government agency that provides policies, training, and education to assure safe and healthful working conditions for employees.

**occupational therapist** A healthcare professional who helps people improve their ability to perform tasks in their daily living and working environments.

**open question** A question that requires an answer that expands beyond "yes" or "no."

**orthosis** A device added to a person's body to support, position, or immobilize a part to correct deformities, assist weak muscles, and restore function.

**outcomes** A step that involves evaluating the effectiveness of the interventions and determining whether the patient's goals have been met or whether any revision is necessary.

# P

**physiatrist** A physical therapy physician specializing in physical medicine and rehabilitation and who sees patients in all age groups and treats problems that touch upon all the major systems in the body. Physiatrists practice in rehabilitation centers, hospitals, and private offices.

**physical abuse** Abuse by grabbing, pinching, shoving, slapping, hitting, hair pulling, or biting; also abuse by denying medical care or forcing alcohol and/or drug use.

**physical therapist (PT)** A healthcare professional who helps patients improve their movement and manage pain through exercises, hands-on therapy, and patient education. Their goal is to restore, maintain, and promote overall fitness and health. PTs must hold a degree in physical therapy and be licensed to practice in their respective states.

**physical therapist assistant (PTA) Caucus** An assembly that represents the PTAs' interests, needs, and issues in the APTA governance. The main purpose was to more fully integrate PTA members into the APTA's governance structure and increase PTAs' influence in the Association.

**physical therapist assistant (PTA)** An educated healthcare professional who aids work under the direction and supervision of PTs.

**physical therapy diagnosis** The use of data obtained by physical therapy examination and other relevant information to determine the cause and nature of a patient's impairments, functional limitations, and disabilities.

**Physical Therapy Political Action Committee (PT-PAC)** A committee vital to the Association's success on Capitol Hill in Washington, DC. PT-PAC committee uses membership donations to influence legislative and policy issues through lobbying efforts directed toward policy decision makers.

**physiotherapists** An allied healthcare professional who helps individuals maintain, restore, and improve movement, activity, and functioning, enabling optimal performance in enhancing health, well-being, and quality of life. There are graduates of physiotherapy schools trained to provide physical therapy services. Initially referred to as physiotherapists, the term was further shortened to PTs to avoid confusion with medical professionals such as physiatrists.

**physiotherapy** A therapy to restore movement and function affected by injury, illness, or disability.

**plan of care (POC)** A list of goals and interventions developed by the PT after evaluating the needs of a patient.

**point-of-service documentation** The practice of recording information about the patient and his or her intervention during the actual treatment of the patient.

**policy** A plan of action chosen from all options to address a particular situation and allow consistency in response to the situation.

**poliomyelitis ("polio")** A viral disease caused by poliovirus in children under 5 years of age, resulting in infantile paralysis.

**preferred provider organization (PPO)** A healthcare plan that allows members to choose any provider, within or outside of the network of professionals. Care provided within the network will be provided at a discounted price, and care outside of the network may require an increased cost incurred by the patient.

**primary care** Type of healthcare practice provided by a PCP, where PTs and PTAs work on an outpatient physical therapy basis. It includes diagnostic, therapeutic (e.g., hypertension, diabetes, or arthritis), or preventive services (e.g., mammograms or vaccinations) for common health issues.

**problem-oriented medical record (POMR)** A medical record that is organized by the patient's impairment and treatment interventions.

**procedure** A series of actions performed in a particular order.

**prognosis** A step that involves predicting the expected outcomes of physical therapy interventions, including the anticipated improvement level in the patient's functional status.

**proprioception** The awareness of posture, movement, and changes in equilibrium and the knowledge of position, weight, and resistance of objects in relation to the body; includes awareness of the joints at rest and with movement.

**prosthesis** An artificial appliance that replaces a limb that has been amputated.

**protected health information (PHI)** Any information about a patient's health, healthcare interventions, or healthcare payments that can be linked to a specific patient.

**psychological abuse** Abuse causing fear by intimidation; threatening physical harm to self, partner, or children; destruction of pets and property; mind games or forcing isolation from friends, family, school, and/or work.

# R

**randomized controlled trials** A research method in which study participants are assigned to a study group by chance and are not specifically chosen for a group. Participants can be assigned to a control group, which does not get the intervention being studied, or to the experimental group, which does get the intervention being studied.

**reconstruction aides** Civilian women who played an influential role in developing physical therapy by providing treatment to enable service members suffering from wounds or battle neurosis to return to the battlefront.

**rigidity** Hypertonicity of muscles offering a constant, uniform resistance to passive movement; the affected muscles are unable to relax and are in a state of contraction even at rest.

# S

**secondary care** Care that is provided to patients requiring more specialized clinical expertise such as orthopedists, cardiologists, urologists, or dermatologists. This level of care may require inpatient hospitalization or ambulatory same-day surgery.

**self-awareness** The understanding of your own personality and character.

**sexual abuse** Abuse by coercing or attempting to coerce any sexual contact without consent, abuse by marital rape, forcing sex after physical beating, attacks on sexual parts of the body, or treating another in a sexually demeaning manner.

**sign** A recognizable indication observed in a patient that demonstrates an illness, disease, or impairment.

**SOAP format** A system of documentation that organizes information into subjective, objective, assessment, and plan.

**source-oriented medical record (SOMR)** A system of recording healthcare information that is organized by the provider that administers the care.

**spasticity** Increase in muscle tone and stretch reflex of a muscle resulting in increased resistance to passive stretch of the muscle and high response to sensory stimulation.

**Special Interest Group (SIG)** Group formed within chapters, sections, or assemblies that has its own governance, activities, and annual programming. Each SIG provides a forum where members can organize themselves into areas of common interest.

**subjective data** Data included in the "S" section of the SOAP note; they include information gathered through an interview of the patient or a representative of the patient; all information gathered by the healthcare provider.

**survey, question, read, recite, and review (SQ₃R)** A system for studying and learning information; made up of Survey, Question, Read, Recite, and Review.

**symptom** A complaint from a patient describing an illness, disease, or impairment.

**systematic reviews** A type of research that summarizes all of the credible research available on a particular topic and provides a level of evidence that is higher than any of the research articles individually.

**systems review** A part of the history that provides additional information about the anatomic and physiological status of the individual's musculoskeletal, genitourinary, cardiovascular/pulmonary, neuromuscular, and integumentary systems and the patient's communication, affect, cognition, learning style, and education needs.

# T

**teaching** The act of imparting information to another person that they were not aware of or did not previously understand.

**tertiary care** Care that involves the management of complex or rare disorders (e.g., major surgical procedures, congenital malformations, or organ transplants) that require high-level care.

**tests and measures** Component of the examination where the procedures are selected by the PT to acquire additional information about the patient's condition, the physical therapy diagnosis, and the necessary therapeutic interventions.

**therapeutic exercises** Physical activities that restore and maintain strength, endurance, flexibility, stability, and balance.

**therapeutic relationship** A relationship that is developed between a patient and a caregiver.

**thermotherapy** Intervention through the application of heat.

# V

**Vision 2020** A movement created in 2000 stating that by 2020, physical therapy will be provided by doctors of physical therapy, recognized by consumers and healthcare professionals.

**Visual Analog Scale (VAS)** A form of quantifying information, such as pain, by using a standardized line that a patient marks.

# W

**World Confederation for Physical Therapy (WCPT)** A confederation that works to move physical therapy forward to be recognized as a global profession for its significant role in improving health and well-being.

# Index